A CD-ROM accompanies this book. Please ensure it is enclosed when the book is returned.

*Every* Decker book is accompanied by a CD-ROM.

www.bcdecker.co...

*Value Added CD-ROM Inside*

BC DECKER IN...

This book is due for return on or before the last date shown below.

...ANIES THIS

...EPT IN THE
...FICE.

PLEASE ASK A MEMBER OF STAFF
FOR ASSISTANCE.

# Chronic Daily Headache for Clinicians

# CHRONIC DAILY HEADACHE FOR CLINICIANS

*Editors*

**Peter J. Goadsby, MD, PhD, DSc, FRACP, FRCP**

Institute of Neurology
The National Hospital for Neurology and Neurosurgery
Queen Square
London, United Kingdom

**Stephen D. Silberstein, MD, FACP**

Director, Jefferson Headache Center
Department of Neurology
Thomas Jefferson University
Philadelphia, Pennsylvania

**David W. Dodick, MD, FRCPC, FACP**

Department of Neurology
Mayo Clinic College of Medicine
Scottsdale, Arizona

2005
BC Decker Inc
*Hamilton • London*

BC Decker Inc
P.O. Box 620, L.C.D. 1
Hamilton, Ontario L8N 3K7
Tel: 905–522–7017; 800–568–7281
Fax: 905–522–7839; 888–311–4987
E-mail: info@bcdecker.com
www.bcdecker.com

05 06 07 08 / WPC / 9 8 7 6 5 4 3 2 1

ISBN 1–55009–265–0

Printed in the United States of America

**Sales and Distribution**

*United States*
BC Decker Inc
P.O. Box 785
Lewiston, NY 14092–0785
Tel: 905–522–7017; 800–568–7281
Fax: 905–522–7839; 888–311–4987
E-mail: info@bcdecker.com
www.bcdecker.com

*Canada*
BC Decker Inc
20 Hughson Street South
P.O. Box 620, LCD 1
Hamilton, Ontario L8N 3K7
Tel: 905–522–7017; 800–568–7281
Fax: 905–522–7839; 888–311–4987
E-mail: info@bcdecker.com
www.bcdecker.com

*Foreign Rights*
John Scott & Company
International Publishers' Agency
P.O. Box 878
Kimberton, PA 19442
Tel: 610–827–1640
Fax: 610–827–1671
E-mail: jsco@voicenet.com

*Japan*
Igaku-Shoin Ltd.
Foreign Publications Department
3–24–17 Hongo

Bunkyo-ku, Tokyo, Japan 113–8719
Tel: 3 3817 5680
Fax: 3 3815 6776
E-mail: fd@igaku-shoin.co.jp

*UK, Europe, Scandinavia, Middle East*
Elsevier Science
Customer Service Department
Foots Cray High Street
Sidcup, Kent
DA14 5HP, UK
Tel: 44 (0) 208 308 5760
Fax: 44 (0) 181 308 5702
E-mail: cservice@harcourt.com

*Singapore, Malaysia, Thailand, Philippines, Indonesia, Vietnam, Pacific Rim, Korea*
Elsevier Science Asia
583 Orchard Road
#09/01, Forum
Singapore 238884
Tel: 65–737–3593
Fax: 65–753–2145

*Australia, New Zealand*
Elsevier Science Australia
Customer Service Department
STM Division
Locked Bag 16
St. Peters, New South Wales, 2044
Australia
Tel: 61 02 9517–8999
Fax: 61 02 9517–2249

E-mail: stmp@harcourt.com.au
www.harcourt.com.au

*Mexico and Central America*
ETM SA de CV
Calle de Tula 59
Colonia Condesa
06140 Mexico DF, Mexico
Tel: 52–5–5553–6657
Fax: 52–5–5211–8468
E-mail:
editoresdetextosmex@prodigy.net.mx

*Brazil*
Tecmedd Importadora E Distribuidora
De Livros Ltda.
Avenida Maurílio Biagi, 2850
City Ribeirão, Ribeirão Preto – SP –
Brasil
CEP: 14021–000
Tel: 0800 992236
Fax: (16) 3993–9000
E-mail: tecmedd@tecmedd.com.br

*India, Bangladesh, Pakistan, Sri Lanka*
Elsevier Health Sciences Division
Customer Service Department
17A/1, Main Ring Road
Lajpat Nagar IV
New Delhi – 110024, India
Tel: 91 11 2644 7160–64
Fax: 91 11 2644 7156
E-mail: esindia@vsnl.net

# Contents

# Foreword

It is easy to imagine the sense of despair that must afflict patients facing day after day of continuing head pain. As treating doctors we share the despair on occasions but also have our moments of therapeutic triumph in breaking through the pain barrier. This art obviously depends on accurate diagnosis and appropriate treatment when possible. There are clearly defined entities with specific treatments that are described here as signposts in management. There are other varieties of headache less clearly understood in which effective treatment awaits further advances in pathophysiology. This book by some of the world's leading authorities on the destructive problem of chronic daily headache will be welcome news for those on each side of the consultation desk.

James W. Lance
May 2005

# Contributors

**Thorsten Bartsch,** MD
Department of Neurology
University of Kiel
Kiel, Germany

**Christopher J. Boes,** MD
Department of Neurology
Mayo Clinic
Rochester, Minnesota

**Nikolai Bogduk,** MD, PhD, DSc, Dip Pain Med
Department of Health Sciences
University of Newcastle
Newcastle, Australia

**James J. Corbett,** MD
Department of Neurology
University of Mississippi Medical Center
Jackson, Mississippi

**Hans-Christoph Diener,** MD, PhD
Department of Neurology
University Hospital Essen
Essen, Germany

**David W. Dodick,** MD, FRCPC, FACP
Department of Neurology
Mayo Clinic College of Medicine
Scottsdale, Arizona

**Stefan Evers,** MD, PhD
Department of Neurology
University of Münster
Münster, Germany

**Arnaud Fumal,** MD
Department of Neurology and Neuroanatomy
University of Liège
Liège, Belgium

**Peter J. Goadsby,** MD, PhD, DSc, FRACP, FRCP
Institute of Neurology
The National Hospital for Neurology and Neuro-surgery
London, United Kingdom

**Steven B. Graff-Radford,** DDS
The Pain Center
Los Angeles, California

**Zaza Katsarava,** MD
Department of Neurology
University Hospital Essen
Essen, Germany

**Joshua B. Khoury,** MD
Department of Neurology
Thomas Jefferson University
Philadelphia, Pennsylvania

**Volker Limmroth,** MD
Department of Neurology
University Hospital Essen
Essen, Germany

**Richard B. Lipton,** MD
Department of Neurology, Epidemiology, and Population Health
Albert Einstein College of Medicine
Bronx, New York

**Manjit S. Matharu,** MRCP
Institute of Neurology
The National Hospital for Neurology and Neuro-surgery
Queen Square, London, England

**Bahram Mokri,** MD
Department of Neurology
Mayo Clinic
Rochester, Minnesota

**Juan A. Pareja,** MD, PhD
Department of Neurology
Fundación Hospital Alcorcón
Juan Carlos I University
Alcorcón-Madrid, Spain

**Julio Pascual,** MD, PhD
Service of Neurology
University Hospital Marqués de Valdecilla
Santander, Spain

**Mario F.P. Peres,** MD, PhD
Department of Neurology
Sao Paulo Headache Center
Sao Paulo, Brazil

**R. Allan Purdy,** MD, FRCPC
Department of Neurology
Dalhousie University
Halifax, Nova Scotia, Canada

**Nabih M. Ramadan,** MD
Department of Neurology
Rosalind Franklin University of Medicine and Science
Chicago, Illinois

**Todd D. Rozen,** MD
Department of Neurology
Michigan Head-Pain and Neurological Institute
Ann Arbor, Michigan

**Maria E. Santiago,** MD
Department of Neurology
GV (Sonny) Montgomery VA Medical Center
Jackson, Mississippi

**Ann I. Scher,** PhD
Department of Preventive Medicine and Biometrics
Uniformed Services University
Bethesda, Maryland

**Jean Schoenen,** MD, PhD
Department of Neurology and Neuroanatomy
University of Liège
Liège, Belgium

**Stephen D. Silberstein,** MD, FACP
Department of Neurology
Thomas Jefferson University
Philadelphia, Pennsylvania

**Walter F. Stewart,** PhD
Outcomes Research Institute
Geisinger Health Systems
Danville, Pennsylvania

**William B. Young,** MD
Department of Neurology
Thomas Jefferson University
Philadelphia, Pennsylvania

# Chronic Daily Headache

# General Principles

# CHAPTER 1

# Introduction and General Remarks

Peter J. Goadsby, MD, PhD, DSc, FRACP, FRCP, David Dodick, MD, FRCPC, FACP,
and Stephen D. Silberstein, MD, FACP

The frequent headache syndromes are among the most challenging disorders that confront clinicians on a routine basis. They at once give the subspecialty of headache a bad name, because they are generally considered difficult to treat, while providing a wonderful opportunity to help many very disabled patients. Clinicians interested in headache will realize that from a practical perspective, frequent headache disorders represent our main priority and responsibility because they occupy such a large part of our clinical workload. Indeed, with a prevalence of 1 in 20, the clinician caring for patients with frequent headache must embrace, understand, and manage these patients. We hope that this book helps with this challenge. The differential diagnosis of frequent headache syndromes is finite, and making a specific diagnosis often leads to clear management strategies. We asked an international group of expert clinicians to review the diagnostic and management issues for the most important and challenging disorders that present with frequent headache. It is also our intent that bringing clinical clarity to these disorders will allow them to be appropriately managed and studied in terms of their primary headache biology.

## HISTORICAL ISSUES IN DAILY HEADACHE

The potential for migraine headache to evolve from a paroxysmal disorder with symptom-free intervals to one characterized by habitual, if not daily, headache has been recognized since the time of Thomas Willis in the seventeenth century. In the decades leading up to the 1980s, many clinical investigators rediscovered frequent migraine. It was recognized that some patients with episodic migraine could progress, alter, or transform over time. The result was a frequent or daily headache disorder with features of both migraine and tension-type headache. Implicit in this concept was the viewpoint that migraine should have some upper limit in

terms of frequency because it became apparent that as migraine attack frequency increases, interval headaches lose some of their migrainous features and begin to resemble tension-type headache. The 1988 International Headache Society diagnostic criteria codified this approach and developed operational diagnostic criteria for chronic tension-type headache. This led to perhaps the most fundamental problem in the approach to and diagnosis of patients with frequent headache: we stopped diagnosing the patient's disorder and started diagnosing primary headache by its attack features alone. Much of what follows is therefore based on the underlying view that the biology of frequent headache is very similar to the corresponding primary headache that was once infrequent, although the frequency of attacks necessitates somewhat different management strategies and may alter the phenotype.

## NOSOLOGIC DIFFICULTIES IN DAILY HEADACHE

Until recently, the nosology of frequent headache disorders has included a bewildering morass of arbitrarily applied terms with no foundation in basic or clinical science. A major problem with the relatively new term, *chronic daily headache* (CDH), has been its confusion with chronic tension-type headache and other commonly used terms for which there have never been operational diagnostic criteria or even informal clinical criteria. The medical literature is replete with examples over the past three decades in which the terms *mixed* headache, *combined* headache, *tension-vascular* headache, and *rebound headache* are used interchangeably. By inference, CDH became synonomous in many clinical settings with chronic tension-type headache with inconvenient vascular or migrainous features or medication overuse. The careless use of the term CDH, not otherwise defined, neither helps the field nor facilitates appropriate treatment strategies.

With the rediscovery that, in clinical settings, many, if not most, of these patients either had episodic migraine at some point in the past or experienced migrainous features with at least some of their headaches, the term *transformed migraine* became increasingly applied to these patients. It needs to be said that transformed migraine, as the term was coined and then later defined, is not the same as *chronic migraine*, as now defined by the International Headache Society. We have used the International Headache Society general principles that to have CDH is to be afflicted on 15 days or more per month. Naturally, this leads to the problem that a patient with 20 headache days per month is described as having daily headache when we mean frequent, not strictly daily. However, this book will attempt to bring some nosologic order to the CDH syndromes by providing a classification that, more than just an academic exercise, will provide a framework for developing a systematic approach to the evaluation and management of these patients. CDH is not an entity itself but an umbrella term. It is broadly speaking a diagnosis, just as anemia is a diagnosis; it invites further clarification. We hope this book provides some part of that clarity.

# CHAPTER 2

# Epidemiology of Chronic Daily Headache

Ann I. Scher, PhD, Walter F. Stewart, PhD, and Richard B. Lipton, MD

Chronic daily headache (CDH) is defined by convention as headache of any type occurring at least 15 days per month. CDH is subdivided into the secondary forms (attributable to an underlying disorder) and the primary forms (not attributable to an underlying disorder). Primary CDH is further subdivided into the short-duration (< 4 hours) and long-duration types. Herein, we focus on primary CDH of long duration. The two most common disorders in this rubric are chronic tension-type headache and transformed migraine; other disorders include hemicrania continua, new daily persistent headache, and various chronic short-duration headaches, such as chronic cluster headache, chronic paroxysmal hemicrania, and hypnic headache.[1] The great majority of CDH sufferers in the population and in subspecialty care have either chronic tension-type headache or transformed migraine.

Although understanding of CDH is increasing owing to recent insights gained from animal models,[2-4] focused clinical studies,[5-11] and epidemiology,[12-15] the development and pathophysiology of most of the frequent headache disorders are incompletely understood. Controlled trials of treatment strategies for CDH are limited.[16-20] Most clinical trials of headache-specific agents specifically exclude CDH. Although recent changes in headache nomenclature have been implemented,[21] continuing uncertainty about the role of medication overuse in the etiology of CDH and diagnostic (and possibly etiologic) overlap between the CDH subtypes continues to make the definition and application of standardized nomenclature of these disorders difficult. In this chapter, we use the Silberstein-Lipton criteria because most published studies use variants of these criteria.[22]

Many chronic headache sufferers do not seek medical care for their headaches and remain undiagnosed.[23,24] Therefore, it is particularly important to study a disorder such as chronic headache in population samples because those in specialty care are likely to differ in important ways from typical chronic headache sufferers. Demographic factors such as gender, income, and place of residence, as well as disease characteristics, comorbid illness, and family history, are factors that likely impact treatment decisions and that also may be mistaken for disease attributes when studies are based on highly selected populations.

This chapter reviews the epidemiology of CDH, including the demographic characteristics of CDH sufferers, risk factors identified in population samples, and prognostic data. We also highlight differences between CDH sufferers in the population and those in subspecialty care.

## DEMOGRAPHIC FACTORS

The epidemiology of CDH has been described in a number of population samples based in Europe, the Far East, and the United States (Table 2–1). The prevalence of CDH is remarkably consistent among studies, at about 4% of the adult and elderly population. In children, epidemiologic data are limited and case definitions are variable, but the prevalence of very frequent headache in late childhood and adolescence may approach the levels seen in adults (Table 2–2). Thus, very frequent headache appears to afflict a relatively constant proportion of the population when examined in very broad age groups (Figure 2–1). In adulthood, CDH is approximately twice as common in women as in men, even in elderly populations.

## CDH SUBTYPES

The CDH population is primarily composed of individuals with chronic tension-type or transformed migraine headaches, but also includes rare headache syndromes, including hemicrania continua and chronic cluster headache, as well as headaches that are

**Table 2–1** Prevalence of Very Frequent Headache in Adult Populations (Ordered by Date of Publication)

| Lead Author (Year of Publication) | Country | N | Case Definition | Age Range, yr | Prevalence, % | | | F:M | Analgesic Overuse, %* |
|---|---|---|---|---|---|---|---|---|---|
| | | | | | Total | CTTH | TM | | |
| Scher (1998)[24] | United States | 13,343 | 15+/mo | 18–65 | 4.1 | 2.2 | 1.3 | 1.8 | |
| Castillo (1999)[41] | Spain | 1,883 | 15+/mo, 4+ h/d | 14+ | 4.7 | 2.2 | 2.4 | 8.7 | 25 |
| Wang (1999)[23] | China | 1,533 | 15+/mo, 6+ mo | 65+ | 3.9 | 2.7 | 1.0 | 3.1 | 25 |
| Hagen (2000)[42] | Norway | 51,383 | 15+/mo | 20+ | 2.4 | | | 1.6 | |
| Ho (2001)[45] | Singapore | 2,096 | > 180/yr | 12+ | 3.3 | | | | |
| Lu (2001)[27] | Taiwan | 3,377 | 15+/mo, 4+ h/d | 15+ | 3.2 | 1.4 | 1.7 | 2.3 | 34 |
| Prencipe (2001)[44] | Italy | 833 | 15+/mo | 65+ | 4.4 | 2.5 | 1.6 | 2.4 | 38 |
| Lantéri-Minet (2003)[43] | France | 10,585 | Daily | 15+ | 3.0 | | | 2.6 | |
| Takeshima (2004)[46] | Japan | 5,758 | CTTH only | 20+ | | 2.1 | | | |

TM = transformed migraine; CTTH = chronic tension-type headache; F:M = female to male prevalence ratio.
*Based on Silberstein and colleagues' criteria.[22]

difficult to classify in population studies. Population studies indicate that the portions of individuals with chronic tension-type headache are roughly equal to those with migrainous features with at least some of their headaches (Figure 2–2). In contrast, the vast majority of CDH patients in subspecialty care begin with a history of migraine or continue to have migraine features; this has led to the perception that CDH is a complication (eg, mediated through medication overuse) or natural progression of episodic migraine.[25,26]

## SOCIOECONOMIC STATUS

CDH appears to be more common in individuals of less education or lower income.[15,23,24,27,28] For example, in a US case-control study, the risk of CDH was more than three times as high in those with less than a high school education relative to those with a graduate-level education (odds ratio [OR] = 3.35 [2.1–5.3]).[15] In a large population study from Norway, Hagen and colleagues compared the risk of CDH in individuals of lower socioeconomic status (measured by educational level, social class based on occupation, and income) with that of higher socioeconomic status.[14] The risk of CDH for those with less than 10 years of education relative to those with 13+ years of education was elevated both for women (relative risk [RR] = 2.4 [1.1–4.9]) and men (RR = 1.6 [1.1–2.1]). Similar results were seen for low social class for women (RR = 2.6 [1.5–4.6]) and men (RR = 1.4 [1.0–2.0]) and for low-income for men (RR = 1.8 [1.2–2.7]) but not for women (RR = 0.9 [0.6–1.4]).

## COMORBID PAIN

In studies based on the previous two population samples from the United States[15] and Norway,[14] CDH sufferers were more likely to report other pain conditions than controls. In Norway, individuals with CDH were more than four times more likely to report musculoskeletal symptoms than those without CDH (RR = 4.6 [1.0–5.3]). Similarly, in the US study, CDH sufferers over age 40 years were considerably more likely to report physician-diagnosed arthritis (OR = 2.41 [1.8–3.3]) than individuals with episodic headache. These findings are in accordance with a body of evidence that chronic pain conditions tend to co-occur.[29]

## MEDICATION USE

Medication overuse for headache may be an aggravating or causal factor for headache progression, a marker of headache intractability, or both. High medication use is less common in population-based samples of CDH sufferers than is seen in patients who consult subspecialty practices, with approximately one-third (25–38%) overusing medication as defined based on Silberstein-Lipton criteria (see Table 2–1).[22] Similar results were reported in a US case-control study[30] and in a recent study from Spain.[31] A somewhat higher proportion of CDH sufferers (41–54%) were found to be overusing medication in a large study from Norway.[32]

**Table 2–2** Prevalence of Very Frequent Headache in Childhood or Adolescence (Ordered by Date of Publication)

| Author (Year of Publication) | Country | N | Case Definition | Age Range, yr | Prevalence, % |
|---|---|---|---|---|---|
| Egermark-Eriksson (1982)[47] | Sweden | 402 | Once or twice a week or daily | 7, 11, 15 | 9.0 |
| Sillanpää (1983)[48] | Finland | 3,784 | 2+ times a week | 13 | 3.4 |
| Sillanpää (1983)[49] | Finland | 2,921 | 2+ times a week | 14 | 4.0 |
| King (1990)[28] | Australia | 900 | Almost all the time | 10–18 | 4.6 |
| Kristánsdóttir (1993)[39] | Iceland | 2,140 | Almost daily or daily | 11–12, 15–16 | 2.5 |
| Sillanpää (1996)[50] | Finland | 1,927 | 2+ times a week | 7 | 0.5 |
| | Finland | 1,433 | 2+ times a week | 7 | 1.0 |
| Rhee (2000)[40] | United States | 6,072 | Almost daily or daily | 11–21 | 7.3 |
| Bandell-Hoekstra (2001)[51] | Netherlands | 2,400 | Few times a week | 10–17 | 13.0 |
| Anttila (2002)[37] | Finland | 1,409 | CTTH | 12 | 0.0 |
| Özge (2003)[52] | Turkey | 5,562 | CTTH | 8–12 | 1.5 |

CTTH = chronic tension-type headache.

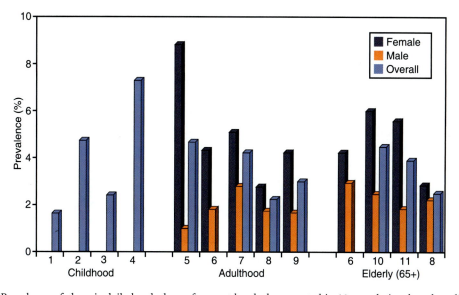

**Figure 2–1** Prevalence of chronic daily headache or frequent headache reported in 11 population-based studies, ordered by the age range of the studied population.

| Study Number | Lead Author |
|---|---|
| 1 | Anttila (2002, Finland)[37] |
| 2 | King (1990, Australia)[38] (headache "almost all the time") |
| 3 | Kristánsdóttir (1993, Iceland)[39] (headache "almost daily or daily") |
| 4 | Rhee (2000, US)[40] (headache "almost every day" or "every day") |
| 5 | Castillo (1999, Spain)[41] |
| 6 | Lu (2001, Taiwan)[27] |
| 7 | Scher (1998, US)[24] |
| 8 | Hagen (2000, Norway)[42] (data extracted) |
| 9 | Lanteri-Minet (2003, France)[43] |
| 10 | Prencipe (2001, Italy)[44] |
| 11 | Wang (2000, Kinmen Island)[23] |

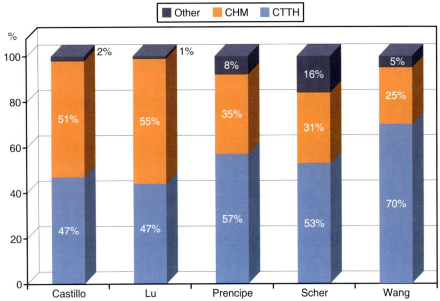

**Figure 2–2** Proportion of chronic daily headache (CDH) sufferers with chronic tension-type headache (CTTH), chronic headache with migraine features (CHM), and other chronic headaches from five population-based studies: Castillo and colleagues,[41] Lu and colleagues,[27] Prencipe and colleagues,[44] Scher and colleagues,[24] and Wang and colleagues.[23]

## SLEEP-RELATED FACTORS

The results from the case-control study revealed that CDH cases were more likely to be habitual (daily) snorers than episodic headache controls.[33] CDH cases were also more likely to report sleep problems and to be either short or long sleepers (unpublished data from[33]). The association between CDH and habitual snoring was not explained by the usual cardiovascular factors associated with sleep-disordered breathing (eg, increased age, male gender, hypertension, body mass index), nor was it explained by other potentially confounding factors that could be associated with both chronic headache and sleep disturbances (eg, caffeine consumption, hypertension, depression). This suggests that if the association is causal, the effect of snoring on very frequent headache is from a different mechanism than sleep apnea or hypopnea.

## STRESSFUL LIFE EVENTS

Specific life changes were found to be associated with CDH onset in a case-control study.[34] Cases and controls were interviewed about the occurrence of specific life events (moves, job changes, child-related changes, changes in marital status, deaths in the family or of close friends, ongoing "extremely stressful" life events) in the time before CDH onset up to the present time. Events were divided into pre- and post-CDH events, with a randomly generated year comparable to CDH onset for the cases used for the controls. Overall, cases reported more pre-CDH events than the controls (2.7 vs 2.0; $p < .001$,

rank sum test). No difference was found for post-CDH events, strengthening a causal interpretation.

A large study based on adolescent students from Taiwan measured the presence of childhood stressors (eg, parental divorce, child abuse) using the Global Family Environment Scale and compared scores between students with CDH and a control group.[12] They found that the CDH students had about a 10% higher score on this scale, suggesting that the presence of these negative life events might be involved in the onset of adolescent CDH.

## PROGNOSIS AND NATURAL HISTORY

The results from three population-based studies suggest that the rates of (presumably) spontaneous remission are high in CDH. In a US-based population sample, more than half (60%) of CDH cases at baseline had remitted to less than 180 headache days per year at follow-up, although remission to a more "normal" headache frequency of < 1 headache per week was much less common (16%).[15] Figures 2–3 and 2–4 from this study illustrate the relationship between headache frequency at baseline and incidence or remission of CDH at 1 year. Figure 2–3 shows that individuals with more frequent headaches at baseline were at higher risk of incident CDH at follow-up and that individuals with less frequent CDH had a higher likelihood of remission at follow-up. Although this finding is somewhat tautologic (because those with more frequent headaches are closer to being cases than those with infrequent headaches), it may be that higher vigilance is warranted

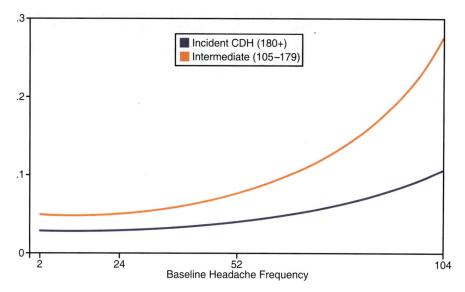

**Figure 2–3** Estimated 1-year *incidence* rate of increased headaches (105–179 headaches/year) (*top line*) and chronic daily headache (CDH) (180+ headaches/year) (*bottom line*) in an episodic headache population (2–104 headaches/year) by baseline headache frequency. Predictions are calculated using multinomial logistic regression and are adjusted for baseline headache frequency and elapsed time between interviews. Reproduced with permission from Scher AI et al.[15]

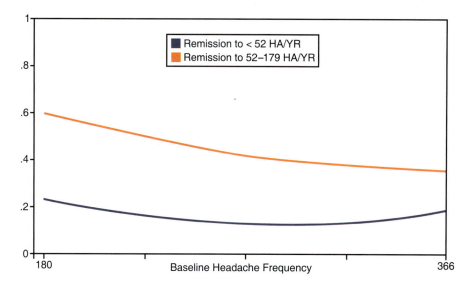

**Figure 2–4** Estimated 1-year *remission* rate to < 180 headaches (HA) per year (*top line*) and < 1 headache per week (*bottom line*) by baseline headache frequency. Predictions are calculated using multinomial logistic regression and are adjusted for baseline headache frequency and elapsed time between interviews. Reproduced with permission from Scher AI et al.[15]

to prevent headache progression in those who are already headache prone. A similar remission rate was reported in Taiwan (65% remitted to fewer than 15 headaches per month after 2 years),[27] although remission was lower in an elderly Chinese population (33% had remitted over a 4-year period).[23] A recent German clinic-based study of migraine sufferers found a 1-year incidence rate for CDH of 14%.[35] Estimates may be higher than in the US study because the clinic-based sample has more severe disease or because migraine itself is a risk factor.

Some prognostic factors were identified in these studies and an additional population-based study from Norway. In the US study, women, whites, those of less educational achievement, and those who were previously married (eg, widowed, divorced, or separated) were at increased risk of CDH at baseline and at reduced risk of remission at follow-up (Table 2–3).[15] Obesity, defined as a body mass-index ≥ 30, was predictive of 1-year CDH incidence in this population. The reason why obesity would predispose individuals to headache progression is

**Table 2–3**   Characteristics Associated with Chronic Daily Headache Prevalence, Incidence, and Remission

| | | Prevalence OR[†] A | Incidence OR[‡] B | Remission OR[§] C |
|---|---|---|---|---|
| Gender | Male | 1.00 | 1.00 | |
| | Female | 1.69 (1.4–2.1)** | 0.94 (0.4–2.4) | |
| Age | Mean age | 0.98 (0.98–0.99)** | 1.00 (0.96–1.04) | |
| | Female × age | | | 1.04 (1.01–1.06)** |
| Race | White | 1.00 | 1.00 | 1.00 |
| | Nonwhite | 0.77 (0.6–1.0)* | 1.28 (0.5–3.2) | 2.05 (1.3–3.2)*** |
| | Missing/refused | 0.82 (0.4–1.6) | — | 1.25 (0.3–4.7) |
| BMI | Normal (< 25) | 1.00 | 1.00 | 1.00 |
| | Overweight | 1.26 (1.0–1.7) | 1.97 (0.4–9.0) | 1.49 (0.9–2.6) |
| | Obese (≥30) | 1.34 (1.0–1.8)* | 5.28 (1.3–21.1)* | 1.58 (0.9–2.8) |
| | Missing/refused | 0.84 (0.7–1.1) | 2.54 (0.7–9.6) | 0.89 (0.5–1.6) |
| Education | < High school | 3.35 (2.1–5.3)** | — | 0.21 (0.1–0.5)** |
| | High school | 1.49 (1.1–2.0)* | 0.36 (0.1–1.3) | 0.57 (0.3–1.1) |
| | Some college | 1.16 (0.8–1.6) | 0.84 (0.3–2.7) | 0.72 (0.4–1.4) |
| | College | 1.10 (0.8–1.5) | 0.45 (0.1–1.8) | 0.63 (0.3–1.2) |
| | Graduate school | 1.00 | 1.00 | 1.00 |
| | Missing/refused | 1.93 (0.4–9.5) | — | — |
| Current marital status | Married | 1.00 | 1.00 | 1.00 |
| | Previously married[ǁ] | 1.45 (1.1–1.9)* | 1.84 (0.6–5.7) | 0.51 (0.3–0.9)* |
| | Never married | 1.05 (0.8–1.4) | 1.30 (0.4–3.9) | 0.99 (0.6–1.6) |
| | Missing/refused | 0.48 (0.3–0.8)** | 2.68 (0.7–10.9) | 0.42 (0.1–1.3) |
| Arthritis diagnosis (age ≥ 40 yr) | No | 1.00 | 1.00 | 1.00 |
| | Yes | 2.41 (1.8–3.3)** | 2.52 (0.7–8.6) | 1.04 (0.6–1.8) |
| | Missing/refused | 5.26 (0.6–47.0) | 1.76 (0.2–18.8) | — |
| Diabetes diagnosis | No | 1.00 | 1.00 | 1.00 |
| | Yes | 1.39 (0.9–2.1) | 3.00 (0.8–11.7) | 2.70 (1.3–5.5)* |
| | Missing/refused | 1.99 (0.9–4.6) | 2.34 (0.6–8.9) | 0.29 (0.03–2.8) |

Adapted from Scher AI et al.[15]

BMI = body mass index; OR = odds ratio.

[†]Adjusted for age, gender, marital status, race, educational level, and BMI.

[‡]Adjusted for BMI and baseline headache frequency squared.

[§]Adjusted for gender, age × female gender, marital status, educational level, race, elapsed time between interviews, and baseline headache frequency (frequency and frequency squared).

[ǁ]Includes widowed, divorced, or separated.

A: Comparing baseline chronic daily headache cases ($n$ = 1,134) with baseline episodic headache controls ($n$ = 798).

B: Among baseline episodic headache controls, comparing new-onset cases ($n$ = 23) with stable controls ($n$ = 726).

C: Among baseline chronic daily headache cases, comparing cases who remitted to < 1 headache/week ($n$ = 153) with stable cases ($n$ = 495).

*$p$ < .05; **$p$ < .005.

unknown. This result suggests the interesting hypothesis that weight reduction in at-risk individuals might reduce the risk of headache progression.

## MEDICATION USE AS A PROGNOSTIC FACTOR

Two prospective studies in Asian populations showed that CDH sufferers with medication overuse had a worse prognosis at follow-up than CDH sufferers without medication overuse. The first study by Lu and colleagues followed a group of 106 CDH sufferers for 2 years, 36 (34%) of whom overused medication at baseline.[27] At follow-up 2 years later, 19 of 70 (27%) nonoverusers had persistent CDH, and 18 of 36 (50%) overusers had persistent CDH, corresponding to an RR of 1.8 (1.1–3.1). Wang and colleagues identified 60 elderly CDH sufferers, 15 (25%) of whom overused medication.[23] At follow-up at least 2 years later, 21 of 37 (57%) nonoverusers had persistent CDH versus 14 of 15 (93%) overusers, corresponding to an RR of 1.6 (1.2–2.3). The previously mentioned German study found that medication overuse predicted incident CDH in episodic migraine specialty patients, even after adjusting for baseline headache frequency.[35] These studies thus support the hypothesis that medication overuse predicts a worse prognosis but do not answer the question of whether medication overuse is itself a risk factor or a marker for headache intractability.

Zwart and colleagues interviewed a large population-based sample of individuals two times over a 10-year period.[36] They found that individuals who used analgesics daily or weekly at baseline were more likely to have chronic pain at follow-up compared with individuals who used analgesics less than weekly. Unfortunately, the reason for medication use at baseline was not known. Therefore, this finding cannot be taken to support the hypothesis that medication overuse predicts CDH incidence because the headache frequency at baseline (and the "at-risk" population for CDH) was not known. For similar reasons, this finding cannot be taken to support the hypothesis that CDH sufferers with medication overuse have a worse prognosis than CDH sufferers without medication overuse because individuals with CDH were not identified in the baseline survey.

## CONCLUSION

CDH is surprisingly common, affecting 1 in 25 adults in several different population samples. The prevalence of very frequent headache may be equally high in late childhood or adolescence, although the data for children are less consistent. CDH is more common in women than men and is inversely related to socioeconomic status. Other identified associations include habitual snoring and other sleep problems, obesity, the occurrence of certain stressful life events, and coexisting arthritis or other musculoskeletal pain.

CDH in the population differs from CDH in subspecialty care, particularly in the relative infrequency of medication overuse and in the substantial rates of (presumably) spontaneous remission.

## REFERENCES

1. Silberstein SD, Lipton RB. Chronic daily headache, including transformed migraine, chronic tension-type headache, and medication overuse. In: Silberstein SD, Lipton RB, Dalessio DJ, editors. Wolff's headache. Oxford (UK): Oxford University Press; 2001. p. 247–82.

2. Srikiatkhachorn A, Suwattanasophon C, Ruangpattanatawee U, Phansuwan-Pujito P. 2002 Wolff Award. 5-HT2A receptor activation and nitric oxide synthesis: a possible mechanism determining migraine attacks. Headache 2002;42:566–74.

3. Srikiatkhachorn A, Tarasub N, Govitrapong P. Effect of chronic analgesic exposure on the central serotonin system: a possible mechanism of analgesic abuse headache. Headache 2000;40:343–50.

4. Srikiatkhachorn A, Tarasub N, Govitrapong P. Acetaminophen-induced antinociception via central 5-HT(2A) receptors. Neurochem Int 1999;34:491–8.

5. Gallai V, Alberti A, Gallai B, et al. Glutamate and nitric oxide pathway in chronic daily headache: evidence from cerebrospinal fluid. Cephalalgia 2003;23:166–74.

6. Sarchielli P, Alberti A, Russo S, et al. Nitric oxide pathway, Ca2+, and serotonin content in platelets from patients suffering from chronic daily headache. Cephalalgia 1999;19:810–6.

7. Sarchielli P, Alberti A, Floridi A, Gallai V. L-Arginine/nitric oxide pathway in chronic tension-type headache: relation with serotonin content and secretion and glutamate content. J Neurol Sci 2002;198:9–15.

8. Welch KM, Nagesh V, Aurora SK, Gelman N. Periaqueductal gray matter dysfunction in migraine: cause or the burden of illness? Headache 2001;41:629–37.

9. Sarchielli P, Alberti A, Floridi A, Gallai V. Levels of nerve growth factor in cerebrospinal fluid of chronic daily headache patients. Neurology 2001;57:132–4.

10. Bahra A, Walsh M, Menon S, Goadsby PJ. Does chronic daily headache arise de novo in association with regular use of analgesics? Headache 2003;43:179–90.

11. Wilkinson SM, Becker WJ, Heine JA. Opiate use to control bowel motility may induce chronic daily headache in patients with migraine. Headache 2001;41:303–9.

12. Juang KD, Wang SJ, Fuh JL, et al. Association between adolescent chronic daily headache and childhood adversity: a community-based study. Cephalalgia 2004;24:54–9.

13. Scher AI, Stewart WF, Lipton RB. Snoring and chronic daily headache: results from the Frequent Headache Epidemiology Study. Neurology 2002;58 Suppl 3:A332.

14. Hagen K, Einarsen C, Zwart JA, et al. The co-occurrence of headache and musculoskeletal symptoms amongst 51 050 adults in Norway. Eur J Neurol 2002;9:527–33.

15. Scher AI, Stewart WF, Ricci JA, Lipton RB. Factors associated with the onset and remission of chronic daily headache in a population-based study. Pain 2003;106:81–9.

16. Saper JR, Lake AE, Cantrell DT, et al. Chronic daily headache prophylaxis with tizanidine: a double-blind, placebo-controlled, multicenter outcome study. Headache 2002;42:470–82.

17. Descombes S, Brefel-Courbon C, Thalamas C, et al. Amitriptyline treatment in chronic drug-induced headache: a double-blind comparative pilot study. Headache 2001;41:178–82.

18. Ondo WG, Vuong KD, Derman HS. Botulinum toxin A for chronic daily headache: a randomized, placebo-controlled, parallel design study. Cephalalgia 2004;24:60–5.

19. Spira PJ, Beran RG. Gabapentin in the prophylaxis of chronic daily headache: a randomized, placebo-controlled study. Neurology 2003;61:1753–9.

20. Mathew NT, Frishberg BM, Gawel M, et al. Botulinum Toxin Type A (BOTOX) for the Prophylactic Treatment of Chronic Daily Headache: A Randomized, Double-Blind Placebo-Controlled Trial. Headache 2005 Apr;45(4):293–307.

21. Headache Classification Subcommittee, International Headache Society. The international classification of headache disorders. Cephalalgia 2004;24 Suppl 1:1–160.

22. Silberstein SD, Lipton RB, Sliwinski M. Classification of daily and near-daily headaches: field trial of revised IHS criteria. Neurology 1996;47:871–5.

23. Wang SJ, Fuh JL, Lu SR, et al. Chronic daily headache in Chinese elderly: prevalence, risk factors, and biannual follow-up. Neurology 2000;54:314–9.

24. Scher AI, Stewart WF, Liberman J, Lipton RB. Wolff Award 1998. Prevalence of frequent headache in a population sample. Headache 1998;38:497–506.

25. Mathew NT, Stubits E, Nigam MP. Transformation of episodic migraine into daily headache: analysis of factors. Headache 1982;22:66–8.

26. Mathew NT, Reuveni U, Perez F. Transformed or evolutive migraine. Headache 1987;27:102–6.

27. Lu SR, Fuh JL, Chen WT, et al. Chronic daily headache in Taipei, Taiwan: prevalence, follow-up and outcome predictors. Cephalalgia 2001;21:980–6.

28. Hagen K, Vatten L, Stovner LJ, et al. Low socio-economic status is associated with increased risk of frequent headache: a prospective study of 22718 adults in Norway. Cephalagia 2002;22(8):672-79.

29. Aaron LA, Buchwald D. A review of the evidence for overlap among unexplained clinical conditions. Ann Intern Med 2001;134(9 Pt 2):868–81.

30. Scher AI, Stewart WF, Lipton RB. Is analgesic use a risk factor for chronic daily headache? Neurology 2001;56:A312.

31. Colas R, Munoz P, Temprano R, et al. Chronic daily headache with analgesic overuse: epidemiology and impact on quality of life. Neurology 2004;62:1338–42.

32. Zwart JA, Dyb G, Hagen K, et al. Analgesic overuse among subjects with headache, neck, and low-back pain. Neurology 2004;62:1540–4.

33. Scher AI, Lipton RB, Stewart WF. Habitual snoring as a risk factor for chronic daily headache. Neurology 2003;60:1366.

34. Stewart WF, Scher AI, Lipton RB. The Frequent Headache Epidemiology study (FrHE): stressful life events and risk of chronic daily headache. Neurology 2001;56:A138–9.

35. Katsarava Z, Schneeweiss S, Kurth T, et al. Incidence and predictors for chronicity of headache in patients with episodic migraine. Neurology 2004;62:788–90.

36. Zwart JA, Dyb G, Hagen K, et al. Analgesic use: a predictor of chronic pain and medication overuse headache: The Head-HUNT Study. Neurology 2003;61:160.

37. Anttila P, Metsahonkala L, Aromaa M, et al. Determinants of tension-type headache in children. Cephalalgia 2002;22:401–8.

38. King NJ, Sharpley CF. Headache activity in children and adolescents. J Paediatr Child Health 1990;26:50–4.

39. Kristánsdóttir G, Wahlberg V. Sociodemographic differences in the prevalence of self-reported headache in Icelandic school-children. Headache 1993;33:376–80.

40. Rhee H. Prevalence and predictors of headaches in US adolescents. Headache 2000;40:528–38.

41. Castillo J, Munoz P, Guitera V, Pascual J. Kaplan Award 1998: epidemiology of chronic daily headache in the general population. Headache 1999;39:190–6.

42. Hagen K, Zwart JA, Vatten L, et al. Prevalence of migraine and non-migrainous headache—Head-HUNT, a large population-based study. Cephalalgia 2000;20:900–6.

43. Lantéri–Minet M, Auray JP, El Hasnaoui A, et al. Prevalence and description of chronic daily headache in the general population in France. Pain 2003;102:143–9.

44. Prencipe M, Casini AR, Ferretti C, et al. Prevalence of headache in an elderly population: attack frequency, disability, and use of medication. J Neurol Neurosurg Psychiatry 2001;70:377–81.

45. Ho KH, Ong BK. Headache characteristics and race in Singapore: results of a randomized national survey. Headache 2001;41:279–84.

46. Takeshima T, Ishizaki K, Fukuhara Y, et al. Population-based door-to-door survey of migraine in Japan: The Daisen Study. Headache 2004;44:8–19.

47. Egermark-Eriksson I. Prevalence of headache in Swedish schoolchildren. A questionnaire survey. Acta Paediatr Scand 1982;71:135–40.

48. Sillanpää M. Prevalence of headache in prepuberty. Headache 1983;23:10–4.

49. Sillanpää M. Changes in the prevalence of migraine and other headaches during the first seven school years. Headache 1983;23:15–9.

50. Sillanpää M, Anttila P. Increasing prevalence of headache in 7-year-old schoolchildren. Headache 1996;36:466–70.

51. Bandell-Hoekstra IE, Abu-Saad HH, Passchier J, et al. Prevalence and characteristics of headache in Dutch schoolchildren. Eur J Pain 2001;5:145–53.

52. Ozge A, Bugdayci R, Sasmaz T, et al. The sensitivity and specificity of the case definition criteria in diagnosis of headache: a school-based epidemiological study of 5562 children in Mersin. Cephalalgia 2003;23:138–45.

# CHAPTER 3

# Diagnostic Evaluation of Chronic Daily Headache

R. Allan Purdy, MD, FRCPC

Although the International Headache Society (IHS) includes new categories of chronic daily headache (CDH) that may present as symptomatic or secondary headaches,[1] there are no evidence-based recommendations available to guide the diagnostic evaluation of patients with CDH. This chapter provides an overview of when and how to investigate patients with CDH from a clinician's perspective based on experience and the available evidence.

## OVERVIEW OF PROBLEM

Primary CDH occurs in approximately 4% of the general population (see Chapter 2, "Epidemiology of Chronic Daily Headache") and represents a very common reason for patients to consult a neurologist. Indeed, approximately 75% of patients seen in tertiary headache centers have CDH. Primary CDH is now classified into disorders in which individual attacks of headache are either of short (< 4 hours) or long (≥ 4 hours) duration. Primary CDH disorders of long duration include chronic tension-type headache, chronic migraine, transformed migraine, new daily persistent headache (NDPH), and hemicrania continua.[2] Cluster headache and other trigeminal autonomic cephalgias (TACs) constitute the majority of those CDH subtypes that are of short duration.

Should all patients with this CDH be investigated, and, if so, what is the most appropriate and efficient diagnostic approach to such patients? At least for episodic headache disorders, because most are not due to an underlying organic cause, it is not surprising that diagnostic testing has a very low yield. One large meta-analysis found only 0.18% of serious etiologies in patients with headache, all types, and normal neurologic examinations,[3] and this has been borne out in many reviews.[4,5] However, similar analyses have not been performed in patients with CDH.

## PRACTICAL CLINICAL DIAGNOSIS

Although CDH is defined as headache occurring on more than 15 days/month, for practical purposes, CDH is a daily or near-daily headache. As indicated, there are various subtypes of CDH, and recent IHS diagnostic criteria (2004) must be applied to make an accurate diagnosis in specific cases. The most important core diagnoses are migraine without aura, tension-type headache, and cluster headache because these underlie the majority of primary chronic headache subtypes. Hemicrania continua is sufficiently different as to warrant separate consideration, and hypnic headache, which occurs primarily in the elderly and exclusively during sleep, is not hard to recognize if the history is carefully taken.

It is important to tease out the diagnosis of migraine characteristics from the patient with a migraine diathesis to determine whether that person has migraine or migrainous headaches or a disorder that mimics migraine. Also note if a transformation has taken place from episodic migraine to chronic migraine and if any part of this transformation was related to the use of medications. Chronic cluster headache is usually not difficult to diagnose, particularly if it transforms from its episodic form, but when chronic from onset, clinicians need to be alert to the presence of any atypical features that might signify that the headache is symptomatic of an underlying cause. Also, cluster headache must be differentiated from other TACs because they each require a different treatment approach.[6–12]

Further there are now many secondary headache disorders that produce CDH, including medication overuse headache, headache owing to cervical spine disease, low and high intracranial pressure, post-traumatic headache, and headache or facial pain associated with temporomandibular joint disorders. All of these disorders are dealt with in detail in subsequent chapters.

## RED FLAGS, ETIOLOGIC CONSIDERATIONS, AND PATTERN RECOGNITION

"Red flags" are still as useful today as they have always been in neurologic diagnosis,[13] so it bears repeating that any patient with CDH who has any of the following red flags needs evaluation for serious or life-threatening causes of headache:

- Any headache that begins suddenly with peak intensity within minutes
- Any headache that is new or different for the patient
- Headache or facial or neck pain that is progressive in nature
- Headache that is associated with fever or other systemic symptoms
- Headache with new neurologic signs
- Precipitation of head pain with the Valsalva's maneuver (by coughing, sneezing, or bending down)
- New headache onset in an adult, especially over 50 years of age

No matter what the ultimate cause of the patient's headache, it is vital to consider a longer differential diagnosis beyond the usual causes of CDH. A list of serious etiologies is helpful to consider in the approach to the patient:

- Space-occupying lesion (eg, tumor, abscess, hematoma)
- Systemic infection, meningitis, encephalitis
- Stroke (infarction, subarachnoid or intracerebral hemorrhage, and cerebral venous sinus thrombosis)
- Systemic disorders (eg, thyroid disease, hypertension, inflammatory disorders)
- Giant cell (temporal) arteritis
- Traumatic head or neck injuries
- Serious cervical spine causes of headache
- Serious ophthalmologic and otolaryngologic causes of headache
- Serious dental or maxillofacial cause of headache and facial pain

When the consideration of red flags and serious etiologies is paired with a complete neurologic examination, most cases of headache can be sorted out clinically. The practice of classic neurologic diagnosis, based on principles of localization, will miss little even before ordering a neuroimaging procedure or another diagnostic test. Some element of the history or neurologic and general examinations will suggest that a particular headache patient is harboring a serious cause of headache. Obviously, any patient with abnormal vital signs or systemic symptoms, cognitive dysfunction, or a focal neurologic sign needs further assessment and investigation.

The heuristic here is simple: if the clinician recognizes a pattern that simply is not in his or her particular experiential database or is atypical or new, then there is a need to proceed with further evaluation and investigation. A side-locked CDH, a change in pattern, progression in severity or frequency, a consultation for a particular headache not usually experienced by the patient, the presence of unusual autonomic signs or tinnitus, or radicular symptoms are clear indications that more evaluation and testing are needed.

## DIAGNOSTIC EVALUATION

### General Comments

There is little doubt that by the time most patients with CDH are seen by specialists, they probably have been investigated, and, in a general sense, the most likely tests have included blood work, neuroimaging, and even electroencephalography (EEG). This is not surprising because following 6 months of any CDH, most patients and their primary care doctors are more than ready to do some "tests"—in large part to ensure that there is no sinister cause of the CDH, particularly a mass lesion.

Even patients with lifelong intermittent migraine frequently ask if they can have a neuroimaging procedure to ensure that they do not have a "brain tumor," so it would not be unusual or unreasonable for a patient with CDH to think in a similar fashion. This is especially important given that brain tumors frequently present with symptoms of primary headache disorders,[14] including tension-type headache and migraine. Forsyth and Posner pointed out in their retrospective review of headache and cerebral neoplasms that headache can be present in 50 to 60% of brain tumors.[15] They also noted that the classic presentation of headache in "brain tumor" as a severe early morning headache associated with nausea and vomiting occurs only in 17% of patients. Most headaches (77%) met the IHS criteria for tension-like headache, some (9%) were migraine-like, and the rest (14%) were mixed. Pain location was not at all useful in separating tumor headache from nontumor headache. New signs or symptoms in a patient with prior headache, a change of headache pattern, or signs of increased intracranial pressure were indications to perform imaging studies.

### Clinical Assessment

The clinical assessment of patients with CDH must be done with great care and patience.

Obviously, using the IHS diagnostic criteria allows the diagnostician to make a diagnosis, and algorithms have been developed to aid in diagnosis,[16] but the history alone will not confirm the presence or absence of organic disease.[17] As noted, various subtypes of CDH are dealt with in other chapters; however, some basic issues should be addressed in the history and physical examination of all patients with CDH that will help in the diagnostic evaluation. Many of these are not important in all patients, but a comprehensive review should take the following into account:

- Do not assume that patients with CDH have a primary headache disorder because some will harbor an underlying secondary cause even in the presence of a clear history of episodic or chronic migraine.[17]

Many patients will have more than one headache type, and it is important to ask, "How many headache types do you have?" Then each headache type needs a separate symptom analysis to determine the usual quality, location, relieving and aggravating factors and triggers, frequency, duration, and temporal sequence of being stable or worsening over time. Postural headache that gets worse as the day goes on may suggest a cerebrospinal fluid (CSF) leak, whereas in patients with chronic migraine, there would usually be a history of intermittent migraine changing over time into two headaches: one with the prior migraine characteristics occurring intermittently and one occurring daily and more phenotypically, such as tension-type headache.[18] Side-locked headache may represent hemicrania continua but could occur as a result of an organic lesion.[19] Frontal headache accompanied by pain in one or more regions of the face, ears, or both may suggest rhinosinusitis.[1]

When there is aura and other symptoms of brain involvement, especially visual symptoms, it is important to spend some time on these symptoms; frequently, there is something that does not fit if a secondary cause is present. A sensory march over 20 minutes would be more in keeping with migraine[1]; seizures usually last a few minutes, in contrast to the absence of a march in transient ischemic attack or stroke, in which symptoms usually last less than 10 minutes.[20]

When dealing with the short-lasting CDHs, take more care to tease out the history. If the suspicion is cluster headache, but the patient does not meet the usual IHS criteria for cluster headache or has any atypical features, then assume that a secondary etiology may be present. In the absence of a secondary cause, either an ayptical cluster headache or another TAC is likely. Sometimes witnesses may be helpful because they will be able to relate whether the patient has cranial autonomic signs during attacks. The use of a witness is unique in these cases but is similar to having a witness describe a seizure because these patients are in severe pain and may not recognize autonomic features or other changes in physical signs or behavior.

Remember that there are many overlooked conditions that can cause CDH, including intracranial hypertension without papilledema; CSF hypovolemia (hypotension) without postural change; enlarging meningioma without localizing signs; Arnold-Chiari malformation (type I) without exertional, cough, or Valsalva's maneuver–induced headache; and cervical pathology without radiculopathy.[17] There are also numerous other conditions that can contribute to frequent headache, including endocrinologic, biochemical, infectious, inflammatory, toxic or metabolic, hematologic, and immunologic disorders.

As a result, ask if there ever was a history of postural headache that at some point was no longer postural (possibly a CSF leak), any history of posterior headache that at one point was worse with coughing or sneezing (possibly a Chiari I malformation), or any radicular history, pulsatile tinnitus, or other "noises" in the head (possibly intracranial hypertension). The general inquiry must be very thorough and directed against numerous other CDH mimics. For example, patients with idiopathic intracranial hypertension (IIH) do not have to be overweight.[21] A detailed neurologic functional inquiry should be done on a neuroanatomic basis, asking about symptoms related to cranial nerves, motor and sensory systems, and stance and gait, as well as behavioral changes.

Get a collateral history from a relative or from the referring doctor, repeat the basic history to the patient to confirm whether it is accurate, and draw simple timeline graphs with plotted attacks to confirm what you are being told. Accept patient records and graphs and insist on diary documentation to support patients' recollections of headache and other symptoms, as well as medication use, because it can be a very important cause of CDH. Pharmacy and office records from the referring physician can be helpful to document medication consumption as well. It is important to ask about all pain-relief medications, especially those taken over the counter, because many patients will not list or recognize those drugs bought off the pharmacy shelf as pertinent.

Repeat pertinent parts of the history during the clinical examination as a useful cross-examination. Generally, it is best to review prior consultant notes after your own history and examination to avoid premature conclusions on any case, although this is not always practical.

Note the presence of comorbid disorders and explore them in sufficient detail to determine the degree and extent to which, if any, they contribute to the headache disorder. These include depression, anxiety disorders, and somatoform or other psychological disorders.[22]

Is the patient overweight (possible IIH), or is there a history of nocturnal headache and snoring (possible obstructive sleep apnea)?

If a patient has a new onset of daily headache, explore the history to see if there are any prior migraine equivalents or other primary headache disorders, and, if not, was there an obvious precipitating event (possibly NDPH or a mimic)?

Fungal (coccidiomycosis), bacterial (Lyme disease, tuberculosis), and parasitic (neurocysticercosis) infections should be considered in susceptible patients. Sphenoid sinusitis can masquerade as daily headache, be unresponsive to analgesics, interfere with sleep, and occur without associated nasal symptoms.[16] If you see a lot of headache patients, then sooner or later you will see one of these cases of rare etiologies. If you live in an area where these infections are endemic, then a high index of suspicion is required. Chronic meningitis and meningeal carcinomatosis can cause daily headache as well. Therefore, lumbar puncture needs to be considered when these diagnoses are suspect because neuroimaging, especially when not contrast or gadolinium enhanced, may well be unrevealing.

Most importantly, take sufficient time to explore the history and examination with these patients in the first instance and, if necessary, bring them back. Some patients can have very long and graphic histories and be very complex, however, and a lower threshold for referral to headache specialists should be exercised with these patients.

Patients with CDH can be difficult to assess and take time, and this can be frustrating for the diagnostician and the patient. This is especially true if the assessment fails to lead to any definitive diagnosis and there is still a concern as to causation, which can occur in patients with CDH. This, however, is not unique in clinical neurology in that many neurologic disorders are hard to deal with during clinical assessment. Nevertheless, full clinical assessment is still the gold standard in such cases.

## Physical Examination

- Remember that a normal examination without focal signs does not rule out serious etiologies for CDH,[17] such as cerebral vein thrombosis, frontal tumor, or a third ventricular colloid cyst, and if the latter is a consideration, then be sure to check for headache and other spells on bending forward.
- Direct the examination toward CDH mimics and look for papilledema; visual field defects; focal, long-tract, or lateralizing neurologic signs; and evidence of any systemic or other neurologic disorder. Examination of the head and neck and temporomandibular joints is necessary, as is a reasonably good ear, nose, and throat examination and a good ophthalmologic assessment.
- Check for tenderness involving the pericranial and paravertebral muscles, temporal mandibular joints, paranasal sinuses, and occipital nerves. Also evaluate the range of motion of the cervical spine and whether any particular motion reproduces or exacerbates the headache. Palpate the temporal arteries for a pulse and evaluate for tenderness, induration, or tortuosity. Listen for cervical, cranial, and orbital bruits and check for abnormal lymph nodes and masses. Abnormal vital signs, such as fever or an abnormal blood pressure or pulse, should not be overlooked.
- If the patient "looks ill" on inspection, he or she is probably ill. This valuable "sign" is frequently overlooked in the presence of a "normal" examination. Apparent weight loss or wasting can be observed only if the patient is examined properly, which implies appropriate gowning.
- Obviously, any problem with mentation, drowsiness, confusion, or disorientation must be viewed as suspicious, along with any obvious speech pattern abnormality. These do not have to be overt symptoms or signs and are not always overt, so listen and observe carefully. Again, a collateral history or observations from a relative or friend may be as valuable as a physical examination in this setting.
- Check the skull, and if any abnormalities are present on inspection or palpation, then be suspicious. Look for changes in range and movement of the spine, particularly the cervical spine. Signs of meningeal irritation can occur in some secondary causes of chronic headache. Test for limitation in flexion or a "catch" because limitation in all directions is less likely.
- The olfactory nerve is usually not tested routinely by most clinicians, but if not tested, then at least ask about smell and taste, recognizing that taste is mainly a seventh nerve function.
- Check the fundi carefully to see if there is any evidence of papilledema, loss of venous pulsations, abnormal cup to disk ratios, retinal emboli, retinal disease, or other abnormalities. The visual fields should be normal to confrontation finger counting, and the acuity should be near-normal, with best corrected vision if glasses are worn. It is easy to miss a visual field defect if not tested. Remember that papilledema may be the only sign in patients with a third ventricular tumor or IIH or that it may be absent in both.
- Check the extraocular muscles, eyelids, and pupils. Look for and ask about diplopia in any direction of gaze, Horner's syndrome (could be cluster headache or something more ominous), upward gaze palsy, or pupillary enlargement or asymmetry. Also look for mild ptosis, which can be present if there is a history of cluster headache.
- Give careful attention to the fifth and seventh cranial nerves. Obvious abnormalities are usually apparent, but do not forget to test facial sen-

sation, corneal reflex, and motor power of the seventh nerve; at least inspect the motor functions of the seventh nerve. The lower cranial nerves must be normal, but in particular look for twelfth nerve abnormalities because it is easy to test the tongue muscles.

- The motor system should be normal. Subtle weakness may demonstrate itself as a drift of one upper limb when both are extended or a gait abnormality. Significant cerebellar abnormalities are usually easy to demonstrate at the bedside, but if they are subtle, then link the examination to the patient's symptom. In other words, if the patient falls to one side or another or has problems with coordination or balance in one limb or another, then test that limb more rigorously and compare it with the normal limb. Any reflex asymmetry, particularly increased reflexes and tone in one limb or on one side of the body, is clearly a red flag, and, of course, look for an upgoing toe (extensor plantar response, Babinski's sign).
- The sensory system examination should not reveal any major abnormalities or asymmetry. There should be no evidence of parietal lobe dysfunction (which is usually present in a parietal lobe lesion but not tested routinely).
- Stance and gait are easy to test, so always see the patient walk normally, in tandem, and on heels and toes. Have the patient stand with eyes closed with both arms away from the side (testing for Romberg's sign). Any abnormality requires an explanation, and if not readily forthcoming, then investigate. Subtleties can be overlooked here, but major abnormalities are easy to discover.
- Ensure that there is no major cardiac or pulmonary disease or evidence of liver or renal disease. Check the skin for significant lesions. Ask yourself at least once during the examination if the patient has thyroid disease or any other endocrine disorder that could be causing the headache.

## Radiologic Assessment

The reasons for imaging patients with headache are quite straightforward, as suggested by Frishberg:

…patients with new-onset headaches, headaches with a progressive course, headaches with a significant change in pattern, headaches that never alternate sides, and headaches associated with any neurological findings or seizures have a substantially higher likelihood of a secondary cause such as tumor, arteriovenous malformation, or

other structural lesion. In these situations, imaging must be considered as part of the workup.[5]

It is hard to escape the fact that neuroimaging is a large part of the evaluation of a patient with CDH. Each case requires individual consideration. Sometimes it is best to make a preliminary diagnosis if the patient appears to have a primary cause of CDH and proceed with treatment. However, if there is not a good response, or if the headache worsens, it would be prudent to reconsider the diagnosis and do a neuroimaging procedure. Ultimately, gadolinium-enhanced magnetic resonance imaging (MRI) would be the best test in most patients, but it may miss some cases of cerebral venous thrombosis or arterial dissection. Nevertheless, it is more sensitive than an enhanced or unenhanced computed tomographic (CT) scan, especially for the evaluation of the posterior fossa, craniocervical junction, leptomeninges, and dura. There are several situations in which the unenhanced CT scan in a patient with chronic headache with a "normal neurologic examination" may be negative or appear normal:

- Temporal arteritis
- Infiltrating glioma
- Ethmoidal or sphenoidal sinusitis
- Central nervous system vasculitis
- Some posterior fossa or craniocervical lesions
- Some aneurysms and vascular malformations
- Venous sinus or cortical vein thrombosis
- Meningitis (including viral, bacterial, or carcinomatous) and encephalitis
- IIH without papilledema
- Bilateral isodense subdural hematomas
- CSF hypovolemia secondary to CSF leak (intracranial hypotension)

Plain CT may be a good screening test in a patient, but enhanced CT will probably yield more, with minimal risk. CT scans should include bone windows and sinus views. Also, a CT scan may be helpful in avoiding nonspecific and nondiagnostic white matter changes seen on MRI. These are common in migraine patients and do not represent a demyelinating disease or vasculitis in the vast majority of patients.[3] Whether they are ischemic in nature and cumulative is yet to be determined; however, for most patients, the results cause more concern than is likely necessary.[23]

One large study looked at the utility of doing magnetic resonance neuroimaging in patients with chronic headache.[24] The authors investigated the use of MRI in adult patients with a complaint of primary chronic headache and no other neurologic symptoms or findings. The medical records and MRIs of 402 adult patients with chronic headache were retrospectively studied. All patients had been evaluated and referred by the neurology service. The findings were categorized as either negative or positive for major abnormality. A detailed analysis was performed, and major abnormalities were found in 15 patients (3.7%), consisting of 7 women (2.4%) and 8 men (6.9%). Major abnormalities were found in 0.6% of those with migraine headaches, 1.4% with tension headaches, none with mixed migraine and tension headaches, 14.1% with atypical headaches, and 3.8% with other types of headaches. Multivariate analysis showed that the atypical headache type was the most significant predictor of major abnormality. The authors concluded that the yield of major abnormalities found with brain MRI in patients with isolated chronic headache is low. However, those patients with atypical headaches have a higher yield of major abnormalities and may benefit from imaging.

Still, questions arise as to whether to investigate some primary CDHs, such as NDPH. The cause of NDPH is uncertain and the literature is sparse, but up to one-third of patients have a history of a flu-like illness. In one retrospective study of 40 patients with NDPH who underwent laboratory testing and neuroimaging, all test results were normal, except for Epstein-Barr virus antibody titers, which were positive in 71% of 7 patients tested, representing past infection.[25]

NDPH needs careful assessment and definite investigation if there is any doubt about the onset or etiology in any individual patient because there are many secondary mimics. The diagnosis is one of excluding the many secondary causes for a clinical picture that resembles NDPH, which is especially critical early in the course of the disease when a secondary etiology is more likely. NDPH mimics include postmeningitis headache, NDPH with medication rebound, neoplasms, temporal arteritis, chronic meningitis, subdural hematoma, post-traumatic headaches, sphenoid sinusitis, hypertension, subarachnoid hemorrhage, low CSF pressure syndrome, cervical artery dissections, idiopathic intracranial hypertension without papilledema (IIHWOP), and cerebral venous sinus thrombosis.[26] Likewise, in patients with suspected IIH with or without papilledema, neuroimaging is indicated prior to lumbar puncture to exclude the presence of a space-occupying lesion.[27] In patients with suspected cortical vein or cerebral venous sinus thrombosis, especially if there is a suspicion of this condition being present as a cause of chronic headache or elevated intracranial hypertension without papilledema, magnetic resonance venography (MRV) could be helpful in a small percentage of patients in whom the abnormality may be missed by routine MRI. In one study, venous thrombosis, detected on MRV, occurred in 9.6% of patients who presented with CDH.[28] About half of the patients with cerebral venous sinus thrombosis had isolated IIHWOP. The authors suggest that MRV may be a useful tool for selecting patients with

CDH who should have lumbar puncture to exclude isolated IIHWOP.

Patients with suspected intracranial hypotension (CSF hypovolemia) do need gadolinium-enhanced MRIs that include the entire central nervous system to determine if there are imaging features consistent with this diagnosis (thickened and enhancing pachymeninges, cerebellar tonsillar descent, enlarged and/or enhancing pituitary gland, subdural hematoma or hygroma, crowded posterior fossa). Patients with definitive CSF leaks and headache owing to CSF hypovolemia may have a normal brain MRI.[29] Therefore, an MRI of the entire spine will sometimes demonstrate the extra-arachnoid fluid collection from a CSF leak, although it often does not localize the site of the leak. Occasionally, pachymeningeal thickening and enhancement and dilation of the epidural venous plexus are also visible on MRIs of the spine in these patients. For these reasons, an MRI of the entire neuraxis is often necessary in these patients. Radionuclide cisternography, via an intrathecal injection, can document the presence of a CSF leak, whereas CT myelography remains the gold standard in identifying the site of the CSF leak.

Cervical spine radiography and cervical CT and MRI are useful if certain disorders are sought, but not for the majority of CDH patients. Good views of the posterior fossa and foramen magnum region are valuable, especially in viewing Chiari type I abnormalities in patients with cough headaches.[30]

## Laboratory Assessment

Because there are many secondary causes of CDH, a vast array of diagnostic tests are available to the clinician. It is therefore important to allow the clinical assessment and differential diagnosis in each case to guide the selection of diagnostic studies.

A complete blood count and differential may suggest the presence of anemia as a result of hematologic or systemic disease, whereas a left-shifted and elevated white blood cell count would suggest infection. An elevated erythrocyte sedimentation rate and/or C-reactive protein in an elderly person may suggest giant cell (temporal) arteritis or some other form of vasculitis or systemic disorder. If giant cell arteritis is suspected, then a temporal artery biopsy (often bilateral) is indicated, even though it may be negative in some cases.

Abnormal liver and renal function tests and a serum chemistry profile give clues to the diagnosis of systemic disorders. In metastatic cancer, the calcium is frequently elevated, whereas low sodium may suggest SIADH (syndrome of inappropriate antidiuretic hormone), which is frequently associated with systemic disease and intracranial abnormalities, including primary and secondary tumors, as well as chronic subdural hematoma.

It may be useful to do a drug screen if there is a concern that the headaches are linked in any way to medications. Blood gases in patients with headache and pulmonary disease may demonstrate low oxygen saturation and elevated carbon dioxide, which can lead to chronic headache. If the patient has a pink color to the skin and the carboxyhemoglobin level is elevated, this would suggest carbon monoxide exposure. In those patients suspected of obstructive sleep apnea, overnight pulse oximetry may demonstrate significant oxygen desaturations during sleep. If positive, or when there is a high index of suspicion, an overnight polysomnogram may be indicated.

Order thyroxine and thyroid-stimulating hormone tests if there is a suspicion that thyroid dysfunction may be causing or contributing to CDH, and in areas where Lyme disease is endemic, do a screening enzyme-linked immunosorbent assay to look for *Borrelia burgoferi* antibodies. Primary and secondary headaches are common in patients with human immunodeficiency virus (HIV) infection and acquired immune deficiency syndrome (AIDS). Therefore, if the diagnosis is suspected, do an HIV titer and possibly a VDRL test (for venereal disease). Tests for hypercoagulability are indicated if headache is related to intracranial thrombosis. Rare familial disorders, such as mitochondrial encephalopathies, including MELAS (mitochondrial encephalomyopathy, lactic acidosis, and stroke-like episodes) and related disorders, which can present with headache, may require other tests, including muscle biopsy.

### Lumbar Puncture and Other Tests

Again, these tests must be done depending on the indication, but especially in those patients suspected of having IIH, CSF hypotension, and chronic meningitis. The observation of Mosek and colleagues, who prospectively measured the CSF opening pressure in 24 patients with CDH and no papilledema, is important to consider.[31] The average CSF opening pressure was 170 $\pm$ 41 mm $H_2O$, and five patients (21%) had an opening pressure of greater than 200 mm $H_2O$. Patients with CDH had a mean CSF opening pressure that was 13 mm $H_2O$ higher than patients without headache after adjusting for body mass index, age, sex, and various nonheadache disorders. The chances of having a CSF opening pressure > 200 mm $H_2O$ was five times greater for patients with CDH than for patients without headache. From this it could be concluded that a subgroup of patients with CDH have elevated intracranial pressure that may be missed if CSF opening pressure is not studied. However, even if such cases were found, it is uncertain how they would be managed.

Unlike in acute headache, in which the utility of EEG is, at best, questionable, patients with CDH can occasionally benefit from such screening, such as when a metabolic derangement is causing both an encephalopathy and CDH syndrome. However, the report of the Quality Standards Subcommittee of the American Academy of Neurology in 1994 made the following recommendation: EEG is not useful in the routine evaluation of patients with headache (guideline).[32] This does not exclude the use of EEG to evaluate headache patients with associated symptoms suggesting a seizure disorder, atypical migrainous aura, or episodic loss of consciousness. Assuming that head-imaging capabilities are readily available, EEG is not recommended to exclude a structural cause of headache (option).

The use of the Minnesota Multiphasic Personality Inventory (MMPI) can detect comorbid psychological problems that are not uncommon in patients with CDH, as suggested by a recent study.[33] However, the presence of comorbid psychological disorders does not rule out serious etiologies for CDH, so psychological testing is ancillary, although helpful in some cases.

## RARE SECONDARY CHRONIC HEADACHE DISORDERS

Structural lesions, particularly involving the brainstem, pituitary gland, or parasellar region, have been described in patients presenting with CDH disorders that closely resemble a TAC, such as chronic paroxysmal hemicrania or SUNCT syndrome (short-lasting, unilateral, neuralgiform headache with conjunctival injection and tearing).[6,10] As well, a case of frontal lobe malignant glioma was found to mimic chronic paroxysmal hemicrania, and an earlier case was described in a patient with a gangliocytoma growing from the sella turcica.[11] Neurologists should therefore exercise caution in making the diagnosis of these rare primary headche disorders without diagnostic testing, especially brain MRI, to exclude underlying structural lesions.

## SUMMARY AND CONCLUSIONS

The diagnostic evaluation of patients with CDH can, no doubt, be challenging, but these patients, who are often significantly disabled, require nothing less than a detailed medical and neurologic evaluation using a methodical and systematic approach. Anything less could leave the patient and physician with an incorrect diagnosis and misguided treatment. The physical examination, although guided by the history, should be complete at the initial evaluation. Laboratory testing and neuroimaging are an important part of the diagnostic evaluation of patients with CDH given the long list of potentially serious underlying conditions that can present with frequent headache or masquerade as primary CDH syndromes. The selection of the most appropriate studies will be guided by the differential diagnosis generated by a thorough history and physical examination.

## REFERENCES

1. Headache Classification Committee, International Headache Society. Classification and diagnostic criteria for headache disorders, cranial neuralgias, and facial pain. Cephalalgia 2004;24 Suppl 1:1–160.

2. Silberstein SD, Lipton RB. Chronic daily headache. Curr Opin Neurol 2000;13:277–83.

3. Evans RW. Diagnostic testing for headache. Med Clin North Am 2001;85:865–85.

4. Frishberg BM. The utility of neuroimaging in the evaluation of headache in patients with normal neurologic examinations. Neurology 1994;44:1191–7.

5. Frishberg BM. Neuroimaging in presumed primary headache disorders. Semin Neurol 1997;17:373–82.

6. Matharu MS, et al. SUNCT syndrome secondary to prolactinoma. J Neurol Neurosurg Psychiatry 2003;74:1590–2.

7. Newman LC, et al. Chronic paroxysmal headache: two cases with cerebrovascular disease. Headache 1992;32:75–6.

8. Goadsby PJ, Lipton RB. A review of paroxysmal hemicranias, SUNCT syndrome and other short-lasting headaches with autonomic feature, including new cases. Brain 1997;120(1 Pt 1):193–209.

9. Massiou H, et al. SUNCT syndrome in two patients with prolactinomas and bromocriptine-induced attacks. Neurology 2002;58:1698–9.

10. van Vliet JA, et al. Trigeminal autonomic cephalalgiatic-like syndrome associated with a pontine tumour in a one-year-old girl. J Neurol Neurosurg Psychiatry 2003;74:391–2.

11. Vijayan N. Symptomatic chronic paroxysmal hemicrania. Cephalalgia 1992;12:111–3.

12. Medina JL. Organic headaches mimicking chronic paroxysmal hemicrania. Headache 1992;32:73–4.

13. Purdy RA. Clinical evaluation of a patient presenting with headache. Med Clin North Am 2001;85:847–63, v.

14. Purdy RA, Kirby S. Headache and brain tumors. Neurol Clin North Am 2004;22:39–43.

15. Forsyth PA, Posner JB. Headaches in patients with brain tumors: a study of 111 patients. Neurology 1993;43:1678–83.

16. Gladstone J, Eross E, Dodick D. Chronic daily headache: a rational approach to a challenging problem. Semin Neurol 2003;23:265–76.

17. Saper JR. Chronic daily headache: a clinician's perspective. Headache 2002;42:538–42.

18. Mathew NT, Reuveni U, Perez F. Transformed or evolutive migraine. Headache 1987;27:102–6.

19. Levy MJ, Matharu MS, Goadsby PJ. Prolactinomas, dopamine agonists and headache: two case reports. Eur J Neurol 2003;10:169–73.

20. Mohr JP, GJ, Pessin MS. Internal carotid artery disease. In: MJ Barnett HJM, Stein B, Yatsu FM, editors. New York: Churchill Livingstone; 1998. p. 355–400.

21. Evans RW, Dulli D. Pseudo-pseudotumor cerebri. Headache 2001;41:416–8.

22. Silberstein SD, Lipton RB, Breslau N. Migraine: association with personality characteristics and psychopathology. Cephalalgia 1995;15:358–69; discussion 336.

23. Kruit MC, et al. Migraine as a risk factor for subclinical brain lesions. JAMA 2004;291:427–34.

24. Wang HZ, et al. Brain MR imaging in the evaluation of chronic headache in patients without other neurologic symptoms. Acad Radiol 2001;8:405–8.

25. Li D, Rozen TD. The clinical characteristics of new daily persistent headache. Cephalalgia 2002;22:66–9.

26. Evans RW. New daily persistent headache. Curr Pain Headache Rep 2003;7:303–7.

27. Evans RW, Silberstein SD. Diagnostic testing for chronic daily headache. Headache 2002;42:556–9.

28. Quattrone A, et al. Cerebral venous thrombosis and isolated intracranial hypertension without papilledema in CDH. Neurology 2001;57:31–6.

29. Mokri B, et al. Absent pachymeningeal gadolinium enhancement on cranial MRI despite symptomatic CSF leak. Neurology 1999;53:402–4.

30. Pascual J, et al. Cough, exertional, and sexual headaches: an analysis of 72 benign and symptomatic cases. Neurology 1996;46:1520–4.

31. Mosek A, SJ, O'Fallon WM, et al. CSF opening pressure in patients with chronic daily headache [abstract]. Cephalalgia 1999;19:323.

32. Practice parameter: the electroencephalogram in the evaluation of headache. Report of the Quality Standards Subcommittee, American Academy of Neurology. Neurology 1994.

33. Bigal ME, et al. MMPI personality profiles in patients with primary chronic daily headache: a case-control study. Neurol Sci 2003;24:103–10.

# Primary Chronic
# Daily Headache

# CHAPTER 4

# Transformed and Chronic Migraine

Stephen D. Silberstein, MD, FACP

Chronic migraine (CM), one of the subtypes of chronic daily headache (CDH), is considered a subtype of migraine in the new International Headache Society (IHS) classification.[1] The term CDH now refers to the headache disorders experienced very frequently (15 or more days a month), including headaches associated with medication overuse. CDH can be divided into primary and secondary varieties.[2] Primary CDH is not related to a structural or systemic illness. Population-based studies in the United States, Europe, and Asia suggest that 4 to 5% of the general population have primary CDH[3–5] and that 0.5% have severe headaches on a daily basis.[6–8] CDH patients account for the most consultations in headache subspecialty practices.[9] Our approach to classifying frequent headache consists of first defining a primary or secondary CDH syndrome and then subclassifying primary CDH on the basis of average daily headache duration ($\geq$ 4 hours or < 4 hours).

Secondary CDH has an identifiable underlying cause, including symptomatic medication overuse, head trauma, cervical spine disorders, vascular disorders, nonvascular intracranial disorders, temporomandibular joint disorders, and sinus infection.[5,10–13] Other causes include chronic meningitis and idiopathic intracranial hypertension (IIH).[3,4,14–16] IIH is easily diagnosed when papilledema is present. Some patients with IIH do not have papilledema, in which case, it can mimic primary CDH. Cervicogenic headache is a unilateral pain disorder that does not switch sides, occurs mainly in women, and may be associated with ipsilateral blurred vision, tinnitus, lacrimation, tingling, difficulty swallowing, photophobia, arm pain, and, when more severe, nausea and anorexia.[17,18] Certain focal dystonias of the head and neck (pharyngeal dystonia, spasmodic torticollis, mandibular dystonia, lingual dystonia, and segmental craniocervical dystonia) are often accompanied by headache.

Once secondary headache (including medication-overuse headache [MOH]) has been excluded, frequent headache sufferers are subdivided into two groups, based on headache duration. When the headache duration is $\geq$ 4 hours, the differential diagnosis includes cluster headache, paroxysmal hemicrania, idiopathic stabbing headache, hypnic headache, and SUNCT syndrome (short-lasting, unilateral, neuralgiform headache with conjunctival infection and tearing). When the headache duration is $\geq$ 4 hours, the major primary disorders to consider are transformed migraine (TM), hemicrania continua (HC), chronic tension-type headache (CTTH), and new daily persistent headache (NDPH) (Table 4–1).[9] CTTH was included in the first IHS classification and inappropriately equated to CDH.[19] CM, NDPH, and HC are primary CDH disorders that are now included in the second IHS classification (see Table 4–1).[1] Transformed migraine is similar but not identical to CM.

## HISTORICAL REVIEW

Many studies found problems with the original criteria mandated by the IHS[19] to classify CDH, one of the most common disorders seen in headache centers.[20–26] These studies showed that CDH was not easily classified within the old IHS system.[22–26] When classified, the headaches were usually placed in the CTTH group. But because the daily headaches often evolve from episodic migraine and the patients had many migrainous features, it was inappropriate to classify them as CTTH. Yet the headaches are too frequent to permit their being classified as migraine.[22]

Migraine and tension-type headache (TTH) have long been considered distinct entities, and the IHS continues this separation.[1,19] However, many clinicians and epidemiologists now believe that the TTH experienced by migraineurs is, in fact, a milder form of migraine.[20] In nonmigraineurs, it is a distinct entity. As

**Table 4–1**    Chronic Daily Headache

| Primary chronic daily headache | Secondary chronic daily headache |
|---|---|
| Headache duration ≥ 4 h | Medication overuse headache |
| Chronic migraine | Post-traumatic headache |
| Chronic tension-type headache | Cervical spine disorders |
| New daily persistent headache | Headache associated with vascular disorders (arteriovenous malformation, arteritis [including giant cell arteritis], dissection, and subdural hematoma) |
| Hemicrania continua | |
| Transformed migraine | Headache associated with nonvascular intracranial disorders (intracranial hypertension, intracranial hypotension, infection [EBV, HIV], neoplasm) |
| Headache duration < 4 h | |
| Cluster headache | Other (temporomandibular joint disorder, sinus infection) |
| Paroxysmal hemicranias | |
| Hypnic headache | |
| Primary stabbing headache | |
| SUNCT | |

EBV = Epstein-Barr virus; HIV = human immunodeficiency virus; SUNCT = short-lasting, unilateral, neuralgiform headache with conjunctival infection and tearing.

headache frequency increases, the clinical distinction between migraine and TTH becomes blurred. As migraine frequency increases, headaches often decrease in severity and associated migrainous features decline in prominence. The headaches occur daily or almost every day, and superimposed on these background headaches may be occasional full-blown migraine attacks. Saper used the term "progressive migraine" for this disorder and referred to the condition as complex headache syndrome because of the presence of comorbidities. Saper credits John Graham as being one of the first physicians who noted the transition from intermittent to daily headache. Mathew and colleagues referred to this disorder as TM.[3] CDH evolving from migraine is another term used to describe this disorder. An older term was "mixed or combined headache."[22,27] The IHS did not use these terminologies. Within the first IHS classification formula, there was no appropriate classification for TM. Nevertheless, at least in the United States, it was a common problem in headache subspecialty practices.[20] The second IHS classification now uses the term CM,[1] which is not identical to TM, and the distinction is important.

Many studies demonstrated that the original IHS system did not adequately classify many patients seen in subspecialty centers. Messinger and colleagues, using the IHS criteria and questionnaire data from two surveys, attempted to classify a clinic-based sample of 410 subjects with a headache history of more than 2 years.[24]

They were unable to classify 35.9% of the patients. Overall, only 9.1% had CTTH, but about 86% of these CTTH patients had two or more migrainous features. Solomon and colleagues evaluated 100 consecutive patients who presented to a tertiary headache center with CDH.[22] Most (61%) had continuous headache; 39% had intermittent headache defined by pain-free intervals of at least 1 hour at least 4 days per week. More than 50% overused acute medication. Although two-thirds of these patients met the criteria for CTTH, many had migrainous features. One-third of the patients could not be classified as having CTTH because they had too many migrainous features. Many of these headaches would be classifiable as migraine were it not for their daily occurrence. Many patients could not be classified in the old IHS system (except as "headache of the tension-type not fulfilling [other] criteria"). The authors pointed out that the IHS criteria did not take into account the historical features of CDH before it becomes daily. Is CDH preceded by episodic migraine or TTH, or do the headaches begin de novo? Past history is an essential part of the headache diagnosis. Solomon and colleagues concluded that the IHS criteria should be modified to include TM (CDH evolving from migraine) and that subtypes with and without medication overuse should be distinguished both for TM and CTTH. They did not propose specific diagnostic criteria for these disorders.

In a less selected sample, Sanin and colleagues attempted to validate the IHS criteria in a headache clinic population.[23] They randomly selected the clinical records of 400 patients and classified them using the IHS criteria. Over 55% of the patients had more than one diagnosis, and 37.7% had CDH. CTTH was diagnosed in 110 patients, 90% of whom also suffered from migraine. They concluded that most patients in their clinic had more than one IHS diagnosis, that CTTH occurring alone is rare, and that chronic headache classification needed revision. Pfaffenrath and Isler investigated the IHS criteria for CTTH in a sample of 211 subjects participating in a clinical trial of antidepressant treatment.[25] Daily headache was present in 56% of patients. Of the remaining 44%, headaches occurred an average of 18 days per month. More than two-thirds met the two major IHS criteria for CTTH (bilateral pain, 79%; pressure or tightening, 72%). Fifty-nine percent met all of the IHS criteria for CTTH. However, many symptoms of migraine were also reported: unilateral headache, 20%; throbbing, 28%; anorexia, 39%; osmophobia, 25%; phonophobia, 60%; nausea, 53%; and increased pain with physical activity, 48%. In total, half of the patients failed to meet one or more of the criteria of migraine. Many patients experienced the symptoms of migraine with headaches of mild intensity. These studies suggested that the IHS criteria need to be revised with respect to the classification of daily headache.

Several studies demonstrate the phenomenon of TM. Mathew reported a series of patients with distinct attacks of migraine whose headaches evolved over the years into a daily or near-daily problem.[26] The majority of women had menstrual aggravation of headache. Patients had features of both migraine and TTH. Most (90%) had migraine without aura. These patients had more triggers, gastrointestinal symptoms, and a family history of headaches than patients with CTTH. Most overused acute medications. Stopping the overused medication frequently resulted in distinct headache improvement.

Saper found that 80% of his CDH patients had prior episodic migraine, with onset between the ages of 26 and 41 years.[16] These patients were typically women. They were frequently clinically depressed and had superimposed acute bouts of migraine. Many of them overused abortive headache medications and had significant long-term improvement following detoxification.

Sandrini and colleagues classified 90 consecutive outpatients with CDH who attended a clinic in Italy.[28] Most (75%) had CDH evolving from migraine, whereas 16.7% began de novo and 7.7% had evolved from episodic tension-type headache (ETTH). They differentiated two subsets of patients with CDH evolving from migraine. "Transformed migraine" referred to those patients who had distinct bouts of migraine that evolved into CDH with the disappearance of typical migraine attacks. "Migraine with interparoxysmal headache" was defined as recurrent bouts of migraine with a constant, low-severity headache between attacks.

Silberstein and colleagues studied 300 patients who had chronic refractory headache and were admitted to an inpatient unit.[29] Most (216) had CDH associated with acute medication overuse. A subset of these patients (50) who overused medication were followed for 2 years. Most had TM (74%), some had NDPH (24%), and only 2% had CTTH with a diagnosis of prior ETTH. Most patients (80%) reverted to episodic headache following detoxification, suggesting that both TM and NDPH associated with medication overuse are perpetuated by drug overuse.

Silberstein and colleagues concluded that (1) the IHS classification was not comprehensive because there was a large subset of patients with daily headache who were not well classified; (2) daily headache is often TM; in this area, the IHS criteria for CTTH may not be valid; and (3) CDH is often associated with medication overuse but may occur without it. They recommended revising the IHS criteria for chronic, frequent primary headache disorders and proposed adding several headache types to the 1988 IHS classification.[9] They defined CDH as a group of several distinct types of primary headaches. CDH includes all of the primary headache disorders, with daily or near-daily headaches lasting more than 4 hours per day untreated. CDH was subdivided into TM, CTTH evolved from ETTH, NDPH, and HC.

Silberstein and Lipton proposed operational criteria for TM in 1994, including it as a subset of migraine (Table 4–2). Its diagnosis depended on a history of IHS-defined migraine and the presence of head pain lasting more than 4 hours a day at least 15 days a month. They elected not to require particular characteristics for the daily or near-daily headaches, in part because these headaches are pleiomorphic; daily headaches may be unilateral or bilateral, mild to severe in intensity, with or without associated migrainous features. They originally required a history of transformation, that is, a period when migraine headaches increased in frequency, whereas the prominence of associated migrainous features decreased. Patients with TM often continue to have episodic superimposed bouts of full-blown migraine. Some patients find that their migraine headaches disappear completely. For this reason, they did not originally use the continuing occurrence of superimposed migraine attacks as part of their definition. TM was subdivided into two categories, one with and one without medication overuse, using a consensus of published reports to define medication overuse. They recommended field-testing their proposed revisions to the IHS criteria to determine whether they served the intended purposes. They prospectively assessed (in a headache subspecialty center) the comprehensiveness of the IHS

**Table 4–2**  Original Proposed Criteria for Transformed Migraine

1.8 Transformed migraine

   A. History of episodic migraine meeting any IHS criteria 1.1 to 1.6

   B. Daily or almost daily (> 15 d/mo) head pain for > 1 mo

   C. Average headache duration of 4 h/d (if untreated)

   D. History of increasing headache frequency with decreasing severity of migrainous features over at least 3 mo*

   E. At least 1 of the following

      1. There is no suggestion of one of the disorders listed in groups 5–11

      2. Such a disorder is suggested but is ruled out by appropriate investigations

      3. Such a disorder is present, but first migraine attacks do not occur in close temporal relation to the disorder

1.8.1 Transformed migraine with medication overuse

1.8.2 Transformed migraine without medication overuse

IHS = International Headache Society.

criteria with and without the addition of the original criteria for TM. They then determined whether subjects could provide the information necessary to assign diagnoses using the revised criteria. They identified subjects who cannot be classified and recommended modifications, based on the results of the field tests.[30]

Silberstein and Lipton confirmed that the old IHS criteria were not comprehensive; they were unable to classify 43% of daily headache sufferers. (This result is concordant with several prior studies conducted at subspecialty centers.[22,24]) Several difficulties with the proposed 1994 revisions to the IHS criteria became apparent. They were still not able to classify 25% of patients. Some patients had difficulty remembering the characteristics of their prior headaches, that is, whether their headaches had escalated, when they had escalated, and how long the process of escalation took. They modified the definition of TM to include subjects with either a history of IHS migraine, a history of escalation over 3 months, or a current headache that, except for duration, met the IHS criteria for migraine (Table 4–3). This allowed the use of both historical and current features of the headache, which are crucial to the diagnosis. Using the 1995 Silberstein and Lipton criteria, 15.3% of patients had CTTH, 78% had TM, none had NDPH, and 6.7% had none of these disorders. To avoid more than one diagnosis for a single headache type, they imposed hierarchical diagnostic rules: patients could not be diagnosed with CTTH if they met the criteria for TM. The focus of their effort was to make the IHS criteria more comprehensive by providing a place for patients with TM. The new IHS classification includes an entity called (CM), which is similar but not identical to TM.[30] In this review, TM, as defined by the Silberstein and Lipton criteria, instead of CM as defined by the

IHS, is used because the latter has not been field-tested and the former has been used as the gold standard in population-based and clinical studies and appears to be more sensitive and relevant to clinical practice.

## TRANSFORMED MIGRAINE

Many studies have described the process and associated features of TM,[3,4,14–16,30] which is similar to what was called transformed or evolutive migraine or mixed headache. Patients with TM often have a past history of episodic migraine that began in their teens or twenties.[4,16,30] Most patients with this disorder are women, 90% of whom have a history of migraine without aura. Patients often report a process of transformation characterized by headaches that become more frequent over months or years, with the associated symptoms of photophobia, phonophobia, and nausea becoming less severe and less frequent.[14,16,31] Patients often develop a pattern of daily or near-daily headaches that phenomenologically resemble a mixture of TTH and migraine. That is, the pain is often mild to moderate and is not always associated with photophobia, phonophobia, or gastrointestinal features. Other features of migraine, including unilaterality, gastrointestinal symptoms, and aggravation by menstruation and other trigger factors, may persist. Attacks of full-blown migraine superimposed on a background of less severe headaches occur in many patients. The term "transformation" has been used to refer to this process.

The term CM is now being used by the IHS as a complication of migraine, in part because a history of transformation may be missing. Eighty percent of patients with TM have depression,[16,26] which often lifts when the pattern of medication overuse and daily

**Table 4–3** Silberstein and Lipton Revised Criteria for Transformed Migraine

A.  Daily or almost daily ($\geq$ 15 d/mo) head pain for $\geq$ 1 mo

B.  Average headache duration of $\geq$ 4 h/d (if untreated)

C.  At least 1 of the following:

    1.  History of episodic migraine meeting any IHS criteria 1.1 to 1.6

    2.  History of increasing headache frequency with decreasing severity of migrainous features over at least 3 mo

    3.  Headache at some time meets IHS criteria for migraine 1.1 to 1.6 other than duration

D.  Does not meet criteria for new daily persistent headache (4.7) or hemicrania continua (4.8)

E.  Not attributed to another disorder

IHS = International Headache Society.

headache is interrupted. Silberstein and Lipton's revised criteria for TM (see Table 4–3) provided three alternative diagnostic links to migraine: (1) a prior history of IHS migraine, (2) a clear period of escalating headache frequency with decreasing severity of migrainous features, or (3) current superimposed attacks of headaches that meet all of the IHS criteria for migraine except duration.[30] Bigal and colleagues used the Silberstein and Lipton criteria to compare the features of TM patients with (TM+) and without (TM−) a history of migraine in a preventive trial of TM.[32] The groups were similar in age (42.5 versus 44.2 years), sex (86.4% versus 78.3% female), monthly migraine days (13.6 versus 12.6), Migraine Disability Assessment Scale (MIDAS) grades, and Beck scores. The groups differed in time of onset (10.6 versus 17.5 years). This suggests that they are the same disorder and supports the Silberstein and Lipton criteria for TM. The difference between the groups is the longer duration of TM−, suggesting that these patients may have forgotten their history of migraine.

Migraine often transforms into CDH as a result of medication overuse (MOH), but transformation occurs without overuse.[3,33] About 80% of CDH patients seen in subspecialty clinics overuse symptomatic medication.[3,4,16,31,34] Headache frequency often increases when medication use increases. Stopping the overused medication usually results in distinct headache improvement, over days to weeks. Many patients have significant long-term improvement after detoxification. Using the 1988 IHS criteria, a diagnosis of headache induced by substance use or exposure requires that the headaches remit after the overused

medication is discontinued.[19] This criterion was difficult to apply reliably, and diagnosis was impossible until it was clear that headache persisted for > 15 days after the overused medication was discontinued.[9] The 2004 IHS criteria attempt to resolve this issue by using the term "probable CM" (see below).

The second IHS classification considers CM to be a subset of migraine (Table 4–4).[1] Its diagnosis requires migraine headache that occurs on 15 or more days a month for more than 3 months without medication overuse. It must not be attributable to another disorder, including HC or NDPH. When medication overuse is present, the diagnosis is unclear until medication has been withdrawn and there has been no improvement. The IHS rule is to code these patients according to the antecedent migraine subtype (usually migraine without aura) plus probable CM plus probable MOH. If the criteria for CM are still fulfilled 2 months after medication overuse has ceased, diagnose CM plus the antecedent migraine subtype and discard the diagnosis of probable MOH. If the CM criteria are no longer fulfilled, change the diagnosis to MOH plus the antecedent migraine subtype and discard the diagnosis of probable CM.[1]

The requirement that the daily headache must meet the criteria for migraine without aura each day remains a concern with the new IHS criteria. Even episodic migraine does not always meet IHS migraine criteria throughout the attack. Some have suggested that the daily headache of CM should meet the criteria of probable migraine (missing one diagnostic feature of migraine) at least half of the time.

**Table 4–4** New International Headache Society Criteria for Chronic Migraine

A.  Headache fulfilling criteria C and D for 1.1 migraine without aura on $\geq$ 15 d/mo for > 3 mo

B.  Not attributed to another disorder

Adapted from Headache Classification Committee, International Headache Society.[19]

Bigal and colleagues applied alternative diagnostic approaches to 638 CDH patients consulting in specialty care.[35] Patients were classified according to both the Silberstein and Lipton and the 2004 IHS classification systems. Patients were predominantly female (65.0%), with ages ranging from 11 to 88 years. Using the Silberstein and Lipton classification, they found eight different diagnoses. The most common diagnosis was TM (87.4%), followed by NDPH (10.8%). Six patients had CTTH. Using the IHS criteria, they found 14 different diagnoses. Migraine was found in 576 (90.2%) patients. CTTH occurred in 621 (97.3%), with only 10 (1.57%) having this as the sole diagnosis. They concluded that both systems allow for the classification of most patients with CDH when daily headache diaries are available. The main difference is that the IHS classification is cumbersome and requires multiple diagnoses. They found that the Silberstein and Lipton system is easier to apply and more parsimonious.

Many researchers have used the Silberstein and Lipton criteria to study the clinical characteristics of TM. Krymchantowski and colleagues retrospectively evaluated 215 CDH patients seen in a headache clinic.[36] Subjects included 158 women and 57 men aged 12 to 83 years (mean age 35 years) who had clear-cut prior IHS migraine attacks (with and/or without aura). Most met the Silberstein and Lipton criteria for TM. All had daily moderate pain, and some had intermittent attacks of severe headache; 46.5% had bilateral pain, 37.1% hemicranial pain, 12.1% diffuse pain, and 26.5% other pain locations. Approximately 41% had throbbing pain, 36.2% tightening pain, 17.2% a combination of throbbing and dull pain, 4.2% burning pain, and 7.4% other types of headache.

Monzón and colleagues classified and analyzed the clinical features of 164 consecutive CDH patients (headache at least 15 days a month during the previous 6 months).[37] CDH had evolved from a previous headache in 151 cases: migraine in 118 (72%) (TM) and ETTH in 33 (20%). CDH was unremitting from onset (NDPH) in 13 cases (8%). Most patients had nonpulsating bilateral pain of moderate intensity, with few associated symptoms. Sixty-five percent overused analgesics or ergots; 18% were men and 82% were women.

## Differentiating TM from Other CDHs

Although most CDHs are due to a primary headache disorder, one must be sure that they are not attributable to another disorder, the most common of which is MOH. Secondary causes of frequent headache include prior trauma (chronic post-traumatic headache), cervical spine disorders, vascular disorders, chronic meningitis, IIH, spontaneous intracranial hypotension secondary to cerebrospinal fluid (CSF) leak, temporomandibular joint disorder, and sinus infection.[2,38] IIH is easily diagnosed when papilledema is present, but if the patient does not have papilledema, intracranial hypertension can mimic primary CDH. Intracranial hypertension may be either idiopathic, with no clear identifiable cause, or symptomatic; underlying etiologies for the latter include venous sinus occlusion, a mass lesion, meningitis, trauma, radical neck dissection, hypoparathyroidism, vitamin A intoxication, systemic lupus, renal disease, or drug side effects (nalidixic acid, danazol, corticosteroid withdrawal). Intracranial hypertension from cerebral venous outflow obstruction can be caused by chronic otitis, head trauma, tumors, hypercoagulable states, or cerebral edema.[39] Increased intracranial pressure consequent to venous outflow hypertension can also occur without obstruction when patients have arteriovenous malformations, cardiac failure, and pulmonary failure. Increased intracranial pressure is not always associated with either headache or papilledema, and there is no direct correlation between the degree of pressure elevation and the presence of headache. IIH, although more common in obese women, can also occur in nonobese women and in men. The presence of transient visual obscurations and intracranial noises provides clues to the diagnosis.

Spontaneous intracranial hypotension secondary to a CSF leak can be missed because the postural relationship may disappear over time. Occasionally, orthostatic headache is never present, and patients may notice that their headaches begin and increase gradually after rising in the morning.[12] Infectious causes, including fungal (coccidiomycosis), bacterial (Lyme disease, tuberculosis), and parasitic (neurocysticercosis) causes, should be considered in high-risk patients. Sphenoid sinusitis can present as an intractable headache that is unresponsive to analgesics and interferes with sleep. It often occurs without associated nasal symptoms. Obstructive sleep apnea can present with daily headaches on awakening. It should be considered when patients have a snoring history, have a large neck size, or are obese. Cervical spine, temporomandibular joint, or dental pathology must be considered when chronic cranial, nuchal, or facial pain is present. Magnetic resonance imaging and magnetic resonance venography (with gadolinium if needed) are the neuroimaging procedures of choice for patients suspected of having a secondary cause for CDH because many of these disorders remain undetected even with contrast-enhanced CT. With a normal physical examination and the absence of red flags or worrisome historical features, secondary causes of TM can usually be eliminated.[40]

Other types of CDH (lasting, on average, $\geq 4$ hours a day) include CTTH, NDPH, and HC. CTTH is described by the IHS as "A disorder evolving from episodic tension-type headache, with daily or very frequent episodes of headache lasting minutes to days. The pain is typically bilateral, pressing or tightening in quality and of mild to moderate intensity, and does not worsen with routine physical activity. There may be mild nausea, photophobia or phonophobia."[25] The new IHS criteria continue to permit only one of mild nausea, photophobia, or phonophobia but exclude moderate or severe nausea or vomiting. Episodic migraine and CTTH can coexist. Guitera and colleagues suggested, based on population-based epidemiologic data, that coexistent CTTH and episodic migraine can coexist if, and only if, the current CTTH has no migrainous features and there is a remote history of migraine.[41]

The introduction of CM into the second edition of "The International Classification of Headache Disorders"[1] creates a problem in the differential diagnosis between CM and CTTH. Both diagnoses require headache (meeting the criteria for migraine or TTH) on at least 15 days a month. Therefore, it is theoretically possible for a patient to have both of these diagnoses. In the Silberstein and Lipton criteria, the diagnosis of one disorder takes precedence over the diagnosis of another.[4,16,30] They suggested that a putative diagnosis of CTTH may not meet the criteria for HC, NDPH, or CM. This would handle the difficulty of the small group of patients who fulfill the IHS diagnostic criteria for both CM and CTTH. This would be possible when two (and only two) of the four pain characteristics are present and the headaches are associated with mild nausea. These cases are most likely CM and have been shown to have elevated levels of calcitonin gene–related peptide (CGRP) (a marker for migraine). They should be coded as CTTH and episodic migraine only if the daily baseline headache has no migrainous features.

NDPH is characterized by the relatively abrupt onset of an unremitting primary CDH.[42,43] The IHS now includes NDPH in its classification. NDPH requires the absence of a history of evolution from migraine or ETTH. In the absence of rapid development, it is coded as CTTH or CM. NDPH may or may not be associated with medication overuse. A diagnosis of NDPH takes precedence over CM and CTTH.

HC[44,45] is a rare, indomethacin-responsive headache disorder characterized by a continuous, moderately severe, unilateral headache that varies in intensity, waxing and waning without disappearing completely.[46] Some patients have photophobia, phonophobia, and nausea. The IHS now includes HC in the classification. It is described as a "persistent strictly unilateral headache responsive to indomethacin."[19] It differs from CM in that it must be unilateral and must respond to indomethacin.

## Medication-Overuse Headache

MOH was previously called rebound headache, drug-induced headache, and medication-misuse headache (Table 4–5). Patients with frequent headaches often overuse analgesics, opioids, ergotamine, and triptans.[47–50] Medication overuse may be both a response to and a consequence of chronic pain, or, in headache-prone patients, it may produce drug-induced headache accompanied by dependence on symptomatic medication. In addition, medication overuse can make headaches refractory to preventive medication.[33,51–56] Although stopping the acute medication may result in the development of withdrawal symptoms and a period of increased headache, subsequent headache improvement usually occurs.[56–60] In American subspecialty centers, most patients with drug-induced headache have a history of episodic migraine that has been converted into CDH (MOH) as a result of medication overuse.[4,5,51,61–63] In European headache centers, 5 to 10% of patients have drug-induced headache.[64] Patients with TTH, HC, and NDPH may also overuse symptomatic medications.

When a new headache occurs for the first time in close temporal relation to substance exposure, it is coded as a secondary headache attributed to the substance. This is true even if the headache has the characteristics of migraine, TTH, or cluster headache.

---

**Table 4–5   New International Headache Society Criteria for Headache Attributed to Medication Overuse**

| | |
|---|---|
| A. | Headache present on ≥ 15 d/mo fulfilling criteria C and D |
| | Characteristics depend on drug |
| B. | Regular overuse for > 3 mo of a medication |
| | Amount depends on drug |
| | Ergotamine, triptans, opioids, and combination analgesics ≥ 10 d/mo |
| | Simple analgesics ≥ 15 d/mo |
| C. | Headache has developed or markedly worsened during medication overuse |
| D. | Headache resolves or reverts to its previous pattern within 2 mo after discontinuation of overused medication |

Adapted from Headache Classification Committee, International Headache Society.[19]

When a preexisting primary headache is aggravated in close temporal relation to substance exposure, there are two possibilities. The patient can either be given only the diagnosis of the preexisting primary headache or both this diagnosis and the diagnosis of headache attributed to the substance. A diagnosis of headache attributed to a substance becomes definite only when the headache resolves or greatly improves after exposure to the substance is terminated. In the case of MOH, an arbitrary period of 2 months after overuse cessation is now stipulated by the IHS; if the diagnosis is to be definite, improvement must occur in that time frame. Prior to cessation, or pending improvement within 2 months after cessation, the diagnosis of probable MOH should be applied. If improvement does not then occur within the 2-month period, the MOH diagnosis is discarded.

Patients with a preexisting primary headache who develop a new type of headache or whose migraine or TTH is made markedly worse during medication overuse should be given the diagnosis of both the preexisting headache and MOH. The headache associated with medication overuse often has a peculiar shifting pattern, even within the same day, from having migraine-like characteristics to having those of TTH (ie, a new type of headache). The diagnosis of MOH is clinically important because patients rarely respond to preventive medications while they are overusing acute medications.

Overuse is now defined in terms of treatment days per month. It is crucial that treatment occur both frequently and regularly, that is, several days each week. For example, the diagnostic criterion of use on 10 or more days a month (15 for simple analgesics) translates into 2 to 3 treatment days every week. Bunching treatment days and having long periods without medication intake, as practiced by some patients, is much less likely to cause MOH. The amount of use that constitutes overuse depends on the drug. Ergotamine-overuse headache requires intake on 10 or more days a month on a regular basis for 3 or more months. The headache is often daily and constant. Triptan-overuse headache is usually frequent, intermittent, and migrainous. Triptan intake (any formulation) on 10 or more days a month may increase migraine frequency to that of CM. Evidence suggests that this occurs sooner with triptan overuse than with ergotamine overuse.[48,49]

## Comorbidity (Psychiatric and Other)

Anxiety, depression, panic disorder, and bipolar disease are more frequent in migraineurs than in nonmigraine control subjects.[65,66] Given that TM is a complication of migraine, one would expect to find a similar profile of psychiatric comorbidity in TM patients. However, many older studies do not clearly differentiate between CDH subtypes. Nevertheless, in clinic-based samples,

depression occurs in 80% of TM patients. The Minnesota Multiphasic Personality Inventory was abnormal in 61% of primary CDH patients compared with 12.2% of episodic migraine patients. Primary CDH patients had significantly higher Zung and Beck Depression Scale scores than did migraine controls.[12,33,51,67] Comorbid depression often improves when the cycle of daily head pain is broken.

Mitsikostas and Thomas found that headache patients had significantly higher average Hamilton rating anxiety and depression scores than did nonheadache controls.[68] Patients with CTTH, mixed headache, or drug-abuse headache had the highest Hamilton rating depression and anxiety scores. Verri and colleagues found current psychiatric comorbidity in 90% of primary CDH patients.[69] Generalized anxiety occurred in 69.3% of patients and major depression in 25%.

Psychiatric comorbidity is a predictor of intractability. The Minnesota Multiphasic Personality Inventory was abnormal in 100% of CDH patients who failed to respond to aggressive management (31% of the primary CDH group) compared with 48% of the responders. Physical, emotional, or sexual abuse, parental alcohol abuse, and a positive dexamethasone suppression test also correlated highly with a poor response to aggressive management. Curioso and colleagues found that 31 of 69 (45%) CDH patients had an adjustment disorder, 16 (23%) had major depression, 12 (17%) were dysthymic, 6 (9%) had generalized anxiety disorder, 1 (2%) was bipolar, and 3 (4%) were normal.[70] The risk of a bad outcome after treatment was significantly greater for patients who had major depression than for those who did not. CDH patients who have major depression or abnormal Beck Depression Inventory scores have worse outcomes at 3 to 6 months compared with patients who are not depressed.

Puca and colleagues evaluated psychopathologic symptoms and psychiatric disorders in 234 adult CDH patients (184 women and 50 men; mean age 43.05 ± 12.90 years).[71] The Structured Clinical Interview for the *Diagnostic and Statistical Manual of Mental Disorders-IV* and the Symptom Check List 90R were used. At least one psychiatric disorder (anxiety disorder, 45%; mood disorder, 33%) was detected in 66% of the sample CDH patients. The prevalence of psychopathologic symptoms was more than 78%. At least one psychosocial stress factor was found in 42% of cases, and 64% of the whole sample overused symptomatic drugs.

Guitera and colleagues analyzed the impact of CDH on quality of life using the Medical Outcome Short Form (SF-36) questionnaire in a population sample of 1,883 individuals, 4.7% of whom met the Silberstein and Lipton criteria for CDH.[30,72] Eighty-nine healthy subjects and 89 episodic migraineurs were control groups. All domains evaluated by the SF-36 were significantly reduced in the CDH patients compared with the healthy subjects. There were no significant differences in quality of life of TM patients compared with CTTH patients. TM patients had a general reduction in quality of life compared with episodic migraine patients (significant for vitality and general and mental health). CDH patients who overused analgesics scored significantly lower than nonoverusers in physical role and bodily pain. The impact of CDH on quality of life depends on the chronicity of the headache disorder rather than on the severity of a given attack. The impact is worse when analgesic overuse is present.

Wang and colleagues looked at the quality of life in 901 headache patients in Taiwan using the SF-36.[73] Using the Silberstein and Lipton CDH criteria, TM was diagnosed in 310 patients and CTTH in 231; 193 had episodic migraine. The patients with TM had the worst SF-36 scores. The scores of those with CTTH and those with migraine were similar.

Juang and colleagues investigated the frequency of depressive and anxiety disorders in 261 consecutive CDH patients seen in a headache clinic.[74] CDH subtypes were classified according to the Silberstein and Lipton criteria. A psychiatrist evaluated the patients according to the structured Mini-International Neuropsychiatric Interview to assess the comorbidity of depressive and anxiety disorders. The mean age was 46 years, and 80% of the patients were women. TM was diagnosed in 152 patients (58%) and CTTH in 92 patients (35%). Seventy-eight percent of patients with TM had psychiatric comorbidity, including major depression (57%), dysthymia (11%), panic disorder (30%), and generalized anxiety disorder (8%). Sixty-four percent of patients with CTTH had psychiatric diagnoses, including major depression (51%), dysthymia (8%), panic disorder (22%), and generalized anxiety disorder (1%). The frequency of anxiety disorders was significantly higher in patients with TM after controlling for age and sex. Both depressive and anxiety disorders were significantly more frequent in women. These results demonstrate that women and patients with TM are at higher risk of psychiatric comorbidity.

CDH also occurs in children. Guidetti and Galli examined the characteristics of childhood- and adolescent-onset CDH, using the Silberstein and Lipton criteria, and the prevalence of psychiatric comorbidity.[75] Eighty-six CDH patients (60 girls, 26 boys; mean age 12.3 years; SD + 2.1 years; range 7 to 18 years) were compared with 100 controls (60 girls, 40 boys; mean age 10.7 years; SD + 2.6 years; range 4 to 18 years). Sixty-four patients had migraine and 36 had ETTH. All subjects had clinical interviews and psychometric tests. CTTH was present in 40% of patients, TTH plus intermittent migraine attacks in 35%, and mixed forms in 25%. Psychiatric comorbidity was present in 90% of CDH patients, 67% of migraine patients, and 25% of TTH patients.

## Other Comorbidities

Fibromyalgia (FM) and TM are common chronic pain disorders. Peres and colleagues estimated the prevalence of FM in 101 TM patients and analyzed its relationship to depression, anxiety, and insomnia.[76] They enrolled 101 consecutive TM patients seen at a headache clinic in São Paulo, Brazil. All had normal neuroimaging and clinical examinations. TM was diagnosed according to the 1996 Silberstein and Lipton criteria.[3] FM was diagnosed according to the American College of Rheumatology diagnostic criteria (1990).[4] FM was diagnosed in 35.6% of cases. FM patients had more insomnia and were older and their headaches were more incapacitating than patients without FM. The mean BDI II score was 21.1. Fifty-seven patients (87.7%) had at least mild depression. Forty-four patients (67.7%) had a state score over 46 and 51 patients (78.5%) had a trait score over 46. The BDI II scores correlated to pain intensity ($p = .002$) and state and trait anxiety scores ($p < .001$). Depression, as measured by the BDI II scores, was also associated with FM ($p = .007$), insomnia ($p = .043$), and disability ($p = .05$). Predictors of FM in patients with TM included insomnia (odds ratio [OR] 10.05, 95% confidence interval [CI] 9.03–13.55) and depression (OR 6.8, 95% CI 4.91–8.68).

Fatigue is a common, frequently reported symptom in many disorders, including headache. Peres and colleagues determined the prevalence of fatigue in 63 TM patients from the São Paulo headache clinic.[77] TM was diagnosed using the Silberstein and Lipton criteria. FM was diagnosed according to the 1990 diagnostic criteria established by the American College of Rheumatology.[78] The Fatigue Severity Scale (FSS)[79] (cutoff of 27 defined fatigue) and the Chalder fatigue scale[80] (Likert scoring[81]) were used. The Chalder fatigue scale has two parts, physical and mental fatigue. Items related to mental fatigue include difficulty concentrating, problems thinking clearly, difficulty finding the correct word, and memory problems. Those related to physical fatigue include tiredness, need to rest more, sleepiness, drowsiness, lack of energy, and weakness or less strength in muscles. Fifty-three patients (84.1%) had FSS scores > 27. Forty-two patients (66.7%) met the criteria for chronic fatigue syndrome established by the Centers for Disease Control and Prevention (CDC). Thirty-two patients (50.8%) met the modified criteria of the CDC, in which headache was eliminated as a criterion of chronic fatigue syndrome. Beck depression scores correlated with FSS and mental and physical fatigue scores. Trait anxiety scores also correlated with fatigue scales. Women had significantly higher FSS scores than men ($p < .05$), and physical fatigue was significantly associated with FM ($p < .05$). Fatigue as a symptom and chronic fatigue syndrome as a disorder were both common in TM patients.

## Epidemiology

In population-based surveys using the Silberstein and Lipton criteria, CDH occurred in 4.1% of Americans, 4.35% of Greeks, 3.9% of elderly Chinese, and 4.7% of Spaniards. Scher and colleagues ascertained the prevalence of CDH in 13,343 individuals aged 18 to 65 years in Baltimore County, Maryland.[6] The overall prevalence of CDH was 4.1% (5.0% women, 2.8% men; 1.8:1 female to male ratio). In both men and women, the prevalence was highest in the lowest educational category. More than half (52% women, 56% men) met the criteria for CTTH (2.2%), almost one-third (33% women, 25% men) met the criteria for TM (1.3%), and the remainder (15% women, 19% men) were unclassified (0.6%). Overall, 30% of women and 25% of men who were frequent headache sufferers met the IHS criteria for migraine (with or without aura). On the basis of chance, migraine and CTTH would co-occur in 0.22% of the population; the fact that TM occurred in 1.3% of this population would suggest that their co-occurrence is more than random.

Castillo and colleagues sampled 2,252 subjects over 14 years of age in Cantabria, Spain.[7] Overall, 4.7% had CDH: none had HC, 0.1% had NDPH, 2.2% had CTTH, and 2.4% had TM. Acute medication overuse occurred in 19% of CTTH and 31.1% of TM patients. Eight patients had a previous history of migraine without aura and now had CDH with only the characteristics of TTH. These headaches met the criteria of TM but could have been migraine and coincidental CTTH.

Wang and colleagues found that 3.9% of elderly Chinese (over 65 years of age) in two townships on Kinmen Island had CDH.[8] Significantly more women than men had CDH (5.6% and 1.8%; $p < .001$). Of the CDH patients, 42 (70%) had CTTH (2.7%), 15 (25%) had TM (1%), and 3 (5%) had other CDH.

Lu and colleagues conducted a two-stage population-based headache survey among subjects aged $\geq 15$ years in Taipei, Taiwan.[82] Subjects who had CDH in the past year were identified, interviewed, and followed up. CDH was defined as headache frequency of more than 15 days per month, with a duration of more than 4 hours per day. Of the 3,377 participants, 108 (3.2%) fulfilled the criteria for CDH, with a higher prevalence in women (4.3%) than in men (1.9%). TM was the most common subtype (55%), followed by CTTH (44%). Thirty-four percent of the CDH subjects overused analgesics.

## Risk Factors

Wang and colleagues ascertained that significant risk factors (Table 4–6) for CDH included analgesic overuse

($OR = 79$), a history of migraine ($OR = 6.6$), and a Geriatric Depression Scale-Short Form score of 8 or above ($OR = 2.6$).[8] At follow-up, patients with persistent primary CDH had a significantly higher frequency of analgesic overuse (33% versus 0%; $p = .03$) and major depression (38% versus 0%; $p = .04$).

Granella and colleagues found that risk factors that were associated with the evolution of migraine without aura into TM included head trauma ($OR 3.3$), analgesic use with every attack ($OR 2.8$), and long duration of oral contraceptive use.[83]

Scher and colleagues described factors that predict CDH onset and remission in an adult population.[84] CDH was more common in women ($OR 1.65$; 95% CI 1.3–2.0), those previously married ($OR 1.5$; 95% CI 1.2–1.9), those with obesity (body mass index $> 30$) ($OR 1.27$; 95% CI 1.0–1.7), and those with less education. Obesity, high baseline headache frequency, high caffeine consumption, habitual daily snoring, and stressful life events were significantly associated with new-onset CDH.[85] Having less than a high school education was associated with a threefold increased risk of CDH ($OR 3.56$; 95% CI 2.3–5.6).

Bigal and colleagues, in a clinic-based study, looked for risk factors associated with CDH and its subtypes.[86] TM without MOH (in comparison with episodic migraine) was associated with allergies, asthma, hypothyroidism, hypertension, and daily caffeine consumption.

Zwart and colleagues examined the relationship between analgesic use at baseline and the subsequent risk of chronic pain ($\geq 15$ days/month) and the risk of analgesic overuse in a population-based study.[87] In total, 32,067 adults reported the use of analgesics from 1984 to 1986 and at follow-up 11 years later (1995 to 1997). The risk ratios (RRs) of chronic pain and anal-

| Table 4–6  Risk Factors for Chronic Daily Headache |
|---|
| High headache frequency |
| Female gender |
| Obesity (body mass index > 30) |
| Snoring |
| Stressful life events |
| High caffeine consumption |
| Acute medication overuse |
| Depression |
| Head trauma |
| History of migraine |
| Less than a high school education |

gesic overuse in the different diagnostic groups (ie, migraine, nonmigrainous headache, and neck pain) were estimated in relation to analgesic consumption at baseline. Individuals who reported use of analgesics daily or weekly at baseline showed significantly increased risk of having chronic pain at follow-up. The risk was most evident for chronic migraine (RR 13.3; 95% CI 9.3–19.1), intermediate for chronic nonmigrainous headaches (RR 6.2; 95% CI 5.0–7.7), and lowest for chronic neck pain (RR 2.4; 95% CI 2.0–2.8). Among subjects with chronic pain associated with analgesic overuse, the RR was 37.6 (95% CI 21.3–66.4) for chronic migraine, 14.4 (95% CI 10.4–19.9) for chronic nonmigrainous headaches, and 7.1 for chronic neck pain (95% CI 5.5–9.2). The RR for chronic headache (migraine and nonmigrainous headache combined) associated with analgesic overuse was 19.6 (95% CI 14.8–25.9) compared with 3.1 (95% CI 2.4–4.2) for those without overuse. Overuse of analgesics strongly predicts chronic pain and chronic pain associated with analgesic overuse 11 years later, especially among those with chronic migraine.

## Pathophysiology of CDH

The trigeminal nucleus caudalis (TNC) of the trigeminal complex, the major relay nucleus for head and face pain, receives nociceptive input from cephalic blood vessels and pericranial muscles (via the trigeminal and upper cervical nerves), as well as inhibitory and facilitatory suprasegmental input. The trigeminal nerve has three divisions: ophthalmic, mandibular, and maxillary. Anterior pain-producing structures are innervated by the ophthalmic (first) division. Posterior regions are subserved by upper cervical nerves.[88] Afferent processes of the trigeminal nerve converge to form the sensory root of the trigeminal nerve, entering the brainstem at the pontine level and terminating in the trigeminal brainstem nuclear complex. The trigeminal brainstem nuclear complex is composed of the principal trigeminal nuclei and spinal trigeminal nuclei (subdivided into the nucleus oralis, the subnuclear interpolaris, and the nucleus caudalis). The brainstem spinal trigeminal nucleus is analogous to the dorsal horn of the spinal canal, the first synapse in the central nervous system (CNS).

Most spinothalamic and trigeminothalamic tract neurons that originate from the dorsal horn and project to ventroposterior lateral and ventroposterior medial nuclei have wide dynamic-range characteristics.[89] The trigeminothalamic tract is analogous to the spinothalamic tract. Second-order neurons from the trigeminal spinal nuclei form the trigeminothalamic tract and project to other midbrain structures, as well as to the thalamic tract.

Most ventroposterior medial nuclei, some with wide dynamic-range characteristics, respond to low-threshold stimuli.[88]

Pain has three spatiotemporal characteristics: (1) as pain intensity increases, the area in which it is experienced often enlarges (radiation); (2) the pain may outlast the evoking stimulus; and (3) repeated nociceptive stimuli may increase the perceived pain intensity, even without increased input (sensitization).[90] Pain has both sensory and affective dimensions. In addition to being physically unpleasant, pain is associated with negative emotional feelings shaped by context, anticipations, and attitudes.[89] Pain unpleasantness is in series with pain sensation intensity.

## Pain in Migraine

Migraine is a primary brain disorder, a form of neurovascular headache in which neural events result in the dilation of blood vessels, neuronal activation, and pain. Migraine most likely results from a dysfunction of the trigeminal nerve and its central connections that normally modulate sensory input. The components involved include (1) the cranial blood vessels and meninges, (2) the trigeminal innervation of the vessels and meninges, (3) the reflex connections of the trigeminal system with the cranial parasympathetic outflow, and (4) local and descending pain modulation. The key pathway for the pain is trigeminovascular input from the meningeal vessels. Brain imaging studies suggest that important modulation of the trigeminovascular nociceptive input stems from the dorsal raphe nucleus, locus ceruleus, and nucleus raphe magnus.[91]

Although the source of pain in CDH is unknown and may depend on the subtype of CDH, recent work suggests several mechanisms that could contribute to the process: (1) increased peripheral nociceptive activation (perhaps owing to chronic neurogenic inflammation) and activation of silent nociceptors; (2) peripheral sensitization; (3) altered sensory neuron excitability owing to changes in ion-channel expression/phosphorylation/accumulation in primary afferents; (4) central sensitization of TNC neurons owing to posttranslational changes in ligand- and voltage-gated ion-channel kinetics, altering the excitability and strength of their synaptic inputs; (5) phenotype modulation owing to alterations in the expression of receptors/transmitters/ion channels in peripheral and central neurons; (6) synaptic reorganization and modification of synaptic connections caused by cell death or sprouting; (7) decreased pain modulation owing to loss of local and descending input[90]; or (8) a combination of these.

## Peripheral Mechanisms/Nociceptor Activation

Although the brain itself is largely insensate, pain can be generated by large cranial vessels, proximal intracranial vessels, or dura mater. The central convergence of the ophthalmic division of the trigeminal nerve and the branches of C2 nerve roots explains the typical distribution of migraine pain over the frontal and temporal regions and the referral of pain to the parietal, occipital, and high cervical regions.[92] During a migraine attack, trigeminal nerve activation is accompanied by the release of vasoactive neuropeptides, including CGRP from the nerve terminals. Intense neuronal stimulation causes induction of c-*fos* (an immediate early gene product) in the TNC of the brainstem. Trigeminal neuropeptides further amplify the trigeminal terminal sensitivity by stimulating the release of bradykinin and other inflammatory mediators from nonneuronal cells.[93] Neurotropins, such as nerve growth factor (NGF), are synthesized locally and can also activate mast cells and sensitive nerve terminals. Prostaglandins and nitric oxide (a diffusible gas that acts as a neurotransmitter)[94] are endogenous mediators that can be produced locally and can sensitize nociceptors. Cortical spreading depression (the physiologic substrate of the migraine aura) can activate the trigeminal system. Repeated episodes of trigeminal activation and sensitization may chronically sensitize the pain pathways and contribute to the development of daily headache.

Sarchielli and colleagues measured CSF levels of NGF, CGRP, and substance P (SP) in patients with TM both with and without medication overuse.[95] Higher NGF, CGRP, and SP levels were found in CSF in both groups of patients compared with controls. A correlation was found between NGF and SP levels. All levels correlated with the duration of the disorder. This study suggests the involvement of NGF and chronic activation of the trigeminal vascular system in TM. NGF production could arise from peripheral trigeminal nerve terminals as well as the TNC and pain-facilitating pathways. Ashina and colleagues compared the interictal plasma levels of CGRP in patients with chronic TTH and healthy control subjects.[96] Patients whose usual headache quality was throbbing had a higher interictal plasma CGRP level than control subjects ($p = .002$), whereas plasma CGRP level was normal in 22 patients with pressing headaches ($p = .36$). This strongly suggests that the patients with an elevated CGRP level had TM and that the trigeminal vascular system is activated as part of the process of TM.

## Sensitization in Migraine

Lance observed that during migraine attacks, patients complain of increased pain to stimuli that would ordinarily be non-nociceptive. These stimuli include hair brushing, wearing a hat, and resting the head on a pillow. This phenomenon of pain being produced by nonpainful stimuli is referred to as allodynia. In a series of now-classic experiments, Burstein and colleagues explored allodynia development in patients with migraine.[97] They measured pain thresholds for hot, cold, and pressure stimuli, both within the region of spontaneous pain and outside it. They found that as an attack progressed in a selected group of migraine sufferers, cutaneous allodynia developed in the region of pain and then outside it (extracephalic locations). They found that 33 of 42 patients (79%) developed allodynia within the first half of the attack in those who eventually developed it.

## Peripheral Sensitization

Sensitization of nociceptors results in an increased spontaneous neuronal discharge rate. Neurons show increased responsiveness to both painful and nonpainful stimuli. The receptor fields expand, and, as a result, pain is felt over a greater part of the dermatome. This results in hyperalgesia (increased sensitivity to pain) and cutaneous allodynia. An example of this is sunburn, with increased sensitivity to temperature (a warm shower feels painfully hot).

How does sensitization occur? Tissue injury and inflammation result in the release of inflammatory mediators, such as prostaglandin $E_2$, bradykinin, and NGF. These substances act on G protein–coupled receptors or tyrosine kinase receptors expressed on nociceptor terminals. This activates intracellular signaling pathways, resulting in phosphorylation of receptors and ion channels. Phosphorylation changes the nociceptor terminals' threshold and kinetics, producing increased sensitivity and excitability, which results in peripheral sensitization.[98] Transcriptional or translational regulation can also contribute to peripheral sensitization. NGF-induced activation of p38 mitogen-activated protein kinase in primary sensory neurons after peripheral inflammation increases the expression and peripheral transport of TRPV1 (a member of the transient receptor potential [TRP] family), exacerbating heat hyperalgesia.[99] (The TRP superfamily consists of cation channels related to the product of the *Drosophila trp* gene. The vanilloid receptor 1 [VR1] forms a distinct subgroup of the TRP family of ion channels. Members of the vanilloid receptor family [TRPV] are activated by a diverse range of stimuli, including heat, protons, lipids, phorbols, phosphorylation, changes in extracellular osmolarity and/or pressure, and depletion of intracellular $Ca^{2+}$ stores. However, VR1 remains the only channel activated by vanilloids, such as capsaicin.)

The normal rhythmic pulsation of the meninges, which are innervated by peripheral trigeminal neurons, can mediate the throbbing pain experienced by migraineurs. With the increase in intracranial neuronal sensitivity that migraine patients experience, the normal rhythmic pulsation is interpreted as painful. Bendtsen and colleagues found evidence for sensitization in CTTH patients.[100] Pericranial myofascial tenderness, evaluated by manual palpation, was considerably higher in patients than in controls ($p < .00001$). The stimulus-response function from highly tender muscle was qualitatively different from that from normal muscle, suggesting that myofascial pain may be mediated by low-threshold mechanosensitive afferents projecting to sensitized dorsal horn neurons.

## Central Sensitization

Central sensitization needs to be differentiated from windup, which is an immediate activity-dependent plasticity characterized by a progressive increase in action potential output from dorsal horn neurons during a conditioning train of repeated low-frequency C-fiber nociceptor stimuli.[101] It results in increased synaptic efficacy, that is, enhanced responses in the conditioning nociceptor pathway (homosynaptic potentiation).[102] C-fiber activation elicits slow synaptic potentials that last several hundred milliseconds.[103,104] Windup results from the summation of these slow synaptic potentials at relatively low afferent input frequencies. This produces a cumulative depolarization that leads to removal of the voltage-dependent $Mg^{2+}$ channel blockade in N-methyl-D-aspartate (NMDA) receptors. Thus, the action potential progressively increases in response to each stimulus in a train of inputs as a result of increased glutamate sensitivity.[105]

Central sensitization, in contrast, refers to an activity- or use-dependent increase in the excitability of nociceptive neurons in the CNS as a result of, and outlasting, a short barrage of nociceptor input. This can take up to 60 minutes to develop. Sensitization results from the activation of multiple intracellular signaling pathways in dorsal horn neurons by the neurotransmitter (glutamate) and the neuromodulators (SP, brain-derived neurotrophic factor, and ephrin-B ligands). Central sensitization is characterized by an increased spontaneous discharge rate, reductions in threshold and an increased responsiveness to both noxious and non-noxious peripheral stimuli, and expanded receptive fields of CNS nociceptive neurons.[106–108] Most dorsal horn neuronal input is subthreshold; the synaptic strength is too weak to evoke an action potential output.[109] After induction of central sensitization, the same input can activate dorsal horn neurons as a result of increases in synaptic efficacy.[110] This is called homosynaptic potentiation. In addition, additional inputs from nonstimulated A-B afferents become activated.[110,111] This is called heterosynaptic facilitation because the Aβ fibers are not the ones that were activated by the nociceptive conditioning stimuli (C fibers must be activated to produce central sensitization). As a result of central sensitization, low-threshold sensory fibers activated by innocuous stimuli, such as a light touch, can activate normally high-threshold nociceptive secondary sensory neurons in the dorsal horn. The increased excitability of CNS neurons results in a reduction in pain threshold (tactile allodynia).

If the stimulus is maintained, central sensitization persists. It can outlast the stimulus for several hours.[107] Clinically, central sensitization contributes to pain hypersensitivity in the skin, muscle, joints, and viscera.[112] Cutaneous allodynic pain is referred to the periphery, but it arises from within the CNS. Does sensitization play a role in headache? Brief chemical irritation of the dura with a cocktail (inflammatory soup) of four inflammatory mediators (histamine, serotonin, bradykinin, and prostaglandin $E_2$) made meningeal perivascular neurons pain sensitive for a period of 1 to 2 hours.[113] This peripheral sensitization can explain the intracranial hypersensitivity (ie, the worsening pain during coughing, bending over, or any head movement) and the throbbing pain of migraine.[114]

Brief dural chemical irritation may also result in central sensitization with changes in the central trigeminal neurons that receive convergent input from the dura and the skin. Their threshold decreases and their excitability increases in response to brushing and heating of the periorbital skin—stimuli to which they showed only minimal or no response prior to chemical stimulation.[115] In addition, the threshold of cardiovascular responses to facial and intracranial stimuli is reduced.[116]

Central sensitization results in muscle tenderness and cutaneous allodynia in patients with migraine. Most migraineurs exhibit cutaneous allodynia inside and outside their pain-referred areas during migraine attacks. Burstein and colleagues studied the development of cutaneous allodynia during migraine by measuring the pain thresholds in the head and forearms of a patient at several points during the migraine attack and compared the pain thresholds in the absence of an attack.[115,117] (Studies in animals show that peripheral nociceptors became sensitized and mediated the symptoms of cranial hypersensitivity ~ 30 minutes after their initial activation.) The barrage of impulses then activated second-order neurons and initiated their sensitization, mediating the development of cutaneous allodynia on the ipsilateral head. Many patients had periorbital cutaneous allodynia ipsilateral to the headache. Patients with allodynia were significantly older than those without cutaneous allodynia, hinting at a possible correlation between age and sensitization. These findings provide a neural basis for the pathophysiology of migraine pain and suggest a basis for continued head pain.

Gallai and colleagues found elevated CSF levels of glutamate and nitrite (a nitric oxide [NO] metabolite) in TM patients with and without medication overuse.[118] The increase in CSF nitrite, a marker for NO production, was accompanied by an increase in cyclic guanosine monophosphate. CGRP, SP, and, to a lesser extent, neurokinin A were also elevated in patients compared with controls. NO plays a crucial role in animal models of sensitization. Its formation is triggered by glutamate receptor activation.

Evidence now exists that central sensitization, defined by the presence of cutaneous allodynia, exists in CDH, including TM with and without medication overuse. Shukla and colleagues studied dynamic brush (mechanical) allodynia in headache patients in an inpatient setting.[119] This study demonstrated that mechanical dynamic brush allodynia is common in hospitalized CDH patients. Of 78 patients, most of whom had TM, 32 (41%) experienced brush allodynia. Allodynia was more common and more severe in V1, indicating the role of central sensitization in its development. Allodynia was significantly more common in patients with unilateral headaches and was usually ipsilateral to the headache.

Creach and colleagues compared heat-pain thresholds in patients with TM with and without medication overuse and patients with episodic migraine.[120] Extracranial, but not face, allodynia was more common in both TM groups (39.5% versus 12.1%). Using a questionnaire, Sobrino found that 56.3% of TM patients had cutaneous allodynia in their pain-referred areas.[121]

## Pain Modulation

The mammalian nervous system contains networks that modulate nociceptive transmission.

The trigeminal brainstem nuclear complex receives monoaminergic, enkephalinergic, and peptidergic projections from regions known to be important in the modulation of nociceptive systems. A descending inhibitory neuronal network extends from the frontal cortex and hypothalamus through the periaqueductal gray (PAG) to the rostral ventromedial medulla (RVM) and the medullary and spinal dorsal horn. The RVM includes the nucleus raphe magnum and the adjacent reticular formation and projects to the outer laminae of the spinal and medullary dorsal horn. Electrical stimulation or injection of opioids into the PAG reduces nociceptive-specific neuron activity. The PAG receives projections from the insular cortex and the amygdala.[88] Stimulation of the RVM can result in inhibition and/or facilitation of nociceptive and non-nociceptive input. The RVM is a relay in descending modulation of nociception.[122] RVM stimulation at relatively high current intensities is both antinociceptive (in the tail-flick test) and responsible for decreased responses of dorsal horn neurons. By contrast, lower current intensity stimulation at the same sites are facilitatory.[123–125] Excitatory neurotransmitters (eg, glutamate, neurotensin) microinjected into the RVM replicated the effects of stimulation, facilitating and inhibiting spinal nociception at lower and higher doses, respectively.[126–129] Microinjection of NMDA into the RVM facilitated the

tail-flick reflex in a dose-dependent manner, an effect blocked by an NMDA receptor antagonist.[130]

Antinociception can be measured by nociceptive reflex inhibition. In the RVM and PAG, three classes of neurons were identified.[131] "Off-cells" pause immediately before the nociceptive reflex, whereas "on-cells" are activated. Neutral cells show no consistent changes in activation.[88] On-cells and off-cells fire in a reciprocating pattern; tail-flick latency was longer during periods of increased off-cell activity and shorter when on-cells were active. Opioids activate off-cells and inhibit on-cells; nociceptive reflexes are inhibited. Naloxone-precipitated opioid withdrawal increases on-cell activity.[132,133] This is abolished by intra-RVM injection of lidocaine.[134,135] Thus, off-cell activity suppresses nociception, whereas on-cell activity enhances the response to noxious stimuli. On- and off-cell activity is modulated by 5-hydroxytryptamine$_1$ receptor agonists.[88] Off-cells and on-cells (descending inhibitory and facilitatory pathways) project from the RVM through both dorsal and ventral parts of the spinal cord to the spinal dorsal horn.[136]

Opioids can paradoxically induce pain and decrease tolerance to nociception. This is similar mechanistically to the abnormal pain that follows peripheral nerve injury. Both are less responsive to the antinociceptive effects of morphine and are reversed by NMDA antagonists.[137] Both activate the RVM descending pain-facilitating pathways. Increased RVM facilitation may be mediated by pronociceptive peptide cholecystokinin (CCK). CCK exists throughout the brain and spinal cord. Immunoreactivity is seen in the PAG and RVM. CCG can contribute to RVM neuron excitability. Intra-RVM CCK produces reversible thermal and tactile hypersensitivity[138] and prevents both the activation of off-cells and the antinociception produced by systemic morphine.[139] Conversely, microinjection of a CCK antagonist into the RVM blocks thermal and tactile hypersensitivity in rats with peripheral nerve injury.[140] CCK antagonists also enhance morphine-induced antinociception and reverse morphine tolerance.[141] The RVM produces descending facilitation by elevating spinal dynorphin expression.[142] Dynorphin acts as an endogenous pronociceptor mediator, resulting in enhanced release of CGRP and SP.[143–145] Dynorphin up-regulation is blocked by lesions in the RVM descending pathways. The lesions also block enhanced CGRP release and abnormal pain. Antibodies to dynorphin also block CGRP release in model systems.[146]

Opioid analgesic tolerance is a pharmacologic phenomenon that occurs after its prolonged administration, in part owing to activation of the NMDA receptor. Excess activation of NMDA receptors can lead to neurotoxicity. Mao and colleagues showed that spinal neuronal apoptosis was induced in rats made tolerant to morphine administered through intrathecal boluses or continuous infusion.[147] The apoptotic cells were predominantly located in the superficial spinal cord dorsal horn. Most apoptotic cells expressed glutamic acid decarboxylase, a key enzyme for the synthesis of the inhibitory neurotransmitter γ-aminobutyric acid (GABA). This was associated with increased nociceptive sensitivity to heat stimulation. Morphine-induced neuronal apoptosis was modulated by spinal glutamatergic activity. Prolonged morphine administration resulted in up-regulation of the proapoptotic caspase 3 and bax proteins but down-regulation of the antiapoptotic bcl-2 protein in the spinal cord dorsal horn. Coadministration with morphine of a pan-caspase inhibitor or a relatively selective caspase 3 inhibitor blocked morphine-induced neuronal apoptosis. These results suggest that opioid-induced neurotoxicity depletes inhibitory GABA interneurons, a mechanism that may have clinical implications in opioid therapy and substance abuse and may account for refractoriness in CM.

The RVM modulates the activity of the TNC and dorsal horn neurons. Increased on-cell activity in the brainstem's pain modulation system could enhance the response to both painful and nonpainful stimuli. Opioid withdrawal results in increased firing of the on-cells, decreased firing of the off-cells, and enhanced nociception.[131,148] Descending facilitatory influences could contribute to chronic pain states and the development and maintenance of hyperalgesia.[149] Headache may be caused, in part, by enhanced neuronal activity in the nucleus caudalis as a result of enhanced on-cell and decreased off-cell activity. Other conditioned stimuli associated with pain and stress also can turn on the pain system and may account, in part, for the association between pain and stress.[131] CDH may result, in part, from enhanced neuronal activity in the TNC as a result of enhanced on-cell and decreased off-cell activity.

Overuse of acute medication can contribute to the transformation of episodic into transformed migraine.[150] Continued high fluctuating doses could result in resetting the pain control mechanisms in susceptible individuals, perhaps by enhancing on-cell activity, enhancing central sensitization through NMDA receptors, or blocking adaptive antinociceptive changes. Chronic opioid use has clearly been shown to activate RVM pain facilitation. Opioid-induced neurotoxicity by depleting inhibitory GABA interneurons may result in headache intractability.

Evidence exists for differences in pain modulation in migraine. Painful stimulation induces two pain sensations: the first acute, short-lasting, and well localized and the second longer but less localized. The second pain intensity increases with repeat stimulation and is enhanced in chronic headaches. Fusco and colleagues evaluated the effect of dextromethorphan and Mg[2+] on temporal summation of second pain in chronic

headache patients, seven with TM and five with other chronic headaches.[151] The pain stimulus consisted of four electrical shocks delivered on the medial forearm at 3-second intervals. The stimulus was repeated 1 hour after a 100 mg oral dose of dextromethorphan, 10 minutes after the end of slow intravenous infusion of Mg[2+], or both. First pain intensity did not change. The exaggerated temporal summation of the second pain in chronic headache was confirmed. Dextromethorphan significantly decreased this. Mg[2+] alone had no effect but did increase the effect of dextromethorphan.

Positron emission tomography (PET) in primary headaches, such as migraine[152] and cluster headache,[153] has demonstrated activations (as measured by increased cerebral blood flow) in brain areas associated with pain, such as the cingulate cortex, insulae, frontal cortex, thalamus, basal ganglia, and cerebellum. These areas are similarly activated when head pain is induced by injecting capsaicin into the forehead of volunteers.[154] Cortical (but not brainstem) activation is reversed by sumatriptan, as is the headache. This area of the brainstem is rich in opioids and includes the pain control centers.[155] Dihydroergotamine (DHE) and centrally penetrant triptans selectively bind to this area of the brainstem. This area of the brainstem may integrate the phenomenon we call migraine, or it could be activated as a result of the migraine attack. If the first explanation is correct, ongoing activity in this area of the brainstem could produce recurrent or daily headache. If this area is responsible for controlling pain, then its failure to activate could explain ongoing headache activity. Acute migraine medications may induce daily headache by preventing the development of adaptive changes and perhaps by maintaining brainstem activation.[152]

In addition, activation of specific brain regions is seen in episodic migraine. Specifically, brainstem areas are activated in episodic migraine,[152] one of which was more clearly localized to the dorsal pons.[156] The underlying pathophysiology of CM is likely to be similar to that of episodic migraine, with perhaps continuous brainstem activation. Matharu and colleagues reported eight patients with the IHS diagnosis of CM who have shown a marked beneficial response to implanted bilateral suboccipital stimulators.[157] Stimulation evoked local paresthesia, the presence of which was a criterion of pain relief. On stimulation, the headache began to improve instantaneously and was completely suppressed within 30 minutes. When the stimulation was switched off, the headache recurred instantly and peaked within 20 minutes. PET scans were performed using regional cerebral blood flow (rCBF) as a marker of neuronal activity. Each patient was scanned in the following three states: (1) stimulator at optimum settings: the patient was pain free but with paresthesia; (2) stimulator off: the patient was in pain but had no paresthesia; (3) stimulator partially activated: the patient had intermediate levels of pain and paresthesia. There were significant changes in rCBF in the dorsal rostral pons, anterior cingulate cortex, and cuneus, correlated to pain scores, and in the anterior cingulate cortex and left pulvinar, correlated to stimulation-induced paresthesia scores. The activation pattern in the dorsal rostral pons is highly suggestive of a role for this structure in the pathophysiology of chronic migraine. The localization and persistence of activity during stimulation are exactly consistent with a region activated in episodic migraine and with the persistence of activation of that area after successful treatment. The dorsal rostral pons may be a locus of neuromodulation by suboccipital stimulation. In addition, suboccipital stimulation modulated activity in the left pulvinar.

Welch and colleagues used high-resolution magnetic resonance techniques to map the transverse relaxation rates R2 $(1/T2)$, R2′ $(1/T2^*-1/T2)$, and R2* $(1/T2^*)$ in the brain, particularly the PAG, red nucleus (RN), and substantia nigra (SN).[158] These measures are sensitive to free iron: R2′ is a measure of nonheme iron in tissues. They evaluated patients with TM, patients with episodic migraine, and nonmigraine controls. In the PAG, there was a significant increase in mean R2′ and R2* values in both the episodic migraine and TM patients. The value increased with disease duration. A decrease in mean R2′ and R2* values in the RN and SN of only the TM group was observed; they attributed this to cerebral blood flow changes owing to head pain. Aurora reported normalization of SN and RN, but not PAG R2′ values following detoxification.[159] The significance of these findings is uncertain and await their duplication.

Contingent negative variation is the surface negative slow-wave potential elicited in expectancy conditions. It represents the excitability of cortical pyramidal neurons. Migraine patients have enhanced negativity and reduced habituation compared with nonmigraine controls. Siniatchkin and colleagues showed that patients with TM also have reduced habituation but significantly lower amplitude than episodic migraine patients.[160] This suggests the presence of a common mechanism in these disorders. TM patients may have lost the compensatory mechanism that is present in episodic patients, leading to chronification and lower negativity of the slow wave. Post and Silberstein suggested the kindling model for epilepsy as a model for nonepileptic progressive disorders, such as mania.[150] They suggested that spontaneous recurrent migraine headaches might be analogous to the low levels of electrical stimulation in the kindling model in the process of headache transformation. Preventive migraine treatment could provide a dual benefit by preventing the occurrence of episodes and blocking the sensitization process that could lead to syndrome progression.

In CM, the hypersensitivity of neurons in the TNC may be a result of supraspinal facilitation. Peripheral nociceptors may be hypersensitive as a result of sensitization. CM may result from a defective interaction between endogenous nociceptive brainstem activity and peripheral input. Physical or psychologic stress can increase the nociception that could trigger or sustain an attack in an individual with altered pain modulation. Emotional mechanisms may also reduce endogenous antinociception. Long-term potentiation of nociceptive neurons and decreased activity in the antinociceptive system could cause primary CDH. Sensitization of the TNC neurons can result in normally nonpainful stimuli becoming painful, producing trigger spots, an overlap in the symptoms of migraine and TTH, and activation of the trigeminal vascular system.

## TREATMENT

### Overview

Patients with CDH can be difficult to treat, especially when the disorder is complicated by medication overuse, comorbid psychiatric disease, low frustration tolerance, and physical and emotional dependency.[4,67] We recommend the following steps. First, exclude secondary headache disorders; second, diagnose the primary headache disorders (CM, CTTH, HC, or NDPH); and third, identify comorbid medical and psychiatric conditions and exacerbating factors, especially medication overuse. Limit all acute medications (with the possible exception of the long-acting nonsteroidal anti-inflammatory drugs [NSAIDs]). Patients should be started on preventive medication (to decrease reliance on acute medication), with the explicit understanding that the drugs may not become fully effective until medication overuse, if present, has been eliminated. Some patients need to have their headache cycle terminated.[161] Outpatient detoxification options, including outpatient infusion in an ambulatory infusion unit, are available. If outpatient treatment proves difficult or is dangerous, hospitalization may be required.[2,162]

In some cases, CM reverts to the episodic variety with initiation of preventive medication and education about limiting acute medication. In other cases, there may be only moderate or no improvement. Patients can have severe exacerbations of their migraine during detoxification. Thus, patients, even if they are on preventive medication, often need additional treatment (which we call headache terminators) to break the cycle of CDH and/or help with the exacerbation that occurs when overused medications are discontinued. Terminators can be given orally, by suppository, or by injection, and some can be given repetitively intravenously. The route of administration depends on both the setting and the intensity of treatment.

Patients need education and continuous support during this process. Disturbances in mood and function are common and require management with behavioral methods of pain management and supportive psychotherapy. Treatment of coexistent psychiatric illness is often necessary before CM comes under control. Chronobiologic interventions, such as encouraging regular habits of sleep, exercise, and meals, are often useful.[161]

Psychophysiologic therapy involves reassurance, counseling, stress management, relaxation therapy, biofeedback, and cognitive behavioral therapy. The use of traditional acupuncture is controversial and has not proved more effective than placebo.[163] Physical therapy consists of modality treatments (heat, cold packs, ultrasonography, and electrical stimulation); improvement of posture through stretching, exercise, and traction; trigger-point injections; occipital nerve blocks; and a program of regular exercise and stretching.[164] It has been my experience that treating painful trigger areas in the neck can result in improvement of intractable CDH.

Patients who are overusing acute medication may not become fully responsive to acute and preventive treatment for 2 to 10 weeks after medication overuse is eliminated. Withdrawal symptoms include severely exacerbated headaches accompanied by nausea, vomiting, agitation, restlessness, sleep disorder, and (rarely) seizures. Barbiturates, opioids, and benzodiazepines, unless replaced with long-acting derivatives, must be tapered to avoid a serious withdrawal syndrome. The washout period may last 3 to 8 weeks; once it is over, there is frequently considerable headache improvement.[29,33,59,165]

Outpatient treatment in an ambulatory infusion unit and home treatment options are available. If outpatient treatment proves difficult or is dangerous, hospitalization may be required. Diener and colleagues were able to detoxify only 1.5% of 200 patients on an outpatient basis.[166] Hering and Steiner, in contrast, successfully used outpatient detoxification in 37 of 46 patients who were taking simple analgesics or ergotamine.[167] A recent consensus paper by the German Migraine Society recommends outpatient withdrawal for highly motivated patients who do not take barbiturates or tranquilizers with their analgesics. Inpatient treatment is recommended for patients who fail outpatient treatment, have high depression scores, or take tranquilizers, codeine, or barbiturates.[168] Hospitalization may be necessary for severe dehydration, for which inpatient parenteral therapy may be necessary; diagnostic suspicion (confirmed by appropriate diagnostic testing) of organic etiology; prolonged, unrelenting headache with associated symptoms, such as nausea and vomiting, which, if allowed to continue, would pose a further threat to the patient's welfare; status migrainosus; dependence on analgesics, ergots, opiates, barbiturates, or tranquilizers; pain that is accompanied by serious adverse reactions or complications from therapy wherein continued use of such therapy aggravates or induces further illness; pain that occurs in the presence of significant medical disease but appropriate treatment of headache symptoms aggravates or induces further illness; failed outpatient detoxification, for which inpatient pain and psychiatric management may be necessary; or treatment requiring copharmacy with drugs that may cause a drug interaction (monoamine oxidase inhibitors and β-blockers), thus necessitating careful observation. We have proposed guidelines for hospitalization (Table 4–7).

## Acute Pharmacotherapy

The choice of acute pharmacotherapy depends on the diagnosis. CM patients, who, by definition, are not overusing acute medication, can treat acute migrainous headache exacerbations with antimigraine drugs, including triptans and DHE, or NSAIDs. These drugs must be strictly limited to prevent superimposed MOH, which will complicate treatment and require detoxification. The risk of MOH is much lower for DHE and triptans than for analgesics, opioids, and ergotamine.

## Preventive Pharmacotherapy

Patients with very frequent headaches should be treated primarily with preventive medications, with the explicit understanding that their medications may not become fully effective until any overused medication has been eliminated. It may take 3 to 6 weeks for treatment effects to develop.

The following principles guide the use of preventive treatment: (1) from among the first-line drugs, choose preventive agents based on their adverse event profiles, comorbid conditions, and specific indications; (2) start at a low dose; (3) gradually increase the dose until you achieve efficacy, until the patient develops side effects, or until the ceiling dose for the drug in question is reached; (4) treatment effects develop over weeks, and treatment may not become fully effective until acute medication overuse is eliminated; (5) if one agent fails and if all other things are equal, choose an agent from another therapeutic class; (6) prefer monotherapy but be willing to use combination therapy; and (7) communicate realistic expectations.[169]

Most preventive agents used for CDH have not been examined in well-designed double-blind studies. Table 4–8 summarizes an assessment of the efficacy, safety, and evidence for a number of agents.[161]

Antidepressants are attractive agents for use in TM because many patients have comorbid depression and anxiety. The most widely used tricyclic antidepressants are nortriptyline (Aventyl, Pamelor); amitriptyline (Elavil), which has been effective in many but not all

**Table 4–7**   Criteria for Hospitalization

Emergency or urgent admission

A. Certain migraine variants (eg, hemiplegic migraine, suspected migrainous infarction, basilar migraine with serious neurologic symptoms such as syncope, confusional migraine, etc)

   1.   When a diagnosis has not been established during a previous similar occurrence

   2.   When a patient's established outpatient treatment plan has failed

B. Diagnostic suspicion of infectious disorder involving central nervous system (eg, brain abscess, meningitis) with initiation of appropriate diagnostic testing

C. Diagnostic suspicion of acute vascular compromise (eg, aneurysm, subarachnoid hemorrhage, carotid dissection) with initiation of appropriate diagnostic testing

D. Diagnostic suspicion of a structural disorder causing symptoms requiring an acute setting (eg, brain tumor, increased intracranial pressure) with initiation of appropriate diagnostic testing

E. Low cerebrospinal fluid headache when an outpatient blood patch has failed and an outpatient treatment plan has failed or no obvious cause

F. Medical emergency presenting with a severe headache

G. Severe headache associated with intractable nausea and vomiting producing dehydration or postural hypotension, or patient is unable to retain oral medication, and patient is unable to be controlled in an outpatient setting or with admission to observation status

H. Failed outpatient treatment of an exacerbation of episodic headache disorder with

   1.   Failure to respond to "rescue" or backup medications or

   2.   Failure to respond to outpatient treatment with IV DHE on a schedule of a minimum of twice daily

Nonemergent admission

A. Coexistent psychiatric disease documented by psychological or psychiatric evaluation with sufficient severity of illness such that a failure to admit could pose a health risk to the patient or impair the implementation of outpatient treatment

B. Coexistent or risk of disease (eg, unstable angina, unstable diabetes, recent transient ischemic attack, myocardial infarction in the past 6 mo, renal failure, hypertension, age > 65 years) necessitating monitoring for treatment of headache significant enough to warrant admission

C. Severe chronic daily headaches involving chronic medication overuse when there is

   1.   Daily use of potent opioids and/or barbiturates

   2.   Daily use of triptans, simple analgesics, or ergotamine in a patient with a documented failed trial of withdrawal of these medications

D. Impaired daily functioning (eg, threatened relationships, many lost days at work or school owing to headache), with a failure to respond to 2 d of outpatient treatment with IV DHE, IV neuroleptics, or IV corticosteroids on a schedule of a minimum of twice-daily or equivalent treatment

Silberstein SD, Young WB, Rozen TD, Lenow J. Personal communication.
DHE = dihydroergotamine; IV = intravenous.

studies[170–182]; and doxepin (Sinequan).[183] Descombes and colleagues assessed the effects of amitriptyline and sudden analgesic withdrawal on headache frequency and quality of life in patients suffering from MOH related to analgesic abuse.[184] Seventeen nondepressed patients with MOH were included in a 9-week, parallel-group, randomized, double-blind, placebo-controlled study. After abrupt analgesic withdrawal, amitriptyline or an active placebo (trihexyphenidyl) was started. The primary efficacy variable was headache frequency recorded on a headache diary in the last 4 weeks of each treatment. Headache frequency decreased by 45% in the amitriptyline group and by 28% in the trihexyphenidyl group. Amitriptyline

**Table 4–8**  Summary of Prophylactic Drugs for Use in Chronic Daily Headache

| Drug | Clinical Efficacy | Side Effects | Clinical Evidence* |
|---|---|---|---|
| **Antidepressants** | | | |
| Amitriptyline | +++ | ++ | +++ |
| Doxepin | +++ | ++ | ++ |
| Fluoxetine | ++ | + | +++ |
| **Anticonvulsants** | | | |
| Divalproex | +++ | ++ | ++ |
| Gabapentin | ++ | ++ | ++ |
| Topiramate | +++ | ++ | ++ |
| **β-Blockers** | | | |
| Propranolol, nadolol, etc | ++ | + | + |
| **Calcium channel blockers** | | | |
| Verapamil | ++ | + | + |
| **Miscellaneous** | | | |
| Methysergide | +++ | +++ | + |

Adapted from Tfelt-Hansen P and Welch KMA.[265]

All categories are rated from + to ++++ based on a combination of published literature and clinical experience.

*Ratings of +++ for clinical evidence indicate at least one double-blind, placebo-controlled study. A rating of ++ indicates open well-designed studies, and + indicates ratings based on clinical experience. A rating of ++++ requires at least two double-blind placebo-controlled trials.

enhanced all of the dimensions of quality of life and significantly improved emotional reaction and social isolation.

Fluoxetine (Prozac), a selective serotonin reuptake inhibitor, is coming into wider use for daily headaches; evidence from a double-blind study demonstrates its efficacy in CDH.[170,185] The combination of fluoxetine and amitriptyline was not more effective than amitriptyline alone. Krymchantowski and colleagues evaluated the efficacy and tolerability of combined treatment with amitriptyline (20 mg twice daily) and fluoxetine (20 mg twice daily) compared with amitriptyline alone for CDH owing to TM.[186] Thirty-nine patients, 26 women and 13 men, aged 20 to 69 years, who fulfilled the Silberstein and Lipton criteria for TM were prospectively studied. The mean difference between the initial and final (9 weeks) headache index was 513.5 ($p < .0005$) for group 1 and 893 ($p < .0017$) for group 2. Fluvoxamine appears to be effective[187] and may have analgesic properties.[188] Other selective serotonin reuptake inhibitors, including paroxetine[189] and monoamine oxidase inhibitors, may have a therapeutic role, but this has not been proven to date.[190]

β-Blockers (propranolol, nadolol) remain a mainstay of migraine therapy[161] and are used for CM.[176,191] Clinicians fear that β-blockers may exacerbate depres-

sion; however, this issue is controversial.[192] β-Blockers are relatively contraindicated in patients who have asthma and Raynaud's disease.

Calcium channel blockers are very well tolerated[161]; anecdotal evidence supports their use for CM. Verapamil (Calan) is the most widely prescribed agent in this family. Diltiazem (Cardizem) and nifedipine (Procardia) may also be considered. Flunarizine[13,161] is widely used in Canada and Europe but is not available in the United States.

**Antiepileptic Drugs**

The anticonvulsant divalproex sodium (Depakote)[193] is effective in migraine prevention, as shown in four double-blind placebo-controlled studies.[193–196] Smaller open studies support its utility in TM.[197] In an open-label study, Edwards and colleagues assessed the possible benefit of sodium valproate in 20 consecutive CDH patients whose headaches were refractory to multiple standard treatments.[198] Eleven (55%) had a response (mild or no headaches within 1 to 4 weeks). The doses ranged from 375 to 1,500 mg/d. Two patients (10%) discontinued medication owing to side effects (nausea and difficulty thinking). Frietag and colleagues assessed the safety and efficacy of divalproex sodium in the long-term treatment of chronic daily headache in a retrospective chart review of 642 current patients treated with divalproex sodium for CDH.[199] The mean improvement was 47%, with an improvement in migraine of about 65%. At least a 50% reduction in headache frequency was reported by 93 of the 138 patients who received treatment with only divalproex sodium. Adverse events occurred in approximately 35% of the patients. None were severe.

Gabapentin, structurally related to GABA, is effective in a number of chronic pain conditions. Wessely and colleagues (reported only in abstract form) did not find it effective in episodic migraine.[200] Mathew and colleagues studied gabapentin in the prophylaxis of episodic migraine.[201] Patients were titrated weekly from 900 mg/d (end of week 1) to 2,400 mg/d (end of week 4). ITT analysis showed that 36% of patients on gabapentin and 16.1% of patients receiving placebo had at least a 50% reduction in the 4-week migraine rate. The most frequently reported adverse events were asthenia, dizziness, somnolence, and infection.

Spira and Beran studied gabapentin in the treatment of CDH in a placebo-controlled study.[202] Gabapentin was significantly superior to placebo for the primary efficacy variable for CDH prophylaxis: a 9.1% difference in headache-free rates. Other measures were also significantly better with gabapentin, including headache-free days/month, severity, and quality of life. However, this study had limitations. First, they did not subclassify CDH. The study preceded the new IHS criteria but did not use the Silberstein and Lipton criteria for the diagnosis of CDH subtypes. Second, the study did not take into account acute medication overuse, which is a major confounding factor in both treatment and interpretation of treatment results. Third, although their results were significant, they were modest (a 9.1% difference in headache-free days) and may not be clinically important. Future CDH studies require subset analysis and control for acute medication overuse.[203]

Topiramate is a D-fructose derivative. In two large, double-blind, placebo-controlled, multicenter trials, topiramate, both 100 and 200 mg, was effective in reducing migraine attack frequency by 50% in half of the patients.[204,205] Topiramate works by blocking voltage-gated $Na^+$ channels. It also modulates the action of GABA on $GABA_A$ receptors by increasing GABA-induced chloride currents.[206] Topiramate has antagonistic properties at the α-amino-3-hydroxy-5-methyl-4-isoxazoleproprionic acid (AMPA)/kainate subtype of glutamate receptors. It inhibits the activity of L-type voltage-activated calcium channels (high voltage-activated calcium channels).[207] It also selectively inhibits carbonic anhydrase (CA) II and IV isozymes, which may be important in its anticonvulsant action.

Shank and colleagues hypothesized that the effects of topiramate occur through protein phosphoryla-tion.[208–212] One or more subunit of each complex is phosphorylated by protein kinase A, protein kinase C, and, possibly, $CA^{2+}$/CaM-activated kinases. Topiramate could modulate the activity of these receptors/ion channels by inhibiting kinase activity, enhancing phosphatase activity, or binding directly to kinase consensus sites, thus preventing their phosphorylation.[213]

Silberstein and colleagues, in the first pivotal placebo-controlled clinical trial of 487 patients, assessed the efficacy and safety of topiramate (50, 100, and 200 mg/d) in the prevention of episodic migraine headaches in a 26-week, multicenter, randomized, double-blind, placebo-controlled study.[214] The 50% responder rates were 52%, 54%, 36%, and 23% for the 200, 100, and 50 mg doses and placebo, respectively ($p = .0001, .0001, .039$ comparing the three drug groups with placebo).

Brandes and colleagues assessed the efficacy and safety of topiramate (50, 100, and 200 mg/d) in migraine headache prevention in the second 26-week, multicenter, randomized, double-blind, placebo-controlled study (MIGR-002, structured identically to the MIGR-001 trial).[215] A significantly greater proportion of patients exhibited at least a 50% reduction in mean monthly migraines in the groups treated with 50 mg/d of topiramate (39%; $p = .009$), 100 mg/d of topiramate (49%; $p < .001$), and 200 mg/d of topiramate (47%; $p < .001$).

Paresthesias occurred in 35% of subjects treated with 50 mg, 50% of subjects treated with 100 mg, and 50% of subjects treated with 200 mg. Paresthesias are mild and often transient and, when bothersome, can be controlled with potassium supplementation.[216] The reported incidence of renal calculi is about 1.5%, representing a two- to fourfold increase over the estimated occurrence in the general population.

Patients taking topiramate often lose rather than gain weight. Subjects in the 50 mg group lost approximately 2.4% of body weight, those in the 100 mg group lost approximately 3.2% of body weight, and those in the 200 mg group lost approximately 4.0% of body weight.

Shuaib and colleagues treated 37 patients who had more than 10 migraine headaches a month with topiramate (25 to 100 mg/d) in an open-label study.[217] Most patients had CDH in addition to migraine; all had failed previous preventive treatment. Over a 3- to 9-month follow-up, 11 patients (30%) had an excellent result (headache frequency decreased by over 60%), 11 patients had a good result (headache frequency decreased 40 to 60%), 3 patients discontinued therapy owing to side effects, and 8 patients had no improvement. This uncontrolled study suggests that topiramate may be useful for CM. Large-scale placebo-controlled trials of CM are under way.

## Other Medications

The ergot derivative methysergide[218] was the first migraine-preventive drug approved by the US Food and Drug Administration. The usual initial dosage of methysergide is 2 mg twice a day. It can be increased to a maximum of 8 mg a day (2 mg four times a day). It is no longer available in the United States.

NSAIDs can be used for both symptomatic and preventive headache treatment. Naproxen sodium is effective in prevention at a dosage of one or two 275 mg tablets twice a day.[219] Other NSAIDs that are effective include tolfenamic acid, ketoprofen, mefenamic acid, fenoprofen, and ibuprofen.[220,221] Aspirin was found to be effective in one study[222] and equal to placebo in another.[223] We believe that the short-acting NSAIDs, such as ibuprofen and aspirin, cause MOH, and their use should be limited. The potential of MOH with the other NSAIDs is uncertain. Indomethacin is the drug of choice for HC, and the response to this medication defines the disorder. In patients with strictly unilateral headaches, we give indomethacin a therapeutic trial to rule out HC, but we otherwise limit the use of NSAIDs. One study found that valdecoxib, a selective cyclooxygenase (COX)-2 inhibitor, was modestly effective in the treatment of episodic migraine. (Merck, data on file).

Although monotherapy is preferred, it is sometimes necessary to combine preventive medications. Antidepressants are often used with β-blockers or calcium channel blockers, and divalproex sodium may be used in combination with any of these medications. Pascual and colleagues found that combining a β-blocker and sodium valproate could lead to an increased benefit in patients with migraine previously resistant to either alone.[224] Fifty-two patients (43 women) with a history of episodic migraine with or without aura and previously unresponsive to β-blockers or sodium valproate in monotherapy were treated with a combination of propranolol (or nadolol) and sodium valproate in an open-label fashion. Fifty-six percent had a > 50% reduction in migraine days. This open trial supports the practice of combination therapy. Controlled trials are needed to determine the true advantage of this combination treatment in episodic and chronic migraine.

### New Treatments

Open trials and placebo-controlled trials have suggested that CDH may improve following injection with botulinum toxin A (Botox); whether this is due to paralysis of muscles or to unknown mechanisms is uncertain. Botulinum toxin has been shown to be effective in decreasing the frequency of migraine attacks.[225,226]

Mauskop used botulinum toxin (50–100 U) to treat 12 refractory CDH patients (5 men, 7 women) who overused acute medications almost daily.[227] Only one patient obtained good relief; she has had repeated injections. The most likely potential cause of the low efficacy of botulinum toxin is acute medication overuse. Eross and Dodick evaluated the effect of BNT-A (25 to 100 U) on reducing disability in 47 patients with either episodic or chronic migraine.[228] Using a well-validated migraine-related disability tool (MIDAS), 58% of all patients reported a decrease in migraine-associated disability. Episodic migraine patients ($n = 12$) appeared to demonstrate the most benefit, with 75% reporting a decrease in migraine frequency compared with 53% of CM patients.

Ondo and Derman conducted a randomized, double-blind, placebo-controlled, parallel clinical trial that examined the effect of BNT-A treatment (200 U or placebo) on patients with CDH, including CTTH and TM.[229] The "follow-the-pain" rationale was used and, at 12 weeks, if the patient consented, a second open-label BNT-A injection. Following the first injection, patients treated with BNT-A had significantly fewer headache days, from weeks 8 to 12 compared with placebo. In addition, 10% of patients treated with BNT-A reported a dramatic improvement and 24% reported a marked improvement compared with 3% and 7%, respectively, in the placebo-treated group. Recent results from a large, randomized, double-blind, placebo-controlled, parallel-group exploratory clinical trial involving 355 patients who suffered from CDH showed that botulinum toxin type A, when compared to placebo, significantly reduced the frequency of headache episodes in migraine patients suffering from CDH starting within 30 days after the first treatment and continuing throughout the nine-month study.[230] The between-group difference on the primary efficacy measure (ie, change from baseline in the number of headache-free days) did not reach statistical significance (botulinum toxin type A6.7 vs. placebo 5.2, p=0.30). Differences on key efficacy measures in favor of botulinum toxin type A were even more evident in a subgroup analysis of study patients who were not taking other prophylactic medications to treat their headaches.[231]

### Opioid Maintenance

The role of maintenence opioids (daily scheduled opioid therapy) for intractable CM is controversial.[232] Some argue that chronic opioid medication is justified[233] and useful[234] when patients have truly intractable headache or alternate treatments are contraindicated (as in the senior population). Until recently, long-term studies of effectiveness, sequelae over several years, predictors of long-term benefit, comparisons of pain-related outcome measures, and the prevalence of problematic drug behavior were not available. Saper and colleagues reported the results of a treatment program of 160 sequential patients, 70 of whom remained on daily scheduled opioid therapy for at least 3 years and qualified for inclusion in an efficacy analysis.[235] The primary clinical efficacy variable was percentage improvement in the severe headache index (frequency × severity of severe headaches/week). Only 41 (26%)

of the original 160 patients had > 50% improvement. Problem drug behavior (dose violations, lost prescriptions, multisourcing) occurred in 50% of patients and usually involved dose violations. Most patients (74%) either failed to show significant improvement or were discontinued from the program for clinical reasons. This study showed that a low percentage of patients had demonstrated efficacy and there was an unexpectedly high prevalence of misuse. Daily scheduled opioid therapy did offer significant benefit for a selected group of intractable headache patients.

## Breaking the Headache Cycle

Patients often need headache terminators to break the cycle of daily headache and/or help with the exacerbation that occurs when overused medications are discontinued. Terminators are given orally, by suppository, or by injection, and some (DHE, neuroleptics [prochlorperazine, chlorpromazine, and droperidol], corticosteroids, valproate sodium, magnesium, and ketorolac) can be given repetitively intravenously. Outpatient home terminators include long-acting NSAIDs, COX-2 inhibitors, short courses of corticosteroids, and typical (eg, prochlorperazine suppositories) and atypical (eg, olanzapine) neuroleptics. We also teach patients to self-inject DHE (subcutaneous or intramuscular DHE [0.25 to 1 mg]), ketorolac, and droperidol.

One of the original headache terminators is DHE. Patients who are not good candidates for DHE or do not respond to it can use repetitive intravenous neuroleptics, such as chlorpromazine, droperidol, prochlorperazine, and/or corticosteroids. These agents may also be used to supplement repetitive intravenous DHE for refractory patients.[29] In the infusion and inpatient units, we typically insert a heplock and administer intravenous fluids and parenteral medications in that way. Our typical hydration mixture is dextrose 5% in water in 0.5 N saline at a rate of 100 to 200 mL/h, which is 3 to 4 L/d.

Repetitive intravenous DHE was effective in eliminating intractable headache in 89% of patients within 48 hours (with or without acute medication overuse). Silberstein and colleagues also found that repetitive intravenous DHE was effective in eliminating prolonged migraine, cluster headache, and CM with or without medication overuse.[29]

Repetitive intravenous DHE is often coadministered with metoclopramide,[165] which helps control nausea and is an effective antimigraine drug in its own right. Following 10 mg of intravenous metoclopramide, DHE 0.5 mg is administered intravenously. Subsequent doses are adjusted based on pain relief and side effects. Promethazine intravenously (0.15 mg/kg diluted in 50 mL of 5% dextrose or normal saline) or ondansetron (a selective 5-hydroxytryptamine₃ receptor antagonist) orally (8 mg tablet) or intravenously (4 to 8 mg) can be used by patients who cannot tolerate metoclopramide because of side effects. Responsiveness may be increased by using other antiemetics and neuroleptics.

We use the neuroleptics chlorpromazine, droperidol, haloperidol, and prochlorperazine, intravenously, intramuscularly, and by suppository, as terminators for nausea, vomiting, and pain. We also use the new atypical neuroleptics, such as olanzapine. Sixteen trials (Agency for Health Care Policy and Research [AHCPR] technical report) compared the efficacy of rectally and parenterally administered antiemetics. Intravenous chlorpromazine and prochlorperazine are effective in controlling intractable headache.[169,236–238] Chlorpromazine was found to be more effective than the combination of meperidine and dimenhydrinate, and prochlorperazine was more effective than placebo in treating emergency department patients.[239] Neuroleptics are locally irritating when given intravenously; they are more effective than when given intramuscularly or by suppository. My colleagues and I have found that intramuscular haloperidol (5 mg), droperidol (1 to 2.5 mg), and thiothixene (5 mg) are effective for severe migraine headache.[29] Intravenous haloperidol and droperidol have also been used successfully.

Prochlorperazine (Compazine), administered intramuscularly, intravenously, or rectally, is relatively safe and effective for the treatment of migraine headache and associated nausea and vomiting. It can be given intravenously (7.5 to 15 mg over 5 to 10 minutes) via a saline drip or "slow push."[238,239] Prochlorperazine suppositories (25 mg) are used as a rescue treatment for headache and nausea and as an outpatient terminator medication. They can be used daily up to three times a day for several days. The drug is not as effective orally. Lu and colleagues retrospectively analyzed the data of refractory chronic daily headache inpatients who received intravenous repetitive prochlorperazine.[240] One hundred thirty-five patients were recruited, including 95 (70%) with analgesic overuse. After intravenous prochlorperazine treatment, 121 (90%) achieved a 50% or greater reduction of headache intensity, including 85 (63%) who became headache free. Compared with DHE, prochlorperazine seemed less effective at achieving "freedom from headache" during hospitalization but had a similar outcome at follow-up.

Chlorpromazine (Thorazine), 10 to 50 mg three to four times a day diluted in 20 to 30 mL of saline, can be administered intravenously by rapid drip or "slow push" over several minutes. It can also be administered intramuscularly, rectally, or orally. The oral dose is 25 to 50 mg. Hypotension may result if the patient is not adequately hydrated prior to intravenous chlorpromazine administration.

Droperidol is a parenteral neuroleptic that was effective in a pilot study of 35 patients with status migrainosus or refractory migraine in an ambulatory infusion center.[241] Droperidol (2.5 mg) was given intravenously every 30 minutes until either three doses were given or the patient was completely or almost headache free. The success rate (headache free or mild headache) was 88% in patients with status migrainosus and 100% in patients with refractory migraine. A double-blind, placebo-controlled, randomized, parallel-group, 22-center study showed intramuscular droperidol to be effective for the acute treatment of migraine with or without aura.[242] More patients in the 2.75, 5.5, and 8.25 mg treatment groups experienced a significant reduction in headache by 2 hours (moderate or severe to none or mild; 87%, 81%, and 84%, respectively) compared with placebo (57%). Adverse events occurring in more than 5% of patients receiving droperidol included asthenia, anxiety, akathisia, somnolence, and injection-site reactions. Most adverse events were mild to moderate. Patients can successfully self-inject droperidol. We now use repetitive intravenous droperidol (1 to 2.5 mg every 6 hours) in combination with intravenous diphenhydramine (25 to 50 mg). One concern with using neuroleptics is a prolonged Q–Tc interval on electrocardiography (ECG). This is more likely to occur with droperidol use than with chlorpromazine or prochlorperazine; it is unlikely with olanzapine. Patients who receive daily repetitive intravenous droperidol should have an ECG before their first dose of the medication and daily thereafter. A Q–Tc that is above 450 is considered a "gray zone" (the drug should be stopped or the dose reduced), and a Q–Tc above 500 is a "red zone" (an absolute contraindication). Bradycardia, an abnormal ECG, and a change in the Q–Tc of more than 60 milliseconds are the other risk factors for torsades de pointes associated with prolonged Q–T syndrome.

Olanzapine, a thienobenzodiazepine, is a new "atypical" antipsychotic drug. Olanzapine's properties suggest that it would be effective for headaches, with a low risk of acute extrapyramidal reactions and tardive dyskinesia. The oral dose is 5 to 10 mg.

Controlled studies have shown corticosteroids to be effective in the treatment of headache associated with altitude sickness.[169,236] Clinical experience suggests that corticosteroids are also effective in the treatment of other headache types. Hydrocortisone or methylprednisolone sodium succinate (Solu-Medrol) can be given intravenously in the following manner: 100 mg via a saline drip over 10 minutes every 6 hours for 24 hours, every 8 hours for 24 hours, every 12 hours for 24 hours, and then a final dose. Dexamethasone (Decadron) can be administered intravenously or intramuscularly, starting at a dose of 8 to 20 mg/day in divided doses, rapidly tapering over 2 to 3 days. Oral dexamethasone, 1.5 to 4 mg twice daily for 2 days with a taper over 3 more days, has also proven useful for less disabled migraineurs with prolonged migraine headache.

At least five different chemical classes of NSAIDs have been used for headache treatment.[243] The major mechanism of action of NSAIDs is the differential inhibition of one of the two subtypes of the enzyme COX (COX-1, the constitutive, and COX-2, the induced form) preventing prostaglandin synthesis.[244] The AHCPR analyzed 33 controlled trials of NSAIDs and other nonopiate analgesics and found that aspirin, ibuprofen, tolfenamic acid, and naproxen sodium were superior to placebo in relieving the pain of migraine. We use naproxen, indomethacin rectal suppositories, and selective COX-2 inhibitors. In addition, we use intramuscular or intravenous ketorolac, especially in situations in which neuroleptics, narcotics, and DHE are relatively contraindicated. When we use intravenous ketorolac, we reduce the risk of gastrointestinal bleeding or renal injury by limiting the days of use (30 mg intravenously every 8 hours, for a maximum of 3 days in a row). We do not use corticosteroids, and we give gastrointestinal protection concurrently.

We occasionally use intravenous valproic acid to treat CDH. In an open-label study, Edwards and colleagues assessed the possible benefit of sodium valproate in 20 consecutive CDH patients who were refractory to multiple standard treatments.[198] Eleven of the 20 patients (55%) had a response to mild or no headaches within 1 to 4 weeks. The dose ranged from 375 to 1,500 mg/day. Two patients (10%) discontinued medication owing to adverse events (difficulty thinking and nausea). In a randomized, double-blind, prospective trial, Tanen and colleagues compared intravenous sodium valproate with intravenous prochlorperazine in the acute treatment of migraine headache in the emergency department.[245] Patients received either 10 mg of prochlorperazine or 500 mg of valproate over 2 minutes. Prochlorperazine was statistically and clinically superior to sodium valproate for the treatment of the pain and nausea of acute migraine headache. In this study, sodium valproate failed to significantly reduce the pain or nausea of acute migraine headache. When we use sodium valproate, we give a 250 to 500 mg intravenous push (one-time dose, which occasionally may be repeated; a recently published protocol of every 8 hours). One can give a 500 to 1,000 mg intravenous drip.

Propofol (2,6-diidopropylphenol) is an intravenous sedative-hypnotic agent used for induction and maintenance of anesthesia or sedation. It is the active ingredient in Diprivan, an injectable emulsion. Propofol's rapid induction of hypnosis—usually within 40 seconds of injection—occurs as a result of the rapid equilibration between the plasma and the highly perfused tissue of the brain. The half-time of the blood-brain equilibration is approximately 1 to 3 minutes.

Krusz and Belanger reported effective treatment of acute headache and other headaches refractory to usual therapy with intravenous propofol.[246] Mendes and colleagues conducted a pilot prospective study using repetitive low-dose boluses of intravenous propofol to treat patients with CDHs refractory to standard medications.[247] Twenty-one trials were conducted on 18 patients. Over 90% of patients had at least some headache relief, with no complications.

Hand and Stark retrospectively surveyed 19 consecutive inpatients, 18 with MOH and 3 with status migrainosus, who were treated with intravenous lignocaine infusion.[248] The 19 patients (16 women) received 27 lignocaine infusions. An ECG was obtained before and 30 to 60 minutes after starting the infusion. Lignocaine was infused at a rate of 2 mg/min by a pump device. The infusion was maintained until the patients were headache free for a minimum of 12 hours or a maximum of 14 days. Preventive medication was permitted and was started during the hospital stay. Seven minor adverse events were noted during four infusions. Eighteen patients had 22 infusions for MOH, with headache resolution in 82% of infusions (17 of the 18 patients responded at least once). The median duration was 5 days. Four patients obtained lasting relief, six returned to their regular manageable pattern of migraine (two of these patients had recurrent CDH after 6 months), four were lost to follow-up, and four had no long-term benefit. Five infusions were given to three patients with status migrainosus, with four of these infusions successfully relieving the headache. Intravenous lignocaine appears to be safe and may be useful in the management of severe intractable CDH and status migrainosus. It is uncertain how much of the improvement was due to the intravenous lignocaine and how much was due to discontinuing the overused acute medication and initiating preventive medication.

## Strategies of Treatment

### Outpatient

There are two general outpatient strategies. One approach is to taper the overused medication. The alternative strategy is to abruptly discontinue the overused drug, substitute a transitional medication to replace the overused drug, and subsequently taper the transitional drug. Serious withdrawal syndromes must be prevented. For example, if high doses of a butalbital-containing analgesic combination are abruptly discontinued, phenobarbital should be used to prevent barbiturate withdrawal syndrome. Similarly, benzodiazepines must be gradually tapered or replaced with long-acting ones. Ergotamine can be replaced with DHE and short-acting NSAIDs with long-acting ones. Terminators are used to stop the headache cycle. Drugs used for this purpose include DHE, NSAIDs, COX-2

inhibitors, corticosteroids, typical and atypical neuroleptics, and triptans.[182,249,250] Outpatient treatment is preferred for motivated patients, but it is not always safe or effective.

Patients who do not need hospital-level care but cannot be safely or adequately treated as outpatients can be considered for ambulatory infusion treatment. Outpatient ambulatory infusion treatment is effective for migraine status and uncomplicated CDH with and without MOH. It must be done in a supervised medical setting in which the patient can be monitored frequently (every 15 minutes). Under these circumstances, repetitive intravenous treatment can be given twice a day for several days in a row. Although ambulatory infusion treatment is better for many patients than outpatient treatment, major concerns still exist. Contraindications to outpatient ambulatory infusion treatment include the likelihood of withdrawal symptoms occurring at night when patients are withdrawn from long-acting or potent drugs, psychiatric disorders that interfere with treatment (these patients cannot be treated aggressively as outpatients), and comorbid medical illnesses that require prolonged monitoring. No long-term observation is available, and many problems manifest themselves in an intensely monitored interactive environment.

### Inpatient

If outpatient treatment fails or is not safe, or significant medical or psychiatric comorbidity is present, inpatient treatment may be needed.[161] The goals of inpatient headache treatment include (1) acute medication withdrawal and rehydration, (2) pain control with parenteral therapy, (3) establishment of effective preventive treatment, (4) termination of the pain cycle, (5) patient education, and (6) establishment of outpatient methods of pain control. Hospitalization is also used as a time for patient education, for introducing behavioral methods of pain control, and for adjusting an outpatient program of preventive and acute therapy.

The experience of my colleagues and I with more than 300 patients has shown that repetitive intravenous DHE is a safe and effective means of rapidly controlling intractable headache.[29] Of 214 patients suffering from MOH, 92% became headache free, usually within 2 to 3 days, with an average hospital stay of 7.3 days. With more aggressive treatment, the average length of stay is now 3 days. Pringsheim and Howse reported similar but less robust results (see below).[251]

## PROGNOSIS

The "natural history" of CDH, and MOH in particular, has never been studied and probably never will be for ethical and technical reasons. Recognition of overuse is probably therapeutic in and of itself and could affect the patient's behavior or the physician's approach. Retrospective analysis suggests that there may be periods of stable drug consumption and periods of accelerated medication use. Patients who are treated aggressively generally improve. There are now literature reports of spontaneous improvement of CDH in population-based studies.[85] Scher and colleagues, in a population-based study, found that the 1-year remission rate to less than one headache per week was 14% and to less than 180 days per year was 57%.[84] This was similar to the rate of remission in a population-based study in Taiwan, which demonstrated a 2-year remission rate of 65% (to less than 180 days per year).[82] The significant predictors for persistent CDH at follow-up included older age ($\geq$ 40 years) (RR 2.4), CDH onset after 32 years (RR 1.8), CDH duration $\geq$ 6 years (RR 2.0), medication overuse (RR 1.8), and daily headache (RR 2.1). Wang and colleagues found that the 4-year remission rate in elderly Chinese was 33%.[8]

My colleagues and I performed follow-up evaluations on 50 hospitalized MOH patients who were treated with repetitive intravenous DHE and became headache free.[252] Once detoxified, treated, and discharged, most patients did not resume daily acute medication use. Seventy-two percent continued to show significant improvement at 3 months and 87% continued to show significant improvement after 2 years. This would suggest at least a 70% improvement at 2 years in the initial group (35 of 50), allowing for patients lost to follow-up.

Our 2-year success rate of 87% is consistent with the long-term success rates reported in the literature.[252] In a series of 22 articles published between 1975 and 1999, the success rate of withdrawal therapy (often accompanied by pharmacologic and/or behavioral intervention) in patients overusing acute medication was between 48 and 91%, with 10 articles reporting the rate as 77% or higher.[10,33,51,58–60,83,166–168,251–263]

Henry and colleagues hospitalized, detoxified, and followed 22 MOH patients for 4 to 24 months.[257] Nine of 15 patients showed marked improvement, one showed slight improvement, and five did not improve. Rapoport and colleagues studied 90 patients with CDH who discontinued analgesics.[60] After 1 month, 30% were significantly improved; 67% were significantly improved within 2 months, 80% after 3 months, and 82% after 4 months. The authors suggested that an "analgesic washout period" exists and may be as long as 3 months for some patients.

Diener and colleagues hospitalized 85 MOH patients.[166] The length of admission was 14 days. They detoxified these patients and followed them for 10 to 75 months (mean 35 months) after discharge. Sixty-nine percent had at least 50% improvement; 29.4% were unchanged, and one had deteriorated. Fifty-four patients with MOH were hospitalized by Baumgartner and colleagues for 2 weeks.[59] They were detoxified and started on a prophylactic drug. At an average of 16.8 months (13.6 months) after treatment and discharge, 38 patients were evaluated; 76.3% had reduced their analgesic intake and 60.5% had experienced a significant relief in headache intensity and frequency.

Lake and colleagues reported on 100 patients who had been hospitalized with severe refractory MOH.[10] At follow-up between 3 months and 1 year after discharge, the mean number of severe headaches was reduced 64% and the mean number of dysfunctional days was reduced 70%. Overall, 87% of patients reported at least a 50% headache reduction.

Hering and Steiner followed 46 migraineurs who developed MOH.[167] Six months after analgesic and ergotamine withdrawal, 80.4% (37) were no longer overusing the agents and no longer had CDH.

Mathew and colleagues studied 200 MOH patients, 58% of whom were taking preventive medication without achieving a benefit.[33,51] At the 3-month follow-up, if the analgesics had been discontinued and preventive medication started or modified, a reduction of approximately 86% in the weekly headache index was achieved, with a dropout rate of 10.3%. If acute medication had been continued, only 21% improvement was achieved. It is interesting to note that merely discontinuing acute medication resulted in 58% improvement.

Schnider and colleagues followed 38 MOH inpatients who had overused ergotamine and/or analgesics and were detoxified.[261] After 5 years, 19 patients had headache 8 or less days a month and 18 had no headache or only mild headache. Outcome was related to headache frequency and duration of drug use. Fifteen patients (39.5%) had relapsed and were again overusing acute drugs.

Pini and colleagues evaluated 102 MOH patients who were overusing ergotamine, analgesics (including butalbital combinations), and/or sumatriptan.[260] Patients were treated as either outpatients or inpatients based on the therapeutic schedule to be followed. Both groups showed equal improvement at 1 and 4 months in the headache index, but there was a higher relapse rate in the outpatients (38%) compared with the inpatients (25%). This suggests that the more complicated and refractory patients were admitted to the hospital.

Pringsheim and Howse detoxified 174 inpatients who were overusing ergotamine, analgesics, and triptans and treated them with repetitive intravenous DHE; 132 patients were followed after 3 months by telephone.[251] Sixty-one percent had an immediate good result. Of these, 56% continued to do well at 3 months and 5% relapsed.

Suhr and colleagues conducted a prospective study of 257 CDH patients allocated to inpatient (147) or outpatient (110) treatment depending on the personal situation of the patient.[263] Only 5% of the patients were headache free at follow-up, which was as long as 5 years after treatment. The total relapse to drug overuse was 20.8%, occurring in 14% of the outpatients and 25% of the inpatients. No baseline analysis of headache days a month or mean pain intensity was given, but there was no significant difference in these outcomes between groups.

Monzón and colleagues prospectively studied the 6- and 12-month outcomes of 164 consecutive CDH patients and analyzed various etiologic causal factors.[264] One hundred eighteen patients (72%) had TM, 33 patients (20%) had CTTH, and 13 patients (8%) had NDPH. One hundred forty-nine patients were treated with outpatient therapy, and 15 refractory patients were admitted to a comprehensive inpatient treatment center. At 6 months, 54 patients had an excellent result, 64 had a good result, and 41 had a fair result; 5 patients continued to have TM. At 12 months, 104 patients were analyzed: 23 had an excellent result, 46 had a good result, and 28 had a fair result; 7 patients continued to have TM. There were no statistically significant differences in evolution when transformation factors were analyzed. Although the differences were not statistically significant, treatment was less efficacious when inpatient therapy was necessary and when patients had a history of analgesic abuse or traumatic life events. This, again, suggests that the more severe and intractable cases were admitted to the hospital.

Lorenzatto and colleagues, using the criteria proposed by Silberstein and colleagues,[30] retrospectively studied 140 patients (101 women and 39 men aged 17 to 83 years) who had MOH.[265] The patients were taken off the overused acute drugs and were treated with preventive medications and education. After 1 month, 23.6% of patients had more than a 50% improvement in headache intensity and frequency, and after 3 months, 56.4% had a similar improvement. Fifty percent improvement after 3 months was observed after 6 months in 70.2% of patients, after 9 months in 82.6%, and after 12 months in 84.6%.

## Why Treatment Fails

When patients fail to respond to therapy or announce that they have already tried everything and nothing will work, it is important to try to identify the reason or reasons that treatment has failed (Table 4–9). The cause of treatment failure may be an incomplete or incorrect diagnosis.[266] For example, (1) an undiagnosed secondary headache disorder is the major source of the head pain, (2) a misdiagnosed primary headache disorder is present (eg, HC is mistaken for CM; episodic paroxysmal hemicrania or hypnic headache is mistaken for cluster), or (3) two or more different headache disorders are present. In addition, pharmacotherapy may have been inadequate or important exacerbating factors, such as medication overuse, may have been missed.

## PREVENTION

Headache sufferers often do not realize that excessive or frequent self-treatment may perpetuate or exacerbate their headaches. Given that most headache sufferers do not seek medical advice until and unless the pain becomes frequent or intense, the physician's opportunity to diagnose and intervene to halt the cycle is often missed. Physicians need to screen CDH patients for analgesic overuse. Headache patients must be informed about the risks of analgesic overuse and rebound headache. Yet, even when patients are aware of the risks, they may still overmedicate. This requires continued vigilance on the part of the treating physician.

Because patients who overuse medication may feel ashamed and out of control, an accurate history may be difficult to obtain. To facilitate this process, the condition of medication rebound should be explained as part of the natural history of migraine. Even if the patient is not rebounding at the time, all symptomatic

**Table 4–9   Why Treatment Fails**

Diagnosis is incomplete or incorrect

   An undiagnosed secondary headache disorder is present

   A primary headache disorder is misdiagnosed

   Two or more different headache disorders are present

Important exacerbating factors may have been missed

   Medication overuse (including over the counter)

   Caffeine overuse

   Dietary or lifestyle triggers

   Hormonal triggers

   Psychosocial factors

   Other medications that trigger headaches

Pharmacotherapy has been inadequate

   Ineffective drug

   Excessive initial doses

   Inadequate final doses

   Inadequate duration of treatment

Other factors

   Unrealistic expectations

   Comorbid conditions complicate therapy

   Inpatient treatment required

Adapted from Lipton RB et al.[266]

headache medications, with the possible exception of the long-acting NSAIDs, should be limited to prevent rebound headache. Patients with MOH, although difficult to treat, often return to a state of intermittent episodic headache after detoxification and treatment with a preventive medication.

## REFERENCES

1. Headache Classification Committee, International Headache Society. The international classification of headache disorders, 2nd edition. Cephalalgia 2004;24 Suppl 1:1–160.

2. Silberstein SD, Lipton RB. Chronic daily headache including transformed migraine, chronic tension-type headache, and medication overuse. In: Silberstein SD, Lipton RB, Dalessio DJ, editors. Wolff's headache and other head pain. New York: Oxford University Press; 2001. p. 247–82.

3. Mathew NT, Stubits E, Nigam MR. Transformation of episodic migraine into daily headache: analysis of factors. Headache 1982;22:66–8.

4. Mathew NT, Reuveni U, Perez F. Transformed or evolutive migraine. Headache 1987;27:102–6.

5. Rapoport AM. Analgesic rebound headache. Headache 1988;28:662–5.

6. Scher AI, Stewart WF, Liberman J, Lipton RB. Prevalence of frequent headache in a population sample. Headache 1998;38:497–506.

7. Castillo J, Munoz P, Guitera V, Pascual J. Epidemiology of chronic daily headache in the general population. Headache 1999;39:190–6.

8. Wang SJ, Fuh JL, Lu SR, et al. Chronic daily headache in Chinese elderly: prevalence, risk factors and biannual follow-up. Neurology 2000;54:314–9.

9. Silberstein SD, Lipton RB, Solomon S, Mathew NT. Classification of daily and near daily headaches: proposed revisions to the IHS classification. Headache 1994;34:1–7.

10. Lake A, Saper J, Madden S, Kreeger C. Inpatient treatment for chronic daily headache: a prospective long-term outcome [abstract]. Headache 1990;30:299–300.

11. Brain WR. Some unsolved problems of cervical spondylosis. BMJ 1963;1:771–7.

12. Mathew NT. Chronic daily headache: clinical features and natural history. In: Nappi G, Bono G, Sandrini G, et al, editors. Headache and depression: serotonin pathways as a common clue. New York: Raven Press; 1991. p. 49–58.

13. Lake AE, Saper JR, Madden SF, Kreeger C. Comprehensive inpatient treatment for intractable migraine: a prospective long-term outcome study. Headache 1993;33:55–62.

14. Mathew NT. Transformed migraine. Cephalalgia 1982;13 Suppl 12:78–83.

15. Olesen J, Tfelt-Hansen P, Welch KMA. The headaches. New York: Raven Press; 1993.

16. Saper JR. Headache disorders: current concepts in treatment strategies. Littleton: Wright-PSG; 1983.

17. Sjaastad O, Saumte C, Hovdahl H. Cervicogenic headache, a hypothesis. Cephalalgia 1983;3:249–56.

18. Sjaastad O. The headache challenge in our time: cervicogenic headache. Funct Neurol 1990;5:155–8.

19. Headache Classification Committee, International Headache Society. Classification and diagnostic criteria for headache disorders, cranial neuralgia, and facial pain. Cephalalgia 1988;8 Suppl 7:1–96.

20. Silberstein SD. Chronic daily headache and tension-type headache. Neurology 1993;43:1644–9.

21. Saper JR. Daily chronic headache. Neurol Clin 1990;8:891–901.

22. Solomon S, Lipton RB, Newman LC. Evaluation of chronic daily headache-comparison to criteria for chronic tension-type headache. Cephalalgia 1992;12:365–8.

23. Sanin LC, Mathew NT, Bellmyer LR, Ali S. The International Headache Society (IHS) headache classification as applied to a headache clinic population. Cephalalgia 1994;14:443–6.

24. Messinger HB, Spierings ELH, Vincent AJP. Overlap of migraine and tension-type headache in the International Headache Society classification. Cephalalgia 1991;11:233–7.

25. Pfaffenrath V, Isler H. Evaluation of the nosology of chronic tension-type headache. Cephalalgia 1993;13 Suppl 12:60–2.

26. Mathew NT. Transformed migraine. Cephalalgia 1993;13 Suppl 12:78–83.

27. Saper JR. Daily chronic headache. Neurol Clin 1990;8:891–901.

28. Sandrini G, Manzoni GC, Zanferrari C, Nappi G. An epidemiologic approach to nosography of chronic daily headache. Cephalalgia 1993;13 Suppl 12:72–7.

29. Silberstein SD, Schulman EA, Hopkins MM. Repetitive intravenous DHE in the treatment of refractory headache. Headache 1990;30:334–9.

30. Silberstein SD, Lipton RB, Sliwinski M. Classification of daily and near-daily headaches: field trial of revised IHS criteria. Neurology 1996;47:871–5.

31. Mathew NT. Transformed or evolutional migraine. Headache 1987;27:305–6.

32. Bigal M, Lipton RB, deGryse R, et al. Similarity of chronic migraine patients with and without a history of migraine [abstract]. Cephalalgia 2003;23:747.

33. Mathew NT, Kurman R, Perez F. Drug induced refractory headache—clinical features and management. Headache 1990;30:634–8.

34. Bigal ME, Sheftell FD, Rapoport AM, et al. Chronic daily headache in a tertiary care population: correlation between the International Headache Society diagnostic criteria and proposed revisions of criteria for chronic daily headache. Cephalalgia 2002;22:432–8.

35. Bigal ME, Sheftell FD, Rapoport AM, et al. Chronic daily headache in a tertiary care population: correlation between the International Headache Society diagnostic criteria and proposed revisions of criteria for chronic daily headache. Cephalalgia 2002;22:432–8.

36. Krymchantowski AV, Barbosa JS, Lorenzatto WS, et al. Clinical features of transformed migraine [abstract]. Cephalalgia 1999;19:336–7.

37. Monzón MJ, Láinez MJ, Morales F, Sancho J. Clinical characteristics of chronic daily headache [abstract]. Cephalalgia 1999;19:410.

38. Bousser MG, Russell RR. Cerebral venous thrombosis. In: Bousser MG, Russell RR, editors. Major problems in neurology. London: Saunders; 1997. p. 175.

39. Wall M, Silberstein SD, Aiken RD. Headache associated with abnormalities in intracranial structure or function: high cerebrospinal fluid pressure headache and brain tumor. In: Silberstein SD, Lipton RB, Dalessio DJ, editors. Wolff's headache and other head pain. New York: Oxford University Press; 2001. p. 393–416.

40. Gladstone J, Eross E, Dodick D. Chronic daily headache: a rational approach to a challenging problem. Semin Neurol 2003;23:265–76.

41. Guitera V, Munoz P, Castillo J, Pascual J. Transformed migraine: a proposal for the modification of its diagnostic criteria based on recent epidemiological data. Cephalalgia 1999;19:847–50.

42. Vanast WJ. New daily persistent headaches: definition of a benign syndrome. Headache 1986;26:317.

43. Li D, Rozen TD. The clinical characteristics of new daily persistent headache. Cephalalgia 2002;22:66–9.

44. Newman LC, Lipton RB, Solomon S. Hemicrania continua: 7 new cases and a literature review. Headache 1993;32:267.

45. Peres MF, Silberstein SD, Nahmias A, et al. Hemicrania continua is not that rare. Neurology 2001;57:948–51.

46. Bordini C, Antonaci F, Stovner LJ, et al. "Hemicrania continua"—a clinical review. Headache 1991;31:20–6.

47. Katsarava Z, Muebig M, Fritsche G, et al. Clinical features of withdrawal headache following overuse of triptans in comparison to other antiheadache drugs. Neurology 2001;57:1694–8.

48. Diener HC, Dahlof CG. Headache associated with chronic use of substances. In: Olesen J, Tfelt-Hansen P, Welch KMA, editors. The headaches. Philadelphia: Lippincott, Williams & Wilkins; 1999. p. 871–8.

49. Limmroth V, Katsarava Z, Fritsche G, et al. Features of medication overuse headache following overuse of different acute headache drugs. Neurology 2002;59:1011–4.

50. Silberstein SD, Lipton RB. Chronic daily headache. In: Goadsby PJ, Silberstein SD, editors. Headache. Newton: Butterworth-Heinemann; 1997. p. 201–25.

51. Mathew NT. Drug induced headache. Neurol Clin 1990;8:903–12.

52. Saper JR. Ergotamine dependence. Headache 1987;27:435–8.

53. Saper JR. Chronic headache syndromes. Neurol Clin 1990;8:891–901.

54. Diamond S, Dalessio DJ. Drug abuse in headache. In: Diamond S, Dalessio DJ, editors. The practicing physician's approach to headache. Baltimore: Williams & Wilkins; 1982. p. 114–21.

55. Wilkinson M. Introduction. In: Diener HC, Wilkinson M, editors. Drug induced headache. Berlin: Springer-Verlag; 1988. p. 1–2.

56. Saper JR. Chronic headache syndromes. Neurol Clin 1989;7:387–412.

57. Saper JR, Jones JM. Ergotamine tartrate dependency: features and possible mechanisms. Clin Neuropharmacol 1986;9:244–56.

58. Andersson PG. Ergotism: the clinical picture. In: Diener HC, Wilkinson MS, editors. Drug induced headache. Berlin: Springer; 1988. p. 16–9.

59. Baumgartner C, Wessly P, Bingol C, et al. Long-term prognosis of analgesic withdrawal in patients with drug-induced headaches. Headache 1989;29:510–4.

60. Rapoport AM, Weeks RE, Sheftell FD, et al. The "analgesic washout period": a critical variable evaluation in

the evaluation of headache treatment efficacy. Neurology 1986;36 Suppl 1:100–1.

61. Kudrow L. Paradoxical effects of frequent analgesic use. Adv Neurol 1982;33:335–41.

62. Diener HC, Dichgans J, Scholz E, et al. Analgesic-induced chronic headache: long-term results of withdrawal therapy. J Neurol 1984;236:9–14.

63. Rasmussen BK, Jensen R, Olesen J. Impact of headache on sickness absence and utilization of medical services. J Epidemiol Community Health 1992;46:443–6.

64. Diener HC, Tfelt-Hansen P. Headache associated with chronic use of substances. In: Olesen J, Tfelt-Hansen P, Welch KMA, editors. The headaches. New York: Raven Press; 1993. p. 721–7.

65. Merikangas KR, Angst J, Isler H. Migraine and psychopathology: results of the Zurich cohort study of young adults. Arch Gen Psychiatry 1990;47:849–53.

66. Breslau N, Davis GC. Migraine, physical health and psychiatric disorders: a prospective epidemiologic study of young adults. J Psychiatr Res 1993;27:211–21.

67. Saper JR. Ergotamine dependency—a review. Headache 1987;27:435–8.

68. Mitsikostas DD, Thomas AM. Comorbidity of headache and depressive disorders. Cephalalgia 1999;19:211–7.

69. Verri AP, Cecchini P, Galli C, et al. Psychiatric comorbidity in chronic daily headache. Cephalalgia 1998;18 Suppl 21:45–9.

70. Curioso EP, Young WB, Shechter AL, Kaiser RS. Psychiatric comorbidity predicts outcome in chronic daily headache patients [abstract]. Neurology 1999;52 Suppl 2:A471.

71. Puca F, Genco S, Prudenzano MP, et al. Psychiatric comorbidity and psychosocial stress in patients with tension-type headache from headache centers in Italy. The Italian Collaborative Group for the Study of Psychopathological Factors in Primary Headaches. Cephalalgia 1999;19:159–64.

72. Guitera V, Muñoz P, Castillo J, Pascual J. Impact of chronic daily headache in the quality of life: a study in the general population [abstract]. Cephalalgia 1999;19:412–3.

73. Wang SJ, Fuh JL, Lu SR, Juang KD. Quality of life differs among headache diagnoses: analysis of SF-36 survey in 901 headache patients. Pain 2001;89:285–92.

74. Juang KD, Wang SJ, Fuh JL, et al. Comorbidity of depressive and anxiety disorders in chronic daily headache and its subtypes. Headache 2000;40:818–23.

75. Guidetti V, Galli F. Chronic daily headache in children and adolescents: clinical features and psychiatric comorbidity [abstract]. Cephalalgia 1999;19:389.

76. Peres MF, Young WB, Kaup AO, et al. Fibromyalgia is common in patients with transformed migraine. Neurology 2001;57:1326–8.

77. Peres MF, Zukerman E, Young WB, Silberstein SD. Fatigue in chronic migraine patients. Cephalalgia 2002;22:720–4.

78. Wolfe F, Smythe HA, Yanus MB. The American College of Rheumatology 1990 criteria for the classification of fibromyalgia: report of the Multicenter Criteria Committee. Arthritis Rheum 1990;33:160–72.

79. Krupp LB, Larocca NG, Muir-Nash J, Steinberg AD. The fatigue severity scale. Application to patients with multiple sclerosis and systemic lupus erythematosus. Arch Neurol 1989;46:1121–3.

80. Chalder T, Berelowitz G, Pawlikowska T, et al. Development of a fatigue scale. J Psychosom Res 1993;37:147–53.

81. Morriss RK, Wearden AJ, Mullis R. Exploring the validity of the Chalder fatigue scale in chronic fatigue syndrome. J Psychosom Res 1998;45:411–7.

82. Lu SR, Fuh JL, Chen WT, et al. Chronic daily headache in Taipei, Taiwan: prevalence, follow-up and outcome predictors. Cephalalgia 2001;21:980–6.

83. Granella F, Cavallini A, Sandrini G, et al. Long-term outcome of migraine. Cephalalgia 1998;18 Suppl 21:30–3.

84. Scher AI, Stewart WF, Ricci JA, Lipton RB. Factors associated with the onset and remission of chronic daily headache in a population-based study. Pain 2003;106:89.

85. Scher AI, Lipton RB, Stewart W. Risk factors for chronic daily headache. Curr Pain Headache Rep 2002;6:486–91.

86. Bigal ME, Sheftell FD, Rapoport AM, et al. Chronic daily headache in a tertiary care population: correlation between the International Headache Society diagnostic criteria and proposed revisions of criteria for chronic daily headache. Cephalalgia 2002;22:432–8.

87. Zwart JA, Dyb G, Hagen K, et al. Analgesic use: a predictor of chronic pain and medication overuse headache: the Head-HUNT Study. Neurology 2003;61:160–4.

88. Messlinger K, Burstein R. Anatomy of central nervous system pathways related to head pain. In: Olesen J, Tfelt-Hansen P, Welch KMA, editors. The headaches. Philadelphia: Lippincott, Williams & Wilkins; 1999. p. 77.

89. Sweatt JD, Weeber EJ, Levenons JM. Central neural mechanisms that interrelate sensory and affective dimensions of pain. Mol Interv 2002;2:393–402.

90. Woolf CJ, Mitchell MB. Mechanism-based pain diagnosis issues for analgesic drug development. Anesthesiology 2001;95:241–9.

91. Goadsby PJ, Lipton RB, Ferrari MD. Migraine-current understanding and treatment. N Engl J Med 2002;346:257–70.

92. Goadsby PJ, Lipton RB, Ferrari MD. Migraine—current understanding and treatment. N Engl J Med 2002;346:257–70.

93. Moskowitz MA. Basic mechanisms in vascular headache. Neurol Clin 1990;8:801–15.

94. Edelman GM, Gally JA. Nitric oxide: linking space and time in the brain. Proc Natl Acad Sci U S A 1992;89:11651–2.

95. Sarchielli P, Alberti A, Floridi A, Gallai V. Levels of nerve growth factor in cerebrospinal fluid of chronic daily headache patients. Neurology 2001;57:132–4.

96. Ashina M, Bendtsen L, Jensen R, et al. Plasma levels of calcitonin gene-related peptide in chronic tension-type headache. Neurology 2000;55:1335–40.

97. Burstein R, Yarnitsky D, Goor-Aryeh I, et al. An association between migraine and cutaneous allodynia. Ann Neurol 2000;47:614–24.

98. Julius D, Basbaum AI. Molecular mechanisms of nociception. Nature 2001;413:203–10.

99. Ji RR, Samad TA, Jin SX, et al. p38 MAPK activation by NGF in primary sensory neurons after inflammation increases TRPV1 levels and maintains heat hyperalgesia. Neuron 2002;36:57–68.

100. Bendtsen L, Jensen R, Olesen J. Qualitatively altered nociception in chronic myofascial pain. Pain 1996;65:259–64.

101. Battaglia G, Rustioni A. Coexistence of glutamate and substance P in dorsal root ganglion neurons of the rat and monkey. J Comp Neurol 1988;277:302–12.

102. Battaglia G, Rustioni A. Coexistence of glutamate and substance P in dorsal root ganglion neurons of the rat and monkey. J Comp Neurol 1988;277:302–12.

103. Murase K, Ryu PD, Randic M. Substance P augments a persistent slow inward calcium-sensitive current in voltage-clamped spinal dorsal horn neurons of the rat. Brain Res 1986;365:369–76.

104. Sivilotti LG, et al. The rate of rise of the cumulative depolarization evoked by repetitive stimulation of small-calibre afferents is a predictor of action potential windup in rat spinal neurones in vitro. J Neurophysiol 1993;69:1621–31.

105. Thompson SW, et al. Activity-dependent changes in rat ventral horn neurones in vitro: summation of prolonged afferent evoked postsynaptic depolarizations produce a D-APV sensitive windup. Eur J Neurosci 1990;2:638–49.

106. Woolf CJ. Evidence for a central component of postinjury pain hypersensitivity. Nature 1983;306:686–8.

107. Woolf CJ, Wall PD. The relative effectiveness of C primary afferent fibres of different origins in evoking a prolonged facilitation of the flexor reflex in the rat. J Neurosci 1986;6:1433–43.

108. Cook AJ, et al. Dynamic receptive field plasticity in rat spinal cord dorsal horn following C primary afferent input. Nature 1987;325:151–3.

109. Woolf CJ, King AE. Subthreshold components of the cutaneous mechanoreceptive fields of dorsal horn neurons in the rat lumbar spinal cord. J Neurophysiol 1989;62:907–16.

110. Woolf CJ, King AE. Dynamic alterations in the cutaneous mechanoreceptive fields of dorsal horn neurons in the rat spinal cord. J Neurosci 1990;10:2717–26.

111. Simone DA, et al. Sensitization of cat dorsal horn neurons to innocuous mechanical stimulation after intradermal injection of capsaicin. Brain Res 1989;486:185–9.

112. Sarkar S, Aziz Q, Woolf CJ, et al. Contribution of central sensitisation to the development of non-cardiac chest pain. Lancet 2000;356:1154–9.

113. Strassman AM, Raymond SA, Burstein R. Sensitization of meningeal sensory neurons and the origin of headaches. Nature 1996;384:560–4.

114. Anthony M, Rasmussen BK. Migraine without aura. In: Olesen J, Tfelt-Hansen P, Welch MA, editors. The headaches. New York: Raven Press; 1993. p. 255–61.

115. Burstein R, Yamamura H, Malick A, Strassman AM. Chemical stimulation of the intracranial dura induces enhanced responses to facial stimulation in brainstem trigeminal neurons. J Neurophysiol 1998;79:964–82.

116. Yamamura H, Malick A, Chamberlin NL, Burstein R. Cardiovascular and neuronal responses to head stimulation reflect central sensitization and cutaneous allodynia in a rat model of migraine. J Neurophysiol 1999;81:479–93.

117. Burstein R, Cutrer MF, Yarnitsky D. The development of cutaneous allodynia during a migraine attack: clinical evidence for the sequential recruitment of spinal and supraspinal nociceptive neurons in migraine. Brain 2001;123:1703–9.

118. Gallai V, Alberti A, Gallai B, et al. Glutamate and nitric oxide pathway in chronic daily headache: evidence from cerebrospinal fluid. Cephalalgia 2003;23:166–74.

119. Shukla P, Richardson E, Young WB. Brush allodynia in an inpatient headache unit [abstract]. Headache 2003;43:542.

120. Creach C, Radat F, Laffitau M, et al. Cutaneous allodynia in transformed migraine with medication overuse [abstract]. Cephalalgia 2003;23:581–762.

121. Sobrino FE. Cutaneous allodynia in chronic migraine [abstract]. Cephalalgia 2003;23:581.

122. Porreca F, Ossipov MH, Gebhart GF. Chronic pain and medullary descending facilitation. Trends Neurosci 2002;25:319–25.

123. Zhuo M, Gebhart GF. Characterization of descending inhibition and facilitation from the nuclei reticularis gigantocellularis and gigantocellularis pars alpha in the rat. Pain 1990;42:337–50.

124. Zhuo M, Gebhart GF. Characterization of descending facilitation and inhibition of spinal nociceptive transmission from the nuclei reticularis gigantocellularis and gigantocellularis pars alpha in the rat. J Neurophysiol 1992;67:1599–614.

125. Zhuo M, Gebhart GF. Biphasic modulation of spinal nociceptive transmission from the medullary raphe nuclei in the rat. J Neurophysiol 1997;78:746–58.

126. Zhuo M, Gebhart GF. Characterization of descending facilitation and inhibition of spinal nociceptive transmission from the nuclei reticularis gigantocellularis and gigantocellularis pars alpha in the rat. J Neurophysiol 1992;67:1599–614.

127. Zhuo M, Gebhart GF. Biphasic modulation of spinal nociceptive transmission from the medullary raphe nuclei in the rat. J Neurophysiol 1997;78:746–58.

128. Urban MO, Gebhart GF. Characterization of biphasic modulation of spinal nociceptive transmission by neurotensin in the rat rostral ventromedial medulla. J Neurophysiol 1997;78:1550–62.

129. Urban MO, Coutinho SV, Gebhart GF. Biphasic modulation of visceral nociception by neurotensin in rat rostral ventromedial medulla. J Pharmacol Exp Ther 1999;290:207–13.

130. Urban MO, Coutinho SV, Gebhart GF. Involvement of excitatory amino acid receptors and nitric oxide in the rostral ventromedial medulla in modulating secondary hyperalgesia produced by mustard oil. Pain 1999;81:45–55.

131. Fields HL, Heinricher MM, Mason P. Neurotransmitters as nociceptive modulatory circuits. Annu Rev Neurosci 1991;219–45.

132. Kim DH, Fields HL, Barbaro NM. Morphine analgesia and acute physical dependence: rapid onset of two opposing, dose-related processes. Brain Res 1990;516:37–40.

133. Bederson JB, Fields HL, Barbaro NM. Hyperalgesia during naloxone-precipitated withdrawal from morphine is associated with increased on-cell activity in the rostral ventromedial medulla. Somatosens Motor Res 1990;7:185–203.

134. Kaplan H, Fields HL. Hyperalgesia during acute opioid abstinence: evidence for a nociceptive facilitating function of the rostral ventromedial medulla. J Neurosci 1991;11:1433–9.

135. Heinricher MM, Roychowdhury SM. Reflex-related activation of putative pain facilitating neurons in rostral ventromedial medulla requires excitatory amino acid transmission. Neuroscience 1997;78:1159–65.

136. Porreca F, Ossipov MH, Gebhart GF. Chronic pain and medullary descending facilitation. Trends Neurosci 2002;25:319–25.

137. Ma QP, Woolf CJ. Noxious stimuli induce an N-methyl-D-aspartate receptor-dependent hypersensitivity of the flexion withdrawal reflex to touch: implications for the treatment of mechanical allodynia. Pain 1995;61:383–90.

138. Kovelowski CJ, Ossipov MH, Sun H, et al. Supraspinal cholecystokinin may drive tonic descending facilitation mechanisms to maintain neuropathic pain in the rat. Pain 2000;87:265–73.

139. Heinricher MM, McGaraughty S, Tortorici V. Circuitry underlying antiopioid actions of cholecystokinin within the rostral ventromedial medulla. J Neurophysiol 2001;85:280–6.

140. Kovelowski CJ, Ossipov MH, Sun H, et al. Supraspinal cholecystokinin may drive tonic descending facilitation mechanisms to maintain neuropathic pain in the rat. Pain 2000;87:265–7.

141. Dourish CT, O'Neill MF, Coughlan J, et al. The selective CCK-B receptor antagonist L-365,260 enhances morphine analgesia and prevents morphine tolerance in the rat. Eur J Pharmacol 1990;176:35–44.

142. Vanderah TW, Gardell LR, Burgess SE, et al. Dynorphin promotes abnormal pain and spinal opioid antinociceptive tolerance. J Neurosci 2000;20:7074–9.

143. Arcaya JL, Cano G, Gomez G, et al. Dynorphin A increases substance P release from trigeminal primary afferent C-fibers. Eur J Pharmacol 1999;366:27–34.

144. Gardell LR, Wang R, Burgess SE, et al. Sustained morphine exposure induces a spinal dynorphin-dependent enhancement of excitatory transmitter release from primary afferent fibers. J Neurosci 2002;22:6747–55.

145. Draisci G, Kajander KC, Dubner R, et al. Up-regulation of opioid gene expression in spinal cord evoked by experimental nerve injuries and inflammation. Brain Res 1991;560:186–92.

146. Gardell LR, Wang R, Burgess SE, et al. Sustained morphine exposure induces a spinal dynorphin-dependent enhancement of excitatory transmitter release from primary afferent fibers. J Neurosci 2002;22:6747–55.

147. Mao J, Sung B, Ji RR, Lim G. Neuronal apoptosis associated with morphine tolerance: evidence for an opioid-induced neurotoxic mechanism. J Neurosci 2002;22:7650–61.

148. Bederson JB, Fields HL, Barbaro NM. Hyperalgesia during naloxone-precipitated withdrawal from morphine is associated with increased on-cell activity in the rostral ventromedial medulla. Somatosens Mot Res 1990;7:185–203.

149. Urban MO, Gebhart GF. Supraspinal contributions to hyperalgesia. PNAS 1999;96:7687–92.

150. Post RM, Silberstein SD. Shared mechanisms in affective illness, epilepsy, and migraine. Neurology 1994;44:S37–47.

151. Fusco BM, Colantoni O, Saturnino C, et al. Altered "second pain" in chronic headaches: pharmacological modulation [abstract]. Cephalalgia 1999;19:399–400.

152. Weiller C, May A, Limmroth V, et al. Brainstem activation in spontaneous human migraine attacks. Nat Med 1995;1:658–60.

153. May A, Bahra A, Buchel C, et al. Hypothalamic activation in cluster headache attacks. Lancet 1998;352:275–8.

154. May A, Kaube H, Buchel C, et al. Experimental cranial pain elicited by capsaicin: a PET study. Pain 1998;74:61–6.

155. Ren K, Dubner R. Descending modulation in persistent pain: an update. Pain 2002;100:1–6.

156. Bahra A, Matharu MS, Buchel C, et al. Brainstem activation specific to migraine headache. Lancet 2001;357:1016–7.

157. Manjit SM, Thorsten B, Ward N, et al. Central neuromodulation in chronic migraine patients with suboccipital stimulators: a PET study [abstract]. Brain 2003;1:220–30.

158. Welch KMA, Nagesh V, Rozell K, et al. Functional MRI of chronic daily headache [abstract]. Cephalalgia 1999;19:462–3.

159. Aurora SK. Imaging chronic daily headache. Curr Pain Headache Rep 2003;7:209–11.

160. Siniatchkin M, Gerber WD, Kropp P, Vein A. Contingent negative variation in patients with chronic daily headache. Cephalalgia 1998;18:565–9.

161. Silberstein SD, Saper JR. Migraine: diagnosis and treatment. In: Dalessio DJ, Silberstein SD, editors. Wolff's headache and other head pain. New York: Oxford University Press; 1993. p. 96–170.

162. Zed PJ, Loewen PS, Robinson G. Medication-induced headache: overview and systematic review of therapeutic approaches. Ann Pharmacother 1999;33:61–72.

163. Tavola T, Gala C, Conte G, Invernizzi G. Traditional Chinese acupuncture in tension-type headache: a controlled study. Pain 1992;48:325–9.

164. Silberstein SD. Treatment of headache in primary care practice. Am J Med 1984;77(3A):65–72.

165. Raskin NH. Repetitive intravenous dihydroergotamine as therapy for intractable migraine. Neurology 1986;36:995–7.

166. Diener HC, Gerber WD, Geiselhart S. Short and long-term effects of withdrawal therapy in drug-induced headache. In: Diener HC, Wilkinson M, editors. Drug-induced headache. Berlin: Springer-Verlag; 1988. p. 133–42.

167. Hering R, Steiner TJ. Abrupt outpatient withdrawal from medication in analgesic-abusing migraineurs. Lancet 1991;337:1442–3.

168. Diener HC, Pfaffenrath V, Soyka D, Gerber WD. Therapie des Medikamenten-induzierten Dauerkopfschmerzes. Münch Med Wschr 1992;134:159–62.

169. Silberstein SD, Lipton RB. Overview of diagnosis and treatment of migraine. Neurology 1994;44 Suppl 7:6–16.

170. Bussone G, Sandrini G, Patruno G, et al. Effectiveness of fluoxetine on pain and depression in chronic headache disorders. In: Nappi G, Bono G, Sandrini G, et al, editors. Headache and depression: serotonin pathways as a common clue. New York: Raven Press; 1991. p. 265–72.

171. Couch JR, Ziegler DK, Hassainein R. Amitriptyline in the prophylaxis of migraine. Arch Neurol 1976;26:121–7.

172. Diamond S, Baltes B. Chronic tension headache treated with amitriptyline: a double blind study. Headache 1971;11:110–6.

173. Low dose amitriptyline prophylaxis in chronic scalp muscle contraction headache. In: Proceedings of the First International Headache Congress. Munich, September. Munich: 1983.

174. Lance JW, Curran DA. Treatment of chronic tension headache. Lancet 1964;i:1236–9.

175. Pluvinage R. Le traitement des migraines et des cephalees psychogenes par l'amitriptyline. Sem Hop 1978;54:713–6.

176. Pfaffenrath V, Kellhammer U, Pollmann W. Combination headache: practical experience with a combination of beta-blocker and an antidepressive. Cephalalgia 1986;6:25–32.

177. Holroyd KA, Nash JM, Pingel JD. A comparison of pharmacologic (amitriptyline HCl) and nonpharmacologic (cognitive-behavioral) therapies for chronic tension headaches. J Consult Clin Psychol 1991;59:387–93.

178. Gobel H, Hamouz V, Hansen C, et al. Chronic tension-type headache: amitriptyline reduces clinical headache-duration and experimental pain sensitivity but does not alter pericranial muscle activity readings. Pain 1994;59:241–9.

179. Pfaffenrath V, Diener HC, Isler H, et al. Efficacy and tolerability of amitriptylinoxide in the treatment of chronic tension-type headache: a multicentre controlled study. Cephalalgia 1994;14:149–55.

180. Cerbo R, Barbanti P, Fabbrini G, et al. Amitriptyline is effective in chronic but not in episodic tension-type headache: pathogenic implications. Headache 1998;38:453–7.

181. Mitsikostas DD, Gatzonis S, Thomas A, Ilias A. Buspirone vs amitriptyline in the treatment of chronic tension-type headache. J Neurol Scand 1997;96:247–51.

182. Bonuccelli U, Nuti A, Lucetti C, et al. Amitriptyline and dexamethasone combined treatment in drug-induced headache. Cephalalgia 1996;16:197–200.

183. Morland TJ, Storli OV, Mogstad TE. Doxepin in the prophylactic treatment of mixed 'vascular' and tension headache. Headache 1979;19:382–3.

184. Descombes S, Brefel-Courbon C, Thalamas C, et al. Amitriptyline treatment in chronic drug-induced headache: a double-blind comparative pilot study. Headache 2001;41:178–82.

185. Saper JR, Silberstein SD, Lake AE, Winters ME. Double-blind trial of fluoxetine: chronic daily headache and migraine. Headache 1994;34:497–502.

186. Krymchantowski AV, Silva MT, Barbosa JS, Alves LA. Amitriptyline versus amitriptyline combined with fluoxetine in the preventative treatment of transformed migraine: a double-blind study. Headache 2002;42:510–4.

187. Manna V, Bolino F, DiCicco L. Chronic tension-type headache, mood depression and serotonin. Headache 1994;34:44–9.

188. Palmer KJ, Benfield P. Fluvoxamine: an overview of its pharmacologic properties and a review of its use in non-depressive disorders. CNS Drugs 1994;1:57–87.

189. Foster CA, Bafaloukos J. Paroxetine in the treatment of chronic daily headache. Headache 1994;34:587–9.

190. Langemark M, Olesen J. Sulpiride and paroxetine in the treatment of chronic tension-type headache. Headache 1994;34:20–4.

191. Mathew NT. Prophylaxis of migraine and mixed headache. A randomized controlled study. Headache 1981;21:105–9.

192. Bright RA, Everitt DE. Beta-blockers and depression: evidence against association. JAMA 1992;267: –1783.

193. Jensen R, Brinck T, Olesen J. Sodium valproate has a prophylactic effect in migraine without aura. Neurology 1994;44:647–51.

194. Mathew NT, Saper JR, Silberstein SD, et al. Migraine prophylaxis with divalproex. Arch Neurol 1995;52:281–6.

195. Hering R, Kuritzky A. Sodium valproate in the prophylactic treatment of migraine: a double-blind study versus placebo. Cephalalgia 1992;12:81–4.

196. Klapper J. Divalproex sodium in the prophylactic treatment of migraine [abstract]. Headache 1995;35:290.

197. Mathew NT, Ali S. Valproate in the treatment of persistent chronic daily headache. An open label study. Headache 1991;31:71–4.

198. Edwards K, Santarcangelo V, Shea P, Edwards J. Intravenous valproate for acute treatment of migraine headaches [abstract]. Cephalalgia 1999;19:356.

199. Freitag FG, Diamond S, Diamond M, Urban G. Divalproex in the long-term treatment of chronic daily headache. Headache 2001;41:271–8.

200. Wessely P, Baumgartner C, Klinger D, et al. Preliminary results of a double-blind study with the new migraine prophylactic drug gabapentin. Cephalalgia 1987;7 Suppl 6:477–8.

201. Mathew NT, Rapoport A, Saper J, et al. Efficacy of gabapentin in migraine prophylaxis. Headache 2001;41:119–28.

202. Spira PJ, Beran RG. Gabapentin in the prophylaxis of chronic daily headache. A randomized, placebo-controlled study for the Australian Gabapentin Chronic Daily Headache Group. Neurology 2003;61:1753–9.

203. Silberstein SD. Gabapentin in the treatment of chronic daily headache (commentary). Neurology 2003;61:1637.

204. Brandes JL, Jacobs DJ, Neto W, Bhattacharaya S. Topiramate in the prevention of migraine headache: a randomized, double-blind, placebo-controlled, parallel study (MIGR-002) [abstract]. Neurology 2003;60 Suppl 1:A238.

205. Mathew NT, Schmit TJ, Jacobs D, Neto W. Topiramate in migraine prevention (MIGR-001): effect on migraine frequency [abstract]. Neurology 2003;60 Suppl 1:A336.

206. White HS, Brown SD, Woodhead JH, et al. Topiramate modulates GABA-evoked currents in murine cortical neurons by a nonbenzodiazepine mechanism. Epilepsia 2000;41 Suppl 1:S17–20.

207. Zhang XL, Velumian A, Jones OT, Carlen PL. Modulation of high voltage-activated calcium channels in dentate granule cells by topiramate. Epilepsia 2000;41 Suppl 1:S52–60.

208. Shank RP, Gardocki JF, Vaught JL, et al. Topiramate: preclinical evaluation of structurally novel anticonvulsant. Epilepsia 1994;35:450–60.

209. Krebs EG. The growth of research on protein phosphorylation. Trends Biochem Sci 1994;19:439.

210. Roche KW, O'Brien RJ, Mammen AL, Huganir RL. Characterization of multiple phosphorylation sites on the AMP receptor GluR1 subunit. Neuron 1996;16:1179–88.

211. Wang JH, Kelly PT. Postsynaptic injection of CA2+/CaM induces synaptic potentiation requiring CaMKII and PKC activity. Neuron 1995;15:443–52.

212. Sigel E. Functional modulation of ligand-gated $GABA_A$ and NMDA receptor channels by phosphorylation. J Receptor Signal Transduction Res 1995;15:325.

213. Shank RP, Gardocki JF, Streeter AJ, Maryanoff B. An overview of the preclinical aspects of topiramate: pharmacology, pharmacokinetics, and mechanism of action. Epilepsia 2000;41 Suppl 1:S3–9.

214. Silberstein SD, Neto W, Schmitt J, et al. MIGR-001 Study Group. Topiramate in migraine prevention: results of a large controlled trial. Arch Neurol 2004;61:490–5.

215. Brandes JL, Saper JR, Diamond M, et al. Topiramate for migraine prevention: a randomized controlled trial. JAMA 2004;291:965–73.

216. Silberstein SD. Control of topiramate-induced paresthesias with supplemental potassium [letter]. Headache 2002;42:85.

217. Shuaib A, Ahmed F, Muratoglu M, Kochanski P. Topiramate in migraine prophylaxis: a pilot study [abstract]. Cephalalgia 1999;19:379–80.

218. Silberstein SD. Methysergide. Cephalalgia 1998;18:421–35.

219. Miller DS, Talbot CA, Simpson W, Korey A. A comparison of naproxen sodium, acetaminophen and placebo in the treatment of muscle contraction headache. Headache 1987;27:392–6.

220. Johnson ES, Tfelt-Hansen P. Nonsteroidal antiinflammatory drugs. In: Olesen J, Tfelt-Hansen P, Welch KMA, editors. The headaches. New York: Raven Press; 1993. p. 391–5.

221. Mylecharane EJ, Tfelt-Hansen P. Miscellaneous drugs. In: Olesen J, Tfelt-Hansen P, Welch KMA, editors. The headaches. New York: Raven Press; 1993. p. 397–402.

222. Kangasniemi PJ, Nyrke T, Lang AH, Petersen E. Femoxetine—a new 5HT uptake inhibitor—and propranolol in the prophylactic treatment of migraine. Acta Neurol Scand 1983;68:262–7.

223. Scholz E, Gerber WD, Diener HC, Langohr HD. Dihydroergotamine vs flunarizine vs nifedipine vs metoprolol vs propranolol in migraine prophylaxis: a comparative study based on time series analysis. In: Scholz E, Gerber WD, Diener HC, Langohr HD, editors. Advances in headache research. London: John Libbey & Co.; 1987. p. 139–45.

224. Pascual J, Leira R, Lainez JM. Combined therapy for migraine prevention? Clinical experience with a beta-blocker plus sodium valproate in 52 resistant migraine patients. Cephalalgia 2003;23:961–2.

225. Smuts JA, Baker MK, Smuts HM, et al. Botulinum toxin type A as prophylactic treatment in chronic tension-type headache [abstract]. Cephalalgia 1999;19:454.

226. Gobel H, Lindner V, Krack P, et al. Treatment of chronic tension-type headache with botulinum toxin [abstract]. Cephalalgia 1999;19:455.

227. Mauskop A. Botulinum toxin in the treatment of chronic daily headaches [abstract]. Cephalalgia 1999;19:453.

228. Eross EJ, Dodick DW. The effects of botulinum toxin type A on disability in episodic and chronic migraine [abstract]. Neurology 2002;58 Suppl 3:A497.

229. Ondo WG, Derman HS. Botulinum toxin A for chronic daily headache: a 60-patient, randomized, placebo-controlled, parallel design study [abstract]. Headache 2002;42:431.

230. Mathew NT, Frishberg BM, Gawel M, et al. Botulinum toxin type A (BOTOX) for the prophylactic treatment of chronic daily headache: A randomized, double-blind, placebo-controlled trial. Headache 2005 Apr;45(4): 293-307.

231. Dodick DW, Mauskop A, Elkind AH, et al. Botulinum toxin type A for the prophylaxis of chronic daily headache: Subgroup analysis of patients not receiving other prophylactic medications (a randomized double-blind, placebo-controlled study). Headache 2005 Apr;45(4):315-324.

232. Harden RN. Chronic opioid therapy: another reappraisal. APS Bull 2002;12(1):1–12.

233. Ziegler DK. Opioids in headache treatment: is there a role? Neurol Clin 1997;15:199–207.

234. Robbins L. Long-acting opioids for severe chronic daily headache. Headache Q 1999;10:135–9.

235. Saper JR, Lake AE, Hamel RL, et al. Daily scheduled opioids for intractable head pain: long-term observations of a treatment program. Neurology 2004. [In press]

236. Silberstein SD, Saper JR, Freitag F. Migraine: diagnosis and treatment. In: Silberstein SD, Lipton RB, Dalessio DJ, editors. Wolff's headache and other head pain. New York: Oxford University Press; 2001. p. 121–237.

237. Bell R, Montoya D, Shuaib A, Lee MA. A comparative trial of three agents in the treatment of acute migraine headache. Ann Emerg Med 1990;19:1079–82.

238. Callaham M, Raskin N. A controlled study of dihydroergotamine in the treatment of acute migraine headache. Headache 1986;26:168–71.

239. Jones J, Sklar D, Dougherty J, White W. Randomized double-blind trial of intravenous prochlorperazine for the treatment of acute headache. JAMA 1989;261:1174–6.

240. Lu SR, Fuh JL, Juang KD, Wang SJ. Repetitive intravenous prochlorperazine treatment of patients with refractory chronic daily headache. Headache 2000;40:724–9.

241. Wang SJ, Silberstein SD, Young WB. Droperidol treatment of status migrainosus and refractory migraine. Headache 1997;37:377–82.

242. Silberstein SD, Young WB, Mendizabal J, et al. Efficacy of intramuscular droperidol for migraine treatment: a dose response study [abstract]. Neurology 2001;56(8 Suppl 3):A64.

243. Pradalier A, Clapin A, Dry J. Treatment review: nonsteroid antiinflammatory drugs in the treatment and long-term prevention of migraine attacks. Headache 1988;28:550–7.

244. Campbell WB. Lipid-derived autocoids: eicosanoids and platelet-activating factor. In: Gilman AG, Rall TW, Taylor P, editors. The pharmacological basis of therapeutics. New York: Pergamon Press; 1990. p. 600–17.

245. Tanen DA, Miller S, French T, Riffenburgh RH. Intravenous sodium valproate versus prochlorperazine for the emergency department treatment of acute migraine headaches: a prospective, randomized, double-blind trial. Ann Emerg Med 2003;41:847–53.

246. Krusz JC, Belanger J. Propofol—a highly effective treatment for acute headaches [abstract]. Cephalalgia 1999;19:358.

247. Mendes PM, Silberstein SD, Young WB, et al. Intravenous propofol in the treatment of refractory headache. Headache 2002;42:638–41.

248. Hand PJ, Stark RJ. Intravenous lignocaine infusions for severe chronic daily headache. Med J Aust 2000;172:157–9.

249. Diener HC, Haab J, Peters C, et al. Subcutaneous sumatriptan in the treatment of headache during withdrawal from drug-induced headache. Headache 1991;31:205–9.

250. Drucker P, Tepper S. Daily sumatriptan for detoxification from rebound. Headache 1998;38:687–90.

251. Pringsheim T, Howse D. Inpatient treatment of chronic daily headache using dihydroergotamine: a long-term followup study. Can J Neurol Sci 1998;25:146–50.

252. Silberstein SD, Silberstein JR. Chronic daily headache: prognosis following inpatient treatment with repetitive IV DHE. Headache 1992;32:439–45.

253. Tfelt-Hansen P, Krabbe AA. Ergotamine. Do patients benefit from withdrawal? Cephalalgia 1981;1:29–32.

254. Schoenen J, Lenarduzzi P, Sianard-Gainko J. Chronic headaches associated with analgesics and/or ergotamine abuse: a clinical survey of 434 consecutive outpatients. In: Rose FD, editor. New advances in headache research. London: Smith-Gordon; 1989. p. 29–43.

255. Isler H. Migraine treatment as a cause of chronic migraine. In: Rose FC, editor. Advances in migraine research and therapy. New York: Raven Press; 1982. p. 159–64.

256. Dichgans J, Diener HD, Gerber WD, et al. Analgetika-induzierter Dauerkopfschmerz. Dtsch Med Wochenschr 1984;109:369.

257. Rose FC, editor. Ergotamine- and analgesic-induced headache. Migraine: proceedings from the Fifth International Migraine Symposium. London: 1984.

258. Andersson PG. Ergotamine headache. Headache 1975;15:118–21.

259. Diener HC, Dichgans J, Scholz E, et al. Analgesic-induced chronic headache: long-term results of withdrawal therapy. J Neurol 1989;236:9–14.

260. Pini LA, Bigarelli M, Vitale G, Sternieri E. Headaches associated with chronic use of analgesics: a therapeutic approach. Headache 1996;36:433–9.

261. Schnider P, Aull S, Baumgartner C, et al. Long-term outcome of patients with headache and drug abuse after inpatient withdrawal: five-year followup. Cephalalgia 1996;16:481–5.

262. Monzon MJ, Lainez MJ. Quality of life in migraine and chronic daily headache patients. Cephalalgia 1998;18:638–43.

263. Suhr B, Evers S, Bauer B, et al. Drug-induced headache: long-term results of stationary versus ambulatory withdrawal therapy. Cephalalgia 1999;19:44–9.

264. Monzón MJ, Lainez MJA, Morales F, Sancho J. Long-term prognosis of chronic daily headache [abstract]. Cephalalgia 1999;19:410.

265. Lorenzatto WS, Cheim CF, Adriano M, et al. Long-term outcome in chronic daily headache [abstract]. Cephalalgia 1999;19:413.

266. Lipton RB, Silberstein SD, Saper J, Goadsby PJ. Why headache treatment fails. Neurology 2003;60(7):1064–70.

267. Tfelt-Hansen P, Welch KMA. Prioritizing prophylactic treatment of migraine. In: Olesen J, Tfelt-Hansen P, Welch KMA, editors. The headaches. Philadelphia: Lippincott Williams & Wilkins; 2000. p. 499–500.

# CHAPTER 5

# Chronic Tension-Type Headache

Arnaud Fumal, MD, and Jean Schoenen, MD, PhD

Tension-type headache (TTH) is an ill-defined and heterogeneous syndrome because its diagnosis is mainly based on the absence of features found in other headache types, such as migraine. It is thus, above all, a "featureless" headache characterized by nothing but pain in the head. The headaches formerly described as "muscular contraction," "psychogenic," "psychomyogenic," "tension," "stress," "essential," or "nonmigrainous" are classified in this group. However, because of the lack of specificity of diagnostic criteria, there is evidence that some patients with migraine are erroneously included.

The term "tension type" was chosen by the first Classification Committee of the International Headache Society (IHS) to offer a new heading underlining the uncertain pathogenesis but indicating, nevertheless, that some kind of mental or muscular tension may play a causative role.[1] Because the exact pathogenesis remains unsolved, this term has been maintained in the second edition of *The International Classification of Headache Disorders* (*ICHD-II*),[2] although it is commonly translated into "tension headache" in many non–Anglo-Saxon countries.

TTH is the most common form of headache but receives much less attention from health authorities, clinical researchers, or industrial pharmacologists than migraine. This may be due to the fact that most subjects with TTH never consult a doctor and treat themselves, if necessary, with over-the-counter analgesics. However, frequent and chronic TTHs constitute a major health problem with an enormous socioeconomic impact.

Despite the meager scientific foundations regarding both mechanisms and treatments of TTH, it is not impossible to manage these patients with some success, even though there has been no major therapeutic breakthrough in recent years.

## CLASSIFICATION

Compared with the first IHS classification, the general diagnostic criteria for TTH in *ICHD-II* are the same (Table 5–1). The only change is the subdivision of TTH into three groups, differing by headache frequency. The division into episodic (ETTH) and chronic (CTTH) subtypes that was introduced in the first edition of the IHS classification has proved useful. The chronic subtype is a serious disease causing greatly decreased quality of life, high disability, and substantial socioeconomic costs. Within the episodic subgroup, however, disability and, most likely, pathophysiology differ between subjects with occasional or frequent episodes of TTH. In *ICHD-II*, it was therefore decided to subdivide ETTH further into an infrequent subtype with headache episodes less than once per month and a frequent subtype (Table 5–2). The infrequent subtype has very little impact on the individual and does not deserve much attention from the medical profession. However, frequent sufferers can encounter considerable disability that sometimes warrants expensive drugs and prophylactic medication.

The first edition of the IHS classification arbitrarily separated TTH patients with (third digit code 1) and without (third digit code 2) so-called "disorder of the pericranial muscles." Because tenderness on manual palpation is the most useful distinguishing criterion,[3,4] patients are now separated according to the presence or not of "increased pericranial tenderness." Pericranial tenderness is easily recorded by manual palpation by small rotating movements and a firm pressure (if possible aided by use of a palpometer) with the second and third fingers on the frontal, temporal, masseter, pterygoid, sternocleidomastoid, splenius, and trapezius muscles. A local tenderness score from 0 to 3 on each muscle can be summated to yield a total tenderness score for each individual.[5] This has proved to be a valid clinical subdivision, but the vast

**Table 5–1   Tension-Type Headache: General Diagnostic Criteria**

| | |
|---|---|
| B. | Headache lasting from 30 min to 7 d |
| C. | At least 2 of the following pain characteristics: |
| | 1.   Bilateral location |
| | 2.   Pressing/tightening (nonpulsating) quality |
| | 3.   Mild or moderate intensity |
| | 4.   Not aggravated by routine physical activity, such as walking or climbing stairs |
| D. | Both of the following: |
| | 1.   No nausea or vomiting (anorexia may occur) |
| | 2.   No more than 1 of photophobia or phonophobia |
| E. | Not attributed to another disorder |

Adapted from *The International Classification of Headache Disorders.*[2]

**Table 5–2   Tension-Type Headache: Specific Diagnostic Criteria**

| | |
|---|---|
| 2.1 | Infrequent episodic tension-type headache |
| | A.   At least 10 episodes occurring on < 1 d/mo (< 12 d/yr) and fulfilling criteria B–D |
| 2.2 | Frequent episodic tension-type headache |
| | A.   At least 10 episodes occurring on ≤ 1 but < 15 d/mo for at least 3 mos (≤ 12 and < 180 d/yr) and fulfilling criteria B–D |
| 2.3 | Chronic tension-type headache |
| | A.   Headache occurring on ≥ 15 d/mo on average for > 3 mo (≤ 180 d/yr)[1] and fulfilling criteria B–D |
| | B.   Headache lasts hours or may be continuous |
| | C.   Both of the following: |
| | 1.   No more than 1 of photophobia, phonophobia, or mild nausea |
| | 2.   Neither moderate or severe nausea nor vomiting |
| 2.4 | Probable tension-type headache |
| | B.   Episodes fulfilling all but one of criteria A–D for 2.1, 2.2, or 2.3 |
| | C.   Episodes do not fulfill criteria for 1.1 migraine without aura |
| | D.   Not attributed to another disorder |

Adapted from *The International Classification of Headache Disorders.*[2]

majority of disabled patients, that is, those with frequent or chronic TTH, have increased pericranial tenderness and thus qualify for third digit code 1.[6] This and the fact that clinical features, pathophysiologic abnormalities, and the response to therapy seem similar between the two subgroups[7] leave open the question of the utility of such subdivision.

The introduction of category 1.5.1 chronic migraine into *ICHD-II* creates a problem in relation to the differential diagnosis between this and 2.3 CTTH. Both diagnoses require headache (meeting the criteria for migraine or TTH, respectively) on at least 15 days a month. Therefore, it is possible, theoretically, that a patient can have both diagnoses. Considering the above, a proposal for new, stricter diagnostic criteria is published under A2 TTH in the appendix of *ICHD-II* (Table 5–3). It is recommended that future studies compare patients diagnosed according to the explicit

| **Table 5–3** Proposal for Stricter General Diagnostic Criteria for Tension-Type Headache (ICHD-II Appendix A2) |
|---|

| | |
|---|---|
| B. | Headache lasting from 30 min to 7 d |
| C. | At least 3 of the following pain characteristics: |
| |    1.    Bilateral location |
| |    2.    Pressing/tightening (nonpulsating) quality |
| |    3.    Mild or moderate intensity |
| |    4.    Not aggravated by routine physical activity, such as walking or climbing stairs |
| D. | No nausea (anorexia may occur), vomiting, photo- or phonophobia |
| E. | Not attributed to another disorder |

ICHD-II = The International Classification of Headache Disorders, second edition.

criteria with others diagnosed according to the appendix criteria. This pertains not only to the clinical features but also to pathophysiologic mechanisms and the response to treatments.

In many patients with CTTH, there may be overuse of acute medication, such as combination analgesics. When this fulfills criterion B (dose and duration of substance intake) for any of the subforms of *ICHD-II* 8.2 medication-overuse headache, the default rule is to code for 2.4.3 probable chronic CTTH, plus 8.2.7 probable medication-overuse headache. When these criteria are still fulfilled 2 months after medication overuse has ceased, 2.3 CTTH should be diagnosed and 8.2.7 discarded. If, at any time sooner, they are no longer fulfilled because improvement has occurred, 8.2 medication-overuse headache should be diagnosed and 2.4.3 discarded.

In most patients, TTH evolves over time from the episodic to the chronic form. However, if the headache fulfills CTTH criteria A to E and, unambiguously, is daily and unremitting within 3 days of its first onset, the patient should receive the diagnostic *ICHD-II* code 4.8 new daily-persistent headache, another heterogeneous entity.

## EPIDEMIOLOGY AND IMPACT

In the Danish Glostrup Population Studies, the most detailed epidemiologic study of headache to date, the 1-year prevalence of ETTH was 63% (56% in men and 71% in women).[8] The prevalence of CTTH was 3% (2% in men and 5% in women). The gender difference was statistically significant, with a male to female ratio of 4:5. The prevalence of TTH decreased with increasing age. The prevalence of chronic daily headache from a survey of the general population in the United States was 4.1%.[9] Half of the sufferers met the criteria for CTTH. In a survey of 2,500 undergraduate students in the United States, the prevalence of CTTH was 2%.[10]

Because of its high prevalence, TTH has a greater socioeconomic impact than any other type of headache. The direct costs include medical costs and social services; indirect costs cause lost production in the economy because of morbidity. Intangible costs include reduced quality of life. Because headache attacks reduce work capability quite significantly, the socioeconomic costs from absenteeism among patients with TTH are quite substantial. The total loss of work days each year because of TTH is 820 days per 1,000 employees compared with 270 days per 1,000 employees as a result of migraine headache.[11] In Denmark, TTH, especially the chronic type, accounts for more than 10% of total disease absenteeism caused by any disease.[11] The individual impact of TTH encompasses physical suffering, loss of quality of life, and economic effect but is more difficult to quantify than the impact on the society. In a study by Holroyd and colleagues, it was demonstrated that CTTH has a profound negative effect on the emotional life of the affected patients; they were seven times more likely than control subjects to be classified as impaired on all of the subscales of the applied quality-of-life instruments, which is similar or even worse than other patients with well-accepted chronic pain diagnosis.[12]

## PATHOPHYSIOLOGY

It is still a matter of debate whether the pain in TTH originates from myofascial tissues or from central mechanisms in the brain. Research progress is hampered by the difficulty of obtaining homogeneous populations of patients because of the lack of specificity of clinical features and diagnostic criteria. The present consensus is nonetheless that peripheral pain mechanisms are most likely to play a role in 2.1 infrequent ETTH and 2.2 frequent ETTH, whereas central pain mechanisms play a more important role in 2.3 CTTH.

There are no data about specific genotypes in TTH, but an increased familial risk was found for CTTH in one study.[13] However, because TTH is an extremely common condition and environmental factors seem to play an important role in triggering headaches, it is unlikely that a single mechanism is responsible for the disorder (see the proposed pathogenic model below).

Is there a model for TTH pathogenesis? Considering the heterogeneity of pathophysiologic abnormalities found in TTH, the following model can be proposed as a working hypothesis.[14] TTH may be the result of an interaction between changes of the descending control of second-order trigeminal brainstem nociceptors and interrelated peripheral changes, such as myofascial pain sensitivity and strain in pericranial muscles. An acute episode of ETTH may occur in many individuals who are otherwise perfectly normal. It can be brought on by physical stress, usually combined with psychological stress or nonphysiologic working positions. In such cases, increased nociception from strained muscles may be the primary cause of the headache, possibly favored by a central temporary change in pain control owing to stress. Emotional mechanisms increase muscle tension via the limbic system and, at the same time, reduce tone in the endogenous antinociceptive system. With more frequent episodes of headache, central changes become increasingly more important. Long-term potentiation and sensitization of nociceptive neurons and decreased activity in the antinociceptive system gradually lead to CTTH. These central changes probably predominate in frequent TTH and in CTTH. The relative importance of peripheral and central factors may, however, vary between patients and over time in the same patient.

The complex interrelation between various pathophysiologic aspects in TTH may explain why this disorder is so difficult to treat. It certainly suggests that various therapeutic approaches should be used in sequence or in combination. In the future, specific trials could be designed to determine whether the relative importance of peripheral and central mechanisms in individual patients might be relevant for the therapeutic choice. Management of TTH should try by all means to prevent chronification.

## TREATMENT

### Acute Treatment

Acute therapy in CTTH should be avoided owing to its potential for causing medication-overuse headache. We found no randomized controlled trial in dedicated literature but found 1 nonsystematic review of 29 observational studies (2,612 people),[15] which maintained that frequent analgesic use (two to three times/week) in people with episodic headache was associated with chronic headache and reduced effectiveness of prophylactic treatment. Many, but not all, people improved over 1 to 6 months following withdrawal of the acute relief medication (73% of 1,101 people, not all of whom had CTTH).

### Prophylactic Pharmacotherapy

The tricyclic antidepressants are the most widely used first-line therapeutic agents for CTTH. Surprisingly, few controlled studies have been performed, and not all of them found an efficacy superior to placebo (Table 5–4). The drawbacks of these studies are small patient numbers, inadequate efficacy parameters, or short duration. Only a few of them can be considered adequate according to the IHS guidelines. One major problem that arises with trials showing statistical differences between placebo and tricyclics is to evaluate whether the observed effect is clinically relevant. In one study, a reduction in average daily headache duration was selected as the primary efficacy parameter.[16] Amitriptyline reduced daily headache duration from 11.1 hours per day to 7.9 hours per day by an average of 3.2 hours. This effect was significantly different from placebo, but the clinical significance of such a reduction is questionable. Nonetheless, in clinical practice, tricyclic antidepressants remain the most useful prophylactic drugs for CTTH or frequent ETTH. Amitriptyline is the most frequently used; clomipramine may be slightly superior but has more side effects. Nortriptyline has fewer side effects. Other antidepressants, such as doxepin, maprotiline, or mianserin, can be used as a second choice.

The initial dosage of tricyclics should be low: 10 to 25 mg of amitriptyline or clomipramine at bedtime. Many patients will be satisfied by such a low dose. The average dose of amitriptyline in CTTH, however, is 75 to 100 mg/d.[17] If a patient is insufficiently improved on this dose, a trial of higher doses of amitriptyline or clomipramine is warranted. If the headache is improved by at least 80% after 4 months, it is reasonable to attempt discontinuation of the medication. Decreasing the daily dose by 20 to 25% every 2 to 3 days may avoid rebound headache.

The mechanism of action of antidepressants in CTTH remains to be determined. Their effect on the headache may be partly independent from their antidepressant effect. Tricyclics have a variety of pharmacologic activities. Serotonin increase by inhibition of its reuptake, endorphin release, or inhibition of N-methyl-D-aspartate receptors, which play a role in pain transmission, may all be relevant for the pathophysiology of TTH.

The more recent generation of antidepressants blocking selectively the reuptake of serotonin (eg, fluoxetine) have not yet been proven to be effective in TTH prophylaxis. Paroxetine (20–30 mg daily), for

**Table 5–4**  Controlled studies of prophylactic pharmacotherapies for tension-type headache.

| References | Drugs tested | No. of subjects | Results | Significance |
|---|---|---|---|---|
| Lance JW, et al. Lancet 1964; 1:1236-1239. | **Amitriptyline** (75 mg/d) Placebo | 27 | > 50% improved 56% 11% | p= 0.01 |
| Diamond S, et al. Headache 1971;11:110-116. | Placebo **Amitriptyline 10** mg (up to 6/day) **Amitriptyline 25** mg (up to 6/day) | 29 28 28 | improvement in headache intensity 33% 54% 38% | p= 0.05 |
| Morland TJ, et al. Headache 1979;19:382-383. | **Doxepin** Placebo | 23 | Headache days decreased 15% by doxepin compared to placebo | p= 0.05 |
| Fogelholm R, et al. *Headache* 1985;25:273-275. | **Maprotiline** (75 mg/day) Placebo | 30 | Headache intensity diminished by 25% and headache free days increased by 40% on Maprotiline | p = 0.001 |
| Langemark M, et al. Headache 1990;30:118-121. | Placebo **Clomipramine** **Mianserine** | 36 28 28 | % intensity improvement (day 43) 49% 57% 54% | Non-significant |
| Pfaffenrath V, et al. Cephalalgia 1991; 11 215-228. | Placebo **Amitriptyline** (50-75 mg/d) **Amitriptylinoxide** (60-90 mg/d) | 64 67 66 | 50% reduction in duration x frequency and in intensity 21.9% 22.4% 30.3% | Non-significant |
| Göbel H, et al. In: Olesen J, Schoenen J (eds). Tension-type headache : classification, mechanisms and treatment. New York: Raven Press, 1993, 275-280. | Placebo **Amitriptyline** (75 mg/d) | 29 24 | Change in mean daily duration -0.28 h -3.2 h | p = 0.001 |
| Bendtsen L, et al. J Neurol Neurosurg Psychiatry. 1996; 61:285-290. | Triple cross-over trial Placebo **Citalopram** (20mg/d) **Amitriptyline** (75mg/d) | 34 | Decrease in AUC (durationxintensity) per 4 weeks 10% 23% 37% | Non-significant p= 0.02 |
| Fogelholm R, et al. Headache 1992;32:509-13. | **Tizanidine** (6-18mg/d) Placebo | | % headache-free days/6 weeks 54.9% 43.7% | p= 0.05 |
| Smuts JA, et al. Eur J Neurol 1999;6:S99-S102. | **Botulinum toxin A** (12 inj; 100U) Isotonic saline | 22 15 | Gain of headache-free days at 3 mths 6 1 | p= 0.05 |
| Rollnik JD, et al. Headache 2000;40:300-305. | **Botulinum toxin A** (10inj of 20U) Isotonic saline | 11 10 | Decrease in pain intensity at 3 mths 12% 23% | Non-significant |

instance, was less effective than sulpiride (200–400 mg daily) in one explanatory crossover study.[18] In another study, it was not useful in CTTH patients who had not responded to tricyclic antidepressants.[19] Citalopram was not superior to placebo in the trial published by Bendtsen and colleagues (see Table 5–4), in which superiority was found for amitriptyline.[20] In clinical practice, selective serotonin reuptake inhibitors may sometimes be tried in subgroups of patients who do not tolerate tricyclics or are overweight.

Tizanidine (6–18 mg/d), the antispastic drug, was just superior to placebo in one crossover trial,[21] but this effect does not seem to be clinically useful in most patients (see Table 5–4).

In recent years, botulinum toxin has been popularized in chronic headache treatment, especially in North America. The enthusiasm manifested by some for this treatment contrasts with the lack of scientific evidence for its use in headache disorders.[22] In CTTH, botulinum toxin A was found superior to isotonic saline in only one small trial (Smuts and colleagues[23]; see Table 5–4), an effect that was not reproduced in the study by Rollnik and colleagues.[24] The large European multicenter trial that was performed after these ambiguous findings with botulinum toxin was not able to show the superiority of the toxin over isotonic saline, but its results are still not published for commercial reasons.

## Nonpharmacologic Treatments

### Psychological and Behavioral Techniques

There is solid scientific support for the usefulness of relaxation and electromyographic (EMG) biofeedback therapies in the management of TTH. Across studies, relaxation training, EMG biofeedback training, and their combination have each yielded a near 50% reduction in headache activity. Improvements are similar for each treatment modality but significantly greater than those observed in untreated patients or patients with false or noncontingent biofeedback.[25] Nonetheless, these treatments do not seem to be interchangeable because some patients who fail to respond to relaxation training may benefit from subsequent EMG biofeedback training.

Cognitive behavioral interventions, such as stress management programs, alone can effectively reduce TTH activity, but they seem to be most useful when added to biofeedback or relaxation therapies in patients with higher levels of daily hassles.

Limited contact treatment based on the patient's guidance at home by audiotapes and written materials with only three or four monthly clinical sessions may be a cost-effective alternative to fully therapist-administered treatment in many patients. Despite this alternative, behavioral therapies are time-consuming for patients and therapists. Although there is no infal-

lible means of predicting treatment outcome, a number of factors have been identified that may have some predictive value. In one study, relaxation producing at least a 50% reduction of EMG activity at the fourth session was predictive of an excellent outcome.[26] Excessive analgesic or ergotamine use limits the therapeutic benefits. Patients with continuous headache are less responsive to relaxation or biofeedback therapies, and patients with elevated scores on psychological tests that assess depression or psychiatric disturbance have done poorly with behavioral treatment in some studies.[27]

Behavioral treatment may produce improvement more slowly than pharmacologic treatment, but improvement is maintained for long periods, up to several years, without monthly burst sessions or contact with the therapist.

It was demonstrated in one study that the combination of stress management therapy and amitriptyline (up to 100 mg/d) or nortriptyline (up to 75 mg/d) was more effective in CTTH than either behavioral or drug treatment alone.[28] There was a reduction in headache index scores of at least 50% in 64% of patients with the combination as opposed to 38% of patients for the tricyclics, 35% for stress management, and 29% for placebo.

### Other Nonpharmacologic Treatments

Various techniques of physical therapy are employed in the treatment of TTH and include positioning, ergonomic instruction, massage, transcutaneous electrical nerve stimulation, heat or cold application, and manipulations. None of these techniques have been proven to be effective in the long term. Physical treatment, such as massage, may be useful for acute episodes of TTH. In the long term, it reduced headache intensity, on average, only by 23% in one study, which was nonetheless superior to acupuncture given as a comparator treatment.[29] More recently, a physical treatment program was found to have some effect in CTTH but not ETTH in a controlled study.[30] The program, however, combined various techniques, such as massage, relaxation, and home-based exercises, and the effect was rather modest. The beneficial effect in this study was 32% on headache days per month, and only 29% of CTTH sufferers were considered to be responders.

Oromandibular treatment may be helpful in selected TTH patients. Unfortunately, most studies claiming efficacy of treatment, such as occlusal splints, therapeutic exercises for masticatory muscles, or occlusal adjustment, are uncontrolled. In one single trial comparing occlusal equilibration or placebo equilibration in 56 TTH patients, the headache frequency was reduced in 80% and the intensity in 47% of patients in the active group compared with 50% and 16% in the placebo group.[31] In another study, headache frequency decreased in 56% of patients treated with occlusal stabilization splints compared with 32% in patients receiving neurologic treatments.[32] Considering the large number of headache-free subjects who display signs and symptoms of oromandibular dysfunction,[33] caution should be taken not to advocate irreversible dental treatments in TTH. A minority of selected patients may, however, benefit from oromandibular treatment.

## CONCLUSION

There is little scientific evidence to guide the selection of treatment modalities in TTH. The best treatment is often found by trial and error. Because the success rates with the different therapeutic strategies (pharmacologic, nonpharmacologic) appear to be very similar, it is of little surprise that the likelihood of dental treatment is much higher if patients see a dentist, that of behavior therapy is higher if they see a psychologist, and that of pharmacologic treatment is higher if they consult a neurologist. This situation is unfortunate because the multifactorial etiopathogenesis of TTH suggests that therapy should be tailored individually to each patient and that a combination of different therapeutic methods, such as the combination of pharmacologic and nonpharmacologic treatments, may yield better results than either treatment by itself. To prove this superior efficacy of combination therapies, multidisciplinary collaborations and large-scale comparative trials are needed.

## REFERENCES

1. Classification Committee, International Headache Society. Classification and diagnostic criteria for headache disorders, cranial neuralgias and facial pain. Cephalalgia 1988;8 Suppl 7:1–96.

2. Headache Classification Subcommittee, International Headache Society. The international classification of headache disorders, 2nd edition. Cephalalgia 2004;24 Suppl 1:1–160.

3. Bendtsen L, Jensen R, Olesen J. Qualitatively altered nociception in chronic myofascial pain. Pain 1996;65:259–64.

4. Jensen R. Mechanisms of spontaneous tension-type headaches: an analysis of tenderness, pain thresholds and EMG. Pain 1996;64:251–6.

5. Jensen K. Quantification of tenderness by palpation and use of pressure algometer. Adv Pain Res Ther 1990;17:165–81.

6. Jensen R, Rasmussen BK, Pedersen B, Olesen J. Muscle tenderness and pressure pain thresholds in headache. A population study. Pain 1993;52:193–9.

7. Schoenen J, Gerard P, De Pasqua V, Sianard-Gainko J. Multiple clinical and paraclinical analyses of chronic tension-type headache associated or unassociated with disorder of pericranial muscles. Cephalalgia 1991;11:135–9.

8. Rasmussen BK, Jensen R, Schroll M, Olesen J. Epidemiology of tension-type headache in a general population. In: Olesen J, Schoenen J, editors. Tension-type headache: classification, mechanisms and treatment. New York: Raven Press; 1993. p. 9–13.

9. Schwartz BS, Stewart WF, Simon D, Lipton RB. Epidemiology of tension-type headache. JAMA 1998;279:381–3.

10. Rokicki LA, Semenchuk EM, Bruehl S, et al. An examination of the validity of the IHS classification system for migraine and tension-type headache in the college student population. Headache 1999;39:720–7.

11. Rasmussen BK, Jenser R, Olesen J. Impact of headache on sickness absence and utilisation of medical services: a Danish population study. J Epidemiol Health 1992;46:443–6.

12. Holroyd KA, Stensland M, Lipchik GL, et al. Psychosocial correlates and impact of chronic tension-type headache. Headache 2000;40:3–16.

13. Östergaard S, Russell MB, Bendtsen L, Olesen J. Increased familial risk of chronic tension-type headache. BMJ 1997;314:1092–3.

14. Olesen J, Schoenen J. Tension-type headache, cluster headache, and miscellaneous headaches. Synthesis of tension-type headache mechanisms. In: Olesen J, Tfelt-Hansen P, Welch KMA, editors. The headaches. 2nd ed. New York: Lippincott Williams & Wilkins; 1999. p. 615–8.

15. Diener H-C, Tfelt-Hansen P. Headache associated with chronic use of substances. In: Olesen J, Tfelt-Hansen P, Welch KMA, editors. The headaches. New York: Raven Press; 1993. p. 721–7.

16. Göbel H, Hamouz V, Hansen C, et al. Effect of amitriptyline prophylaxis on headache symptoms and neurophysiological parameters in tension-type headache. In: Olesen J, Schoenen J, editors. Tension-type headache: classification, mechanisms and treatment. New York: Raven Press; 1993. p. 275–80.

17. Couch JR, Micieli G. Tension-type headache, cluster headache, and miscellaneous headaches: prophylactic pharmacotherapy. In: Olesen J, Tfelt-Hansen P, Welch KMA, editors. The headaches. New York: Raven Press; 1993. p. 537–42.

18. Langemark M, Olesen J. Sulpiride and paroxetine in the treatment of chronic tension-type headache. An explanatory double-blind trial. Headache 1994;34:20–4.

19. Holroyd KA, Labus JS, O'Donnell FJ, Cordingley G. Treating tension-type headache not responding to amitriptyline hydrochloride with paroxetine hydrochloride: evaluation. Headache 2003;43:999–1004.

20. Bendtsen L, Jensen R, Olesen J. A non-selective (amitriptyline), but not a selective (citalopram), serotonin reuptake inhibitor is effective in the prophylactic treatment of chronic tension-type headache. J Neurol Neurosurg Psychiatry 1996;61:285–90.

21. Fogelholm R, Murros K. Tizanidine in chronic tension-type headache: a placebo controlled double-blind crossover study. Headache 1992;32:509–13.

22. Evers S, Rahmann A, Vollmer-Haase J, Husstedt IW. Treatment of headache with botulinum toxin A—a review according to evidence-based medicine criteria. Cephalalgia 2002;22:699–710.

23. Smuts JA, Baker MK, Smuts HM, et al. Prophylactic treatment of chronic tension-type headache using botulinum toxin type A. Eur J Neurol 1999;6 Suppl 4:S99–102.

24. Rollnik JD, Tanneberger O, Schubert M, et al. Treatment of tension-type headache with botulinum toxin type A: a double-blind, placebo-controlled study. Headache 2000;40:300–5.

25. Holroyd KA, Penzien DB. Client variables and behavioral treatment of recurrent tension headaches: a meta-analytic review. J Behav Med 1986;9:515–36.

26. Schoenen J, Pholien P, Maertens de Noordhout A. EMG biofeedback in tension-type headache: is the 4th session predictive of outcome? Cephalalgia 1985;5:132–3.

27. Holroyd KA. Tension-type headache, cluster headache, and miscellaneous headaches: psychological and behavioral techniques. In: Olesen J, Tfelt-Hansen P, Welch KMA, editors. The headaches. New York: Raven Press; 1993. p. 515–20.

28. Holroyd KA, O'Donnell FJ, Stensland M, et al. Management of chronic tension-type headache with tricyclic antidepressant medication, stress management, and their combination: a randomized controlled trial. JAMA 2001;285:2208–15.

29. Carlsson J, Fahlcrantz A, Augustinsson L-E. Muscle tenderness in tension headache treated with acupuncture or physiotherapy. Cephalalgia 1990;10:131–41.

30. Torelli P, Jensen R, Olesen J. Physiotherapy for tension-type headache: a controlled study. Cephalalgia 2004;24:29–37.

31. Forsell H, Kirveskari P, Kangasniemi P. Changes in headache after treatment of mandibular dysfunction. Cephalalgia 1985;5:229–36.

32. Schokker RP, Hansson TL, Ansink BJ. The results of treatment of the masticatory system of chronic headache patients. J Craniomandib Disord Facial Oral Pain 1990;4:126–30.

33. Jensen R, Rasmussen BK, Pedersen B, et al. Oromandibular disorders in a general population. J Craniomandib Disorders Facial Oral Pain 1993;7:175–82.

# CHAPTER 6

# Chronic Cluster Headache

David W. Dodick, MD, FRCPC, FACP

Cluster headache is an uncommon yet well-defined primary neurovascular headache syndrome occurring in both episodic and chronic forms. Chronic cluster headache (CCH) is a rare condition; approximately 20% of cluster headache sufferers experience recurrent attacks without periods of significant remission.[1] The International Headache Society developed operational diagnostic criteria for cluster headache, distinguishing it from migraine and other primary headache disorders (Table 6–1).[2]

CCH may be unremitting from onset or evolve from episodic cluster headache (ECH). The evolution to CCH has been reported to occur in 3.8 to 12.9% of ECH sufferers.[3–5] The mean age at onset of CCH is approximately 30 years compared with 26 years for ECH.[6] Several studies have reported a tendency for CCH patients to develop cluster headache at an older age. This appears to be especially true for women and for those who develop CCH from onset.[6–9] Interestingly, women have been reported to experience a more rapid evolution of ECH into the chronic stage.[6] Other factors that have been reported to be predictive of this evolution from ECH to CCH include a high frequency of cluster periods, the presence of sporadic attacks, cluster periods lasting more than 8 weeks, especially in men, remission periods lasting less than 6 months, and the presence of four to eight accompanying symptoms.[6,7] It has also been reported that patients with CCH behave differently from patients with ECH in the extent to which they indulge in nonessential consumption habits, such as smoking and alcohol consumption.[6,10–15] These factors, in addition to the higher prevalence of head injury in patients with CCH, may play a role in worsening the clinical prognosis of ECH.[6,16,17] Once CCH has developed, whether de novo or after evolution from the episodic form, it may persist for years, even into old age, although long-term follow-up has shown that up to 50% of affected individuals eventually revert to or switch to an episodic form.[4,5]

## CLINICAL FEATURES

In large samples of cluster headache patients who were carefully evaluated clinically, few clinical differences were observed between ECH and CCH and between males and females. Cluster headache is characterized by strictly unilateral first division trigeminal pain, which is predominantly retro-orbital and temporal. There are accompanying ipsilateral autonomic features characterized by cranial parasympathetic activation and sympathetic hypofunction (see Table 6–1). The most common associated features are lacrimation (90%), conjunctival injection (77%), nasal congestion (75%), rhinorrhea (72%), and ptosis (74%). Motor restlessness and agitation are also highly diagnostic features of this disorder.[18] However, the sine qua non of the syndrome is its periodicity with a cyclic pattern of discrete and relatively short-lived attacks. The attacks generally last 60 to 180 minutes and occur from one to eight times daily. In patients with ECH, attacks occur during discrete bouts lasting approximately 2 months each year.

## DIFFERENTIAL DIAGNOSIS

Although cluster headache is clinically very distinctive, the mean time to diagnosis, although improving over the past few decades, is still approximately 2.6 years, and a mean of three primary care physicians are seen before a diagnosis is made.[18] Unfortunately, this diagnostic delay results in a substantial proportion of cluster headache sufferers (40%) experiencing a delay in effective therapy and unnecessary invasive procedures. Early neurologic referral is therefore important in patients with a suspected diagnosis of cluster headache so that management can be optimized and unnecessary procedures avoided.

**Table 6–1**   International Headache Society Criteria for Cluster Headache

3.1 Cluster headache

   A.  At least 5 attacks fulfilling criteria B–D.

   B.  Severe, unilateral, orbital, supraorbital, and/or temporal pain lasting 15–180 min untreated

   C.  Headache is associated with at least 1 of the following:

       1.   Ipsilateral conjunctival injection and/or lacrimation

       2.   Ipsilateral nasal congestion and/or rhinorrhea

       3.   Ipsilateral eyelid edema

       4.   Ipsilateral forehead and facial sweating

       5.   Ipsilateral miosis and/or ptosis

       6.   A sense of restlessness or agitation

   D.  Attacks have a frequency of 1 every other day to 8 per day

   E.  Not attributed to another disorder

3.1.1 Episodic cluster headache

   A.  Attacks fulfilling criteria A–E for 3.1 cluster headache

   B.  At least 2 cluster periods lasting 7–365 d and separated by pain-free remission periods of ≥ 1 mo

3.1.2 Chronic cluster headache

   A.  Attacks fulfilling criteria A–E for 3.1 cluster headache

   B.  Attacks recur over > 1 yr without remission periods or with remission periods lasting < 1 mo

Dentists and ENT physicians are the most frequently consulted specialists, prior to neurologists, because of a mistaken diagnosis of sinus headache or dental pathology. The short-lasting discrete attacks that recur daily and lack the systemic and clinical features of infection make differentiating between cluster headache and acute infectious rhinosinusitis quite straightforward. Other possibilities should be considered in the differential diagnosis. Migraine may present with recurrent unilateral headache associated with ipsilateral autonomic symptoms, particularly during severe attacks. However, the periodicity of cluster headache is often stereotyped for a given patient, and the attacks of cluster headache are short-lived (45 to 90 minutes), often nocturnal, exclusively unilateral, and associated with restlessnes, agitation, and more robust cranial autonomic symptoms and signs. Furthermore, cluster attacks may and often do recur several times per day and are usually not associated with aura, nausea, vomiting, or photophobia.

Trigeminal neuralgia is characterized by paroxysmal electric shock-like jabs of unilateral pain lasting seconds, often triggered by stimulation of limited areas of facial skin or oral mucosa, and, unlike cluster headache, is not associated with significant cranial autonomic features and is most commonly limited to the distribution of the second and/or third divisions of the trigeminal nerve. Other disorders to be considered are dissection of the cervicocephalic arteries (carotid or vertebral), giant cell arteritis, glaucoma, intracranial aneurysms, tumors or arteriovenous malformations, and even cervical cord lesions (meningioma) or infarction. In most of these instances, however, the history and examination disclose features that are worrisome for a secondary cause, the history lacks the typical stereotyped circadian or circannual rhythmicity of cluster attacks, or the response to conventional medications used to treat cluster headache is lacking.[19]

Finally, there are a number of primary headache syndromes that may closely resemble cluster headache, such as chronic paroxysmal hemicrania and SUNCT syndrome (short-lasting, unilateral, neuralgiform headache with conjunctival infection and tearing) (Table 6–2). Collectively, these disorders have been referred to as trigeminal autonomic cephalgias because of the trigeminal distribution of pain and the associated autonomic signs.[20] Like cluster headache, they are characterized by discrete, short-lasting, episodic attacks of intense, unilateral, orbitotemporal headache associated with prominent ipsilateral autonomic signs. These

**Table 6–2** Trigeminal Autonomic Cephalgias

| Feature | Cluster | CPH | SUNCT |
|---|---|---|---|
| Gender, M:F | 4:1 | 1:3 | 4:1 |
| Attack duration | 15–180 min | 2–45 min | 5–250 s |
| Attack frequency | 1–8/d | 1–40/d | 1/d to 30/h |
| Autonomic features | ++ | ++ | ++ |
| Alcohol ppt | ++ | + | + |
| Indomethacin effect | - | ++ | - |

CPH = chronic paroxysmal hemicrania; SUNCT = short-lasting, unilateral, neuralgiform headache with conjunctival infection and tearing.

syndromes may also be precipitated by alcohol and associated with nocturnal attacks. However, these disorders differ from cluster headache mainly in the higher frequency and shorter duration of individual attacks, with an almost inverse relationship across these disorders as the attack frequency increases, the attack duration tends to decrease.[21] The distinction between cluster headache and other paroxysmal hemicranias is important because of the differential response to therapy. The paroxysmal hemicranias and hemicrania continua often respond in a dramatic fashion to indomethacin, whereas patients with SUNCT syndrome derive no benefit from indomethacin or the drugs typically used to treat cluster headache, and are more likely to respond to newer anticonvulsants, such as lamotrigine, gabapentin, or topiramate.[22]

## PATHOGENESIS

A unifying pathophysiologic explanation of cluster headache must account for the three major features of the syndrome: the trigeminal distribution of pain, the ipsilateral autonomic features, and the tendency for attacks to cluster with striking circadian and circannual consistency, which is the signature feature of cluster headache.

### Pain and Autonomic Features

In humans, evidence for activation of the trigeminovascular system in cluster headache has been highlighted by a marked increase in the level of calcitonin gene–related peptide in the cranial venous circulation during attacks of cluster headache.[23,24] In addition, evidence of parasympathetic activation in humans has been corroborated by the finding of significantly elevated levels of vasoactive intestinal polypeptide during attacks in which ipsilateral autonomic features are robust.[23,24] These findings support the integral involvement of the trigeminovascular and cranial parasympathetic systems in cluster headache and provide the anatomic and physiologic basis for the expression of first division trigeminal pain and ipsilateral autonomic symptoms, which occur during cluster attacks.

### Periodicity

The signature feature of cluster headache is the circadian and circannual periodicity of the disorder. This distinctive periodicity has strongly implicated a disturbance in the biologic clock or pacemaker, which, in humans, is located in the hypothalamic gray matter in an area known as the suprachiasmatic nucleus. Hypothalamic regulation of the endocrine system involves rhythmic and phasic modulation of the hypophyseal hormones and melatonin to maintain homeostasis. Substantially lowered concentrations of plasma testosterone during cluster headache periods in men provided the first evidence of hypothalamic involvement in the pathogenesis of cluster headache. This finding was followed by reports of alterations in the production of a wide range of secretory circadian rhythms involving luteinizing hormone, cortisol, and prolactin, as well as altered responses in the production of cortisol, luteinizing hormone, follicle-stimulating hormone, prolactin, growth hormone, and thyroid-stimulating hormone to diverse challenges in cluster headache.[25]

Melatonin is the most sensitive surrogate marker of circadian function in humans, and its rhythmic secretion is under the control of the suprachiasmatic nucleus.[26] The principal environmental stimulus for the entrainment and rhythmic secretion of melatonin is light intensity. Photic information reaches the suprachiasmatic nucleus from a direct retinal-hypophyseal pathway. In humans, the circadian rhythm for the release of melatonin from the pineal gland is closely synchronized with the habitual hours of sleep. Therefore, melatonin levels are normally low during the day and increase during the hours of darkness and sleep. In patients with cluster headache, the 24-hour production of melatonin is reduced, the nocturnal peak in melatonin concentration is blunted during cluster periods, and the acrophase (the time from midnight to the moment of peak hormone level) is moved forward.[27] Pain-induced stress cannot explain this decrease because stress causes a release in endogenous norepinephrine, which is known to increase melatonin production.

The most direct and convincing evidence for the role of the hypothalamus in the pathogenesis of cluster headache has come from functional and morphometric neuroimaging. Using positron emission tomography (PET) to detect areas of functional activation, marked activation in the ipsilateral ventral hypothalamic gray matter during attacks of acute cluster headache induced by nitroglycerin has been demonstrated.[28] This finding appears to be specific for cluster headache and perhaps other related trigeminal autonomic cephalgias because the same pattern of activation in this region of the hypothalamus has been demonstrated in a patient with SUNCT syndrome.[29] This pattern of activation has not been seen during attacks of migraine or experimentally induced ophthalmic (first division) pain after capsaicin injection into the forehead of control subjects.[30]

In addition, a voxel-based morphometric analysis of the structural $T_1$-weighted magnetic resonance images (MRIs) of 25 right-handed patients with cluster headache revealed a significant difference in hypothalamic gray matter density between these patients and 29 right-handed healthy male volunteers.[31] This difference consisted of an increase in volume and was present for the entire cohort. This structural difference was bilateral in the diencephalon, coinciding with the inferior posterior hypothalamus. In terms of the stereotaxic coordinates, it was almost identical to the area of activation seen during an acute cluster headache attack with PET. The colocalization of morphologic and functional changes within a discrete hypothalamic region may identify the precise anatomic location for the central nervous system "generator" of cluster headache and explains the circadian signature of this syndrome. The demonstration that continuous stimulation of this brain region can completely suppress attacks in patients with medically intractable CCH lends more credence to the hypothesis that the posterior hypothalamic gray matter is integral to the pathogenesis of cluster headache.

## MANAGEMENT

CCH is often a challenging disorder to treat effectively with preventive medications. The medications used to treat both ECH and CCH are similar, although certain medications and combinations may be more effective for CCH. The successful treatment of both ECH and CCH will require both acute (symptomatic) therapy and the daily use of preventive medications, which are designed to decrease the frequency of or completely eliminate attacks.

## ACUTE THERAPY

Because of the rapid onset and short time to peak pain intensity of cluster attacks, a fast-acting symptomatic therapy is imperative. Oxygen and subcutaneous sumatriptan provide the most rapid, effective, and reliable relief for attacks of cluster headache.

### Oxygen

Oxygen inhalation has been the standard of care for the symptomatic relief of cluster headache since it was introduced as an effective therapy in the 1950s. If delivered at the onset of an attack via a non-rebreathing facial mask at a flow rate of 10 to 12 L/min for 15 minutes, approximately 70% of patients will obtain relief within 15 minutes.[32] In some patients, flow rates up to 15 L/min may be necessary to achieve relief. In some patients, oxygen is most effective if taken when the pain is at maximal intensity, whereas in others, the attack is delayed for minutes to hours. Oxygen therapy has obvious practical limitations in that treatment is not always readily available, and although small portable cylinders are available for use at work or when out of the house, some patients find this to be cumbersome and inconvenient.

In a recent study evaluating hyperbaric oxygen (HBO) for the treatment of cluster headache, 16 patients (12 with ECH, 4 with CCH) were randomly selected to start with one of two different hyperbaric treatments in a double-blind, placebo-controlled, crossover study design.[33] Both gases were administered by a mask inside a multiplace hyperbaric chamber for 70 minutes at 250 kPa (2.5 ATA) in two sessions 24 hours apart. Active treatment was 100% oxygen (HBO treatment), whereas placebo treatment was 10% oxygen in nitrogen (hyperbaric normoxic placebo = sham treatment), corresponding to breathing air at sea level. HBO was found not to be effective in reducing the headache intensity or interrupting the cluster headache period when given in a well-established cluster period or in patients with CCH.

### Sumatriptan

Subcutaneous sumatriptan is the most effective self-administered medication for the symptomatic relief of cluster headache. In a placebo-controlled study, 6 mg of sumatriptan delivered subcutaneously was significantly more effective than placebo, with 74% of patients having complete relief by 15 minutes compared with 26% of patients treated with placebo.[34] In long-term open-label studies, sumatriptan is effective in 76 to 100% of all attacks within 15 minutes, with no evidence of tachyphylaxis or rebound even after repetitive daily use for several months.[35,36] However, sumatriptan is not effective when used before an expected attack in an attempt to prevent an oncoming attack, nor is it useful when used in a preventive fashion with scheduled daily dosages. The overall efficacy of sumatriptan has been reported to be slightly less in patients with CCH than in patients with ECH.[36] Although generally well tolerated, sumatriptan is contraindicated in patients with ischemic heart disease, variant angina, cerebrovascular and peripheral vascular disease, and uncontrolled hypertension. In this sense, caution must be exercised in patients with cluster headache because the disorder is more common in middle-aged males who often have other risk factors for cardiovascular disease, particularly tobacco abuse, which is present in up to 88% of cluster headache sufferers.

Sumatriptan nasal spray has also recently been demonstrated to be effective and well tolerated for the acute treatment of cluster headache attacks of at least 45 minutes duration.[37] In a double-blind, placebo-controlled, randomized trial involving 118 patients with ECH or CCH who treated 154 attacks of at least 45 minutes duration with 20 mg sumatriptan nasal spray, the responder rate at 30 minutes was 57% for sumatriptan and 26% for placebo ($p = .002$). Pain-free rates at 30 minutes were 47% for sumatriptan and 18% for placebo ($p = .003$). Sumatriptan was also superior to placebo, considering the initial response, in terms of meaningful relief and relief of associated symptoms. The nasal spray may offer a viable alternative for some patients, particularly those who are averse to self-injection or when subcutaneous administration is accompanied by intolerable side effects.

## Octrotide

Somatostain has been shown to inhibit the release of calcitoxin gene-related peptide and vasoactive intestinal polypeptide. Based on the results of two small randomized, double-blind trials that suggested efficacy of intravenous somatostatin in cluster headache[38,39] a recent randomized double-blind placebo-controlled crossover study evaluated the use of octrotide, a somatostatin analogue for the acute treatment of cluster headache.[40]

Patients were instructed to treat two attacks of at least moderate pain severity, with at least a 24-hour break, using subcutaneous octreotide 100 µg or matching placebo. The primary end point was the headache response defined as very severe, severe, or moderate pain becoming mild or none, at 30 minutes. A total of 57 patients were recruited of whom 46 provided efficacy data on attacks treated with octreotide and 45 with placebo. The headache response rate with subcutaneous octreotide was 52% compared to a placebo-response rate of 36% ($p < .01$). Octreotide was well tolerated with no reports of serious side effects. The main side effect observed was gastrointestinal upset in eight patients treated with octreotide compared with four patients treated with placebo. All side effects

resolved spontaneously and were generally short-lived and mild in nature.

## Dihydroergotamine

Dihydroergotamine (DHE) is available in the United States in injectable and intranasal formulations. DHE-45 administered intravenously provides prompt and effective relief of cluster headache within 15 minutes. The intramuscular and subcutaneous routes of administration provide slower relief because of the lower bioavailability and delayed absoprtion time. Because of the rapid peak intensity and relatively short duration of each cluster headache attack, DHE is a less attractive option than sumatriptan because of the necessity of having to get to an emergency department or physician's office to have an intravenous line placed. In addition, it is not a feasible long-term solution for these with CCH who experience daily attacks.

A double-blind crossover trial compared intranasal DHE (1 mg) with placebo and found no effect on headache frequency or duration, but the pain intensity was significantly reduced with DHE compared with placebo.[41] The effect, however, was not dramatic. It has been suggested that the dose used (1 mg) was lower than the recommended dose for migraine and less than what is currently available in commercial preparations of DHE nasal spray (2 mg). Therefore, DHE at a dose of 2 mg may be more effective than 1 mg, but this has not been studied in a controlled fashion.

## Zolmitriptan

Zolmitriptan is an effective oral agent for the acute treatment of migraine. Recently, a double-blind controlled trial compared the efficacy of 5 and 10 mg oral zolmitriptan with placebo for the treatment of acute cluster headache attacks in patients with ECH and CCH.[42] With headache response defined as a 2-point reduction on a 5-point pain intensity scale, at 30 minutes, response rates following placebo and 5 and 10 mg of zolmitriptan were 29%, 40%, and 47%, respectively. The difference reached statistical significance for 10 mg zolmitriptan compared with placebo. In addition, significantly more patients reported mild or no pain 30 minutes after treatment with 5 and 10 mg zolmitriptan (57% and 60%, respectively) than following placebo (42%).

Zolmitriptan nasal spray may prove to be a more useful alternative than the tablet in patients with cluster headache. The pharmacokinetics of zolmitriptan nasal spray are consistent with a fast onset of action; following intranasal administration, zolmitriptan is detected in the plasma at 2 minutes post-dose and in the brain at 5 minutes post-dose.[43–46] Intranasal absorption has been shown to account for approximately 70% of the total exposure to zolmitriptan in the first hour post-dose.[47] Correspondingly, in a recent single-blind observation trial involving five patients who treated 36 attacks of cluster headache with 5 mg zolmitriptan nasal spray, a pain-free response was observed in 27 of 36 attacks at 15 minutes.[48] Conclusive evidence for the efficacy and safety of zolmitriptan nasal spray will, however, await the results from a randomized placebo-controlled trial which is currently in progress.

## Lidocaine

Because cocainization of the sphenopalatine ganglion has been helpful in aborting cluster headache attacks, intranasal lidocaine has been used as an adjunctive therapy. However, in general, whether applied via a spray bottle or by dropping 4% viscous lidocaine in the nostril ipsilateral to the pain, this therapy achieves only a moderate reduction in pain in less than one-third of patients. Therefore, it may be useful as adjunctive but not as "stand-alone" therapy for relief of acute cluster attacks.

## PREVENTIVE PHARMACOTHERAPY

The importance of an effective preventive regimen, especially in patients with CCH, cannot be overstated. Patients have daily or near-daily attacks of cluster headache, which often occur daily, and at times up eight times per day. Treating frequent daily attacks with acute therapy alone may result in overmedication or toxicity and unnecessarily prolong the misery of having to suffer repeated attacks every day. Furthermore, acute therapies may be contraindicated, ineffective, not tolerated or may simply delay the attack.

The primary goals of preventive therapy are to produce a rapid suppression of attacks and to maintain the patient in remission. Secondary objectives are to reduce the headache frequency, as well as attack severity and duration. To achieve these primary goals, preventive therapy can best be thought of in terms of transitional and maintenance prophylaxis (Table 6–3).

## TRANSITIONAL PROPHYLAXIS

### Ergotamine

Both ergotamine tartrate (2 mg) and DHE-45 (1 mg) are effective agents for achieving rapid suppression of attacks when administered daily for a short period of time. Patients often tolerate these medications for a period of 2 to 3 weeks, and there appears to be less risk of medication-overuse (rebound) headache in this group of patients. Ergotamine tartrate is more convenient because of its oral route of administration and may be particularly useful when given 1 to 2 hours prior to bedtime for attacks that occur predominantly or exclusively during sleep. Both agents may also be administered in divided daily doses (not to exceed 4 mg ergotamine

| Table 6–3   Preventive Treatment for Cluster Headache |
|---|
| Transitional |
|   Prednisone 60 mg daily for 3 d, then 10 mg decrements every 3 d (18 d) |
|   Ergotamine tartrate 1–2 mg orally/suppository daily (hs or divided dosage) |
|   DHE-45 0.5–1.0 mg subcutaneously/intramuscularly every 8–12 h |
|   Occipital nerve blockade (eg, 3–5 cc 0.5% bupivicaine + 10–20 mg methylprednisolone) |
| Maintenance |
|   1st-line    Verapamil 80 mg tid or 240 sustained release; up to 720 mg/d |
|   2nd-line |
|        Valproic acid 500–2,000 mg/d in divided dosages |
|        Topiramate 50–200 mg in divided daily dosages |
|        Gabapentin 300 – 3600 mg three divided daily dosages |
|   3rd-line |
|        Methysergide 2 mg tid; up to 12 mg/d |
|        Lithium carbonate 150–300 mg tid or 450 mg sustained release |
| Adjunctive |
|   Melatonin 10 mg orally daily |

DHE = dihydroergotamine.

tartrate or 3 mg DHE) when attacks are multiple or occur throughout the day. Both agents are contraindicated in patients with peripheral vascular disease, coronary artery disease, uncontrolled hypertension, and during pregnancy. They should not be used for the duration of the cluster period and are not intended for long-term preventive use. They also limit the long-term preventive and acute options available because their use is contraindicated within 24 hours of using sumatriptan, and they are generally not administered concomitantly with methysergide because of the risk of potentiating the vasoconstrictive effects of each drug.

In a recent report, 63 patients with either ECH or CCH underwent 97 outpatient treatment sessions consisting of 3 consecutive days with combined intravenous and subcutaneous or intranasal administration of DHE.[49] At 1 month, for the treatment of ECH, there was complete resolution in 44 (73%) of 60 cases, partial resolution in 9 cases (13%), and failure in 7 cases (12%). For treatment of CCH, there was complete resolution in 17 (46%) of the 37 cases, partial resolution in 4 cases (11%), and 16 failures (43%). The authors concluded that outpatient intravenous DHE is a useful treatment for refractory cluster headache, more effective for ECH, and has a rapid onset of action. It did not change the evolution of the episodic form, but of the 17 patients with CCH to achieve complete suppression of attacks at 1 month, 3 patients reverted to an episodic pattern.

### Corticosteroids

Corticosteroids (prednisone and dexamethasone) are the most rapid-acting of the prophylactic agents. They represent a very effective initial preventive option to rapidly suppress attacks during the time required for the longer-acting maintenance prophylactic agents to take effect because the maximum benefit from other preventive drugs may not be realized until 2 weeks after treatment is begun. Although the data are limited and uncontrolled, the largest open-label study reported marked relief of cluster headache in 77% of 77 patients with ECH and partial relief in another 12% of patients treated with prednisone.[50] Treatment is usually initiated with 60 mg/d for 3 days followed by 10 mg decrements every 3 days over an 18-day period.

Prednisone is useful primarily for inducing a rapid remission in patients with ECH, and although it may provide a brief respite for patients with CCH, its long-term use in these patients is generally discouraged.

### Greater Occipital Nerve Blockade

Several open-label studies have suggested that corticosteroid injection in the greater occipital nerve region may be an effective short-term treatment option for patients with cluster headache. In a recent double-blind placebo-controlled study involving 23 patients with ECH and 7 patients with CCH, 92% of patients who received an injection of betamethasone 9.06 mg/dL and 0.3 mL 2% xylocaine in the region of the greater occipital nerve on the side ipsilateral to the pain experienced at least a 50% reduction in attack frequency in the first postinjection week compared with the preinjection week, whereas only 1 patient in the placebo group had a similar improvement ($p = .0004$).[51] Four weeks after the injection, 9 patients who received the corticosteroid injection, including 3 patients with CCH, were attack free, without any other preventive therapies. The authors concluded that a single suboccipital corticosteroid injection significantly suppresses attacks in ECH and CCH, inducing a temporary remission in 70% of patients.

## MAINTENANCE PROPHYLAXIS

Maintenance prophylaxis refers to the use of preventive medications throughout the anticipated duration of the cluster period. For those with CCH, preventive treatment is used for an indefinite period of time or until the patient has been in remission without attacks for 6 months. Preventive medications are often used in conjunction with a transitional agent and are usually used in combinations, especially in patients with CCH. It is worth noting that the preventive treatment of cluster headache is largely based on clinical experience, and few randomized controlled clinical trials have been performed. The following is a brief review of the currently accepted preventive treatments for cluster headache based on open and controlled studies.

### Verapamil

Verapamil is the preventive therapy of choice in both ECH and CCH. It is generally well tolerated and can be used safely in conjunction with sumatriptan, ergotamine, corticosteroids, and other preventive agents. A double-blind placebo-controlled trial evaluated the efficacy of verapamil 360 mg (three divided dosages) over a 14-day period in 26 patients with ECH. A statistically significant reduction in headache frequency and analgesic consumption was seen in the verapamil-treated patients, with a greater reduction in the second week of treatment.[52]

The initial starting daily dosage is usually 80 mg three times daily or 240 mg sustained release per day. The dosages employed range from 240 to 720 mg/d in divided dosages. Both the regular and extended-release preparations have been shown to be useful, but no direct comparative trials are available. Delayed-release verapamil at dosages up to 720 mg may be effective in cases of refractory cluster headache. Because of this apparent dose-response relationship, a total daily dosage of between 480 and 720 mg is recommended before the medication is deemed a failure. Constipation is the most common side effect, but dizziness, edema, nausea, fatigue, hypotension, and bradycardia may also occur. Electrocardiography (ECG) should be performed on all patients prior to starting therapy to determine whether there is evidence of atrioventricular conduction delay or block and to serve as a baseline against which follow-up ECGs can be compared if and when the dosage is escalated.

## Lithium Carbonate

Although the beneficial results of lithium carbonate therapy for cluster headache prevention have been derived mainly from open clinical trials, this drug has and continues to be used as an effective agent for cluster headache prevention. Collectively, in over 28 clinical trials involving 468 patients, good to excellent results were found in 78% of 304 patients with CCH.[53] The efficacy of lithium in patients with CCH also appears to be durable up to 4 years after treatment. On interruption or cessation of therapy with lithium in this group, a transition from CCH to ECH has been recognized.[53] Although somewhat less robust than the response in patients with CCH, lithium has been shown to induce a remission in 63% of 164 patients with ECH.[53] A double-blind crossover study comparing verapamil (360 mg daily) and lithium (900 mg daily) in 30 patients claimed equal efficacy for the two drugs.[54] On the other hand, a single double-blind placebo-controlled trial failed to show the superiority of lithium (800 mg sustained release) over placebo.[55] However, this study was terminated 1 week after treatment began, and there was an unexpectedly high placebo response rate of 31%. The treatment period was therefore too short to be conclusive.

The initial starting daily dosage is either 300 mg three times daily or 450 mg sustained release. Again, trials comparing the two formulations are not available, but a long half-life affords the option of a once-daily dose regimen, which is simpler and may enhance compliance.

Lithium is often effective at serum concentrations (0.4 to 0.8 mEq/L) less than that usually required for the treatment of bipolar disorder. Most patients will benefit from doses between 600 and 900 mg/d.

Lithium has the potential for many side effects and has a narrow therapeutic window. The serum concentration should be measured 12 hours after the last dose and should not exceed more than 1.0 mEq/L. Renal and thyroid function must be measured prior to and during treatment; side effects, such as tremor, diarrhea, and polyuria, must be monitored; and caution must be exercised when other drugs are prescribed, such as diuretics and nonsteroidal anti-inflammatory drugs.

## Methysergide

Methysergide is a potent preventive drug for the treatment of cluster headache, but because of the potential for fibrotic complications, it is not commonly employed for long periods of time (> 6 months) in patients with CCH. In patients with ECH, good to excellent results have been demonstrated in up to 70% of patients, but the drug appears to lose its effectiveness with repeated use in up to 20% of patients. The efficacy of methysergide in CCH has been questioned because of low efficacy rates of 20 to 26% in open-label studies.[10,56] Methysergide is metabolized to an active metabolite, methylergometrine. This metabolite, used as add-on therapy in a low dose of 0.6 to 0.8 mg/d, demonstrated efficacy in 19 of 20 subjects with ECH who were said not to be responding satisfactorily to preventive treatments.[57]

Because of the active metabolite methylergometrine, methysergide should be used with caution in patients receiving other ergotamine derivatives, a triptan, or other vasoconstrictive drugs. The short-term side effects include nausea, muscle cramps, abdominal pain, and pedal edema. Long-term side effects include fibrosis of the retroperitoneum or pleural and pericardial lining. The daily dose employed is usually 2 mg in three divided dosages, but up to 12 mg may be used if tolerated. It is recommended that patients be screened for fibrotic complications and undergo a 1-month drug holiday every 6 months. This screening process should include echocardiography, computed tomography or MRI of the chest and abdomen, urinalysis, and sedimentation rate. The drug is no longer distributed in the United States.

## Valproic Acid

An open-label study in 15 patients with cluster headache demonstrated the efficacy of valproic acid (600 to 2,000 mg) with a 73% favorable response rate.[58] Nine of 15 patients had complete suppression of attacks, and the time to pain relief was brief, ranging from 1 to 4 days. Treatment was well tolerated, with only nausea reported, but weight gain, hair loss, tremor, and lethargy are other potential side effects. It has been suggested that patients whose cluster headaches are accompanied by migrainous features, such as nausea, vomiting, photophobia, and phonophobia, may preferentially respond to valproic acid.

A recent double-blind placebo-controlled study of 1,000 to 200 mg/d of sodium valproate in the prophylaxis of 96 patients with cluster headache (77% ECH) was reported.[59] After a 7-day run-in period, patients were treated for 2 weeks. The primary efficacy criterion was the percentage of patients successfully improved (≥ 50% reduction in the average number of attacks per week between the run-in period and the last week of treatment). There was no difference between the two groups: 50% of subjects in the sodium valproate group and 62% in the placebo group were successfully improved (*p* = .23). This high success rate observed in the placebo group, which is likely to be due to the spontaneous remission of the episode, does not allow any valid conclusion to be drawn with regard to the true efficacy of sodium valproate in the prophylaxis of cluster headache.

Based on this limited and conflicting data, valproic acid may be considered as add-on therapy in refractory CCH patients until valid controlled experience becomes available. The medication is usually started in divided dosages of 250 mg twice daily, and 250 mg increments per dose are recommended to find the lowest effective dose so as to minimize side effects. Pancreatitis, platelet dysfunction, thrombocytopenia, and hepatic dysfunction have been described with this medication, thereby necessitating baseline and follow-up complete blood counts and liver function testing.

## Topiramate

In an open-label study, treatment with topiramate was associated with rapid improvement in 10 cluster headache patients.[60] Cluster headache period remission occurred in 1 to 3 weeks in nine patients, two of whom had CCH. All patients responded to relatively small dosages ranging between 50 and 125 mg/d in two divided dosages. In another open-label study, 26 patients with ECH (*n* = 12) or CCH (*n* = 14) were treated with topiramate 25 mg once a day, and the dose was titrated every 3 to 7 days to a maximum of 200 mg, according to clinical response and tolerability.[61] Topiramate rapidly induced cluster headache remission in 15 patients, reduced the number of attacks more than 50% in 6 patients, and reduced the cluster headache period duration in 12 patients. The mean time to remission was 14 days (range 1 to 27 days), but in 7 patients, remission was obtained within the first days of treatment with very low doses (25 to 75 mg/d). Tolerability was good within the lower range of doses used. Six patients discontinued treatment owing to side effects (all with daily doses over 100 mg) or a lack of efficacy.

However, less optimistic findings were reported in a study of 33 patients with ECH (*n* = 23) or CCH (*n* = 10) in which the median number of daily attacks did not differ between the run-in and treatment periods.[62] In seven patients (21%), the daily number of attacks was reduced by > 50%; six of these patients (26%) had the episodic form and one patient (10%) had the chronic form. Six of these responders received 100 mg/d and one received 150 mg/d during the treatment period. The seven patients who received 200 mg/d or more for 15 days experienced no improvement. There was no significant change in headache frequency following administration of topiramate in this study. In seven patients (21%), six of whom had ECH,

there was a > 50% reduction in the number of daily attacks during the treatment period, but this reduction did not seem to be dose related.

In view of the limited number of patients treated in these studies, the open-label design, and the conflicting results, it can be safely concluded that controlled studies with longer treatment periods are required to establish the efficacy of topiramate as first-line treatment for cluster headache prophylaxis. However, until such studies become available, topiramate may be considered as add-on therapy in patients with CCH who are refractory to monotherapy with verapamil.

Starting at low dosages and making small increments can minimize both the total daily dosage and the potential for side effects. Somnolence, dizziness, ataxia, and cognitive symptoms are the most common side effects reported by patients. Additionally, because of the weak carbonic anhydrase inhibition of this drug, renal calculi and paresthesias have been reported. Acute angle-closure glaucoma is a rare but potentially adverse event that is idiosyncratic and has occurred in approximately 100 patients worldwide.

## Gabapantin

Although currently limited, clinical data showing the effectiveness of gabapentin for the prevention of cluster headache is available. In a small open-label trial, 12 patients (8 with episodic and 4 with chronic cluster headache) previously shown to be refractory to other preventive therapies were treated with gabapentin initiated at a dosage of 900 mg per day. All patients were pain free after a maximum of 8 days following the initiation of gabapentin.[1] During this study, two patients reported mild drowsiness. In one case study, a 28-year-old man with chronic cluster headache responded to gabapentin when other treatments had failed. The patient was started on 300 mg/d gabapentin with an increment of 300 mg/d every third day. He noticed improvement at 1,200 mg/d gabapentin and reported being symptom free on a dose of 1,800 mg/d.[63] In another case study, a 38-year-old man diagnosed with episodic cluster headache was effectively treated with 300 mg of twice daily bid gabapentin. The only side effect was initial drowsiness, which disappeared after 3 doses.[64]

Given the relative paucity of data, it is currently difficult to make general recommendations on how to use gabapentin for the prevention of cluster headache. However, given the relative lack of drug interactions and relatively good tolerability of this drug, adjunctive treatment in patients with CCH is quite reasonable. Further studies are warranted to verify that the effectiveness of gabapentin for the prevention of cluster headache.

## Melatonin

The efficacy of 10 mg of oral melatonin has been evaluated in a double-blind placebo-controlled trial.[65]

Cluster headache remission within 3 to 5 days was achieved in 5 of 10 patients who received melatonin compared with 0 to 10 patients who received placebo. Similar observations were made in two patients with medically intractable CCH who responded to melatonin 9 mg with complete cessation of attacks during a 6- to 8-month follow-up. However, in another placebo-controlled crossover study involving nine patients (six with CCH, three with ECH) with cluster headache, no significant differences in any outcome measure were demonstrated when comparing 1 month on melatonin 2 mg controlled release with a 1-month baseline or 1-month placebo treatment period.[66] Taken together, given the recalcitrant nature of this disorder and the benign side-effect profile of melatonin, it is not unreasonable to use melatonin as an adjunctive treatment in patients with otherwise intractable CCH.

### Pizotifen

Pizotifen has modest efficacy for the preventive treatment of cluster headache. A review of seven small studies demonstrated a 38% (21 of 56) response rate.[67] In one single-blind trial of pizotifen in ECH, however, a response rate of 57% was found.[68] Pizotifen is not available in the United States but is available in Europe and Canada and may be useful in some patients with cluster headache.

### Indomethacin

Although several other trigeminal autonomic cephalgias, such as chronic and episodic paroxysmal hemicrania, respond in an absolute way to indomethacin, the weight of evidence appears to support its lack of effectiveness in cluster headache. Recently, the effect of indomethacin treatment in a group of 18 patients with ECH (3 females and 15 males) was evaluated.[69] From day 8 of the active period, indomethacin 100 mg intramuscularly was administered every 12 hours, for 2 consecutive days, in an open fashion. The mean daily attack frequency before the test (1.6 ± 0.6) was not statistically different from that on day 1 (2.1 ± 0.9) and day 2 (1.9 ± 0.8) after indomethacin administration. The mean interval between indomethacin injection and the following attack (days 1 and 2) was 4.6 + 1.1 hours. The authors did not observe any refractory period in any patient after indomethacin. They concluded that there is no therapeutic effect of indomethacin in cluster headache.

### Others

A number of other agents have been reported in small open-label studies or within case reports to have demonstrated efficacy in patients with cluster headache. These include methylphenidate, antispasticity drugs (tizanidine and baclofen), clonidine, diltiazem, flunarizine, histamine, somatostatin, and intranasal capsaicin. These is a paucity of clinical experience with these drugs, and because of the lack of data, further evidence is needed before recommendations can be made to support their routine use in cluster headache. However, consideration of all medical options should be given in patients with treatment-resistant cluster headache before an ablative surgical procedure is attempted.

## REFRACTORY CCH

### Medical Therapy

Approximately 15 to 20% of patients develop CCH that does not respond to monotherapy. In addition, patients with ECH with frequent cluster periods may develop resistance, intolerance, or contraindications to preventive and/or acute medications and may require a more definitive surgical procedure for pain control.

Before considering surgery, it is important to realize that some patients may do best with drugs used in combination rather than maximal dosages of one drug as monotherapy. At the 9th International Headache Research Seminar held in Copenhagen, Denmark, in 1999, a consensus was reached among a group of headache specialists with a special interest in cluster headache and the drugs of choice for ECH and CCH, as well as the optimal combinations for patients with more refractory disease (Table 6–4).[70] It should be noted that alternative adjunctive medications, such as melatonin, topiramate, divalproex sodium, and gabapentin, have shown some promise, at least in open-label or small randomized controlled trials. These drugs may be considered in combination-drug regimens, particularly given their lack of toxicity relative to more conventional medications, such as lithium and methysergide.

### Surgical Treatment

For the most intractable patients who have failed maximal medical therapy or for those with contraindications or intolerance that limits the use of effective medications, surgery may be a feasible option in carefully selected patients. Only patients whose headaches have been exclusively unilateral should be considered for surgery because patients whose attacks have alternated sides are at risk of a contralateral recurrence after surgery.

### Trigeminal Rhizotomy

With no remission periods and an often incomplete response to medications, many patients with CCH are considered for surgical intervention. Because CCH is arguably the most disabling of the primary headache disorders, investigators have allowed their threshold for defining a worthwhile therapy to include lower percentages of responders and higher percentages of potential adverse events.

Historically, surgical options aimed at the sensory trigeminal nerve for CCH have included radiofrequency

**Table 6–4**  Drugs of Choice for Preventive Treatment of Episodic and Chronic Cluster Headache

| Single Drugs | Combination of Drugs |
|---|---|
| Episodic cluster headache | |
| Verapamil | Verapamil + prednisone |
| Prednisone | Verapamil + ergotamine |
| Ergotamine | Verapamil + lithium |
| Methysergide | |
| Lithium | |
| Pizotifen | |
| Chronic cluster headache | |
| Verapamil | Verapamil + lithium |
| Lithium | Verapamil + ergotamine |
| Methysergide | Verapamil + methysergide |
| Pizotifen | Verapamil + lithium + ergotamine |

Based on consensus obtained at the 9th International Headache Research Seminar.[64]

thermocoagulation of the trigeminal ganglion, glycerol gangliorhizolysis, alcohol injection into the gasserian ganglion or the supraorbital or infraorbital nerve, gamma-knife radiosurgery, microvascular decompression, and trigeminal root section (Table 6–5).[71] Procedures directed at autonomic pathways include sectioning or dividing the greater superficial petrosal nerve or nervus intermedius and sectioning or cocainization of the sphenopalatine ganglion.[72,73] Sectioning the trigeminal nerve is traditionally reserved as a procedure of last resort for a desperate patient.

Percutaneous radiofrequency rhizolysis has been reported to be effective for the relief of cluster headache in patients with medically refractory disease. Fair to excellent results have been reported for 12 of 22 (55%) patients and poor results were observed in 10 of 22 (45%) patients after an initial radiofrequency procedure[74] In that study, 10 other patients underwent trigeminal root section. Six of these patients (60%) had excellent results, and 40% failed to respond. Interestingly, 6 of the 10 patients with poor results from their initial radiofrequency procedure went on to have a sensory rhizotomy, and 5 of these 6 (83%) patients had excellent pain relief. This was confirmed in another study in which 9 of 17 (53%) patients who failed radiofrequency thermocoagulation had long-term complete or near-complete relief after trigeminal nerve section.[75]

The overall results of radiofrequency rhizotomy suggest that, at least initially, approximately 75% of patients have good to excellent results. The recurrence rate, however, appears to be at least 20%, but some patients have been reported to remain free of cluster headache even 20 years after the procedure.[76] The best results may require complete analgesia or dense hypalgesia. If the pain is primarily orbital in location, V1 and V2 lesions appear to be adequate, but if the pain also involves the temporal or auricular region, a V3 lesion may also be necessary for optimal results. Indeed, in those patients whose pain is primarily located around the ear, temple, or cheek, an ablative trigeminal procedure may not be curative or as successful. Transient complications may include diplopia, hyperacusis, ice-pick pain, and jaw deviation, whereas longer-term complications include corneal anasthesia and, in less than 4% of cases, anasthesia dolorosa. Aggressive long-term ophthamic follow-up and eye care are critically important.

Microvascular decompression of the trigeminal nerve with or without microvascular decompression or section of the nervus intermedius was reported to be effective in CCH.[77] In this series, 28 patients, 2 of whom had bilateral cluster headache, underwent 39 operations for microvascular decompression of the trigeminal nerve, alone or combined with microvascular decompression or section of the nervus intermedius. Twenty-two of the 30 first-time procedures resulted in 50% relief or better, but long-term follow-up (average 5.3 years) showed a fall in good to excellent relief to 46%. Repeat procedures were ineffective. Three patients who responded with pain reduction of > 50% with microvascular decompression of the trigeminal

**Table 6–5**  Surgical Procedures for Cluster Headache

Procedures directed toward the sensory trigeminal nerve

    Radiofrequency trigeminal rhizotomy

    Retrogasserian glycerol injection

    Alcohol injection into supra- or infraorbital nerve, gasserian ganglion

    Trigeminal nerve root sections

    Microvascular decompression ± section or MVD of nervus intermedius

Procedures directed toward autonomic pathways

    Section of greater superficial petrosal nerve or nervus intermedius

    Section or cocainization of sphenopalatine ganglion

Gamma-knife radiosurgery

Deep brain stimulation

Occipital nerve stimulation

MVD = microvascular decompression.

nerve improved to better than 90% after a microvascular decompression or section of the nervus intermedius. These procedures require the skill of a very experienced surgical team and a craniotomy. Further experience with this combined approach is needed.

The long-term effectiveness and safety of percutaneous retrogasserian glycerol rhizolysis (PRGR) in the treatment of medically refractive CCH were recently analyzed.[78] This technique is sometimes considered as an alternative to radiofrequency rhizotomy because it may result in a lower rate of both corneal and facial anesthesia. In a prospective, consecutive series, 18 patients with intractable CCH were followed for a mean of 5.2 years (range 40 to 78 months) after they had undergone PRGR. Fifteen patients (83%) obtained immediate pain relief after one or two injections. Cluster headache recurred in seven patients (39%) over the course of the study. Two of these patients responded to a second injection. The overall daily headache frequency decreased from 3.5 ± 0.3 attacks per day preoperatively to 0.6 ± 0.2 attacks per day at last follow-up. The severity of these headaches, as assessed by verbal pain scales, also decreased from 10 preoperatively to 4.4 ± 1.4 at follow-up. None of the patients, including those who required a second procedure, experienced corneal anesthesia or facial dysesthesia. The authors concluded that this study lent support to both the safety and long-term efficacy of this procedure and that further investigations are needed to compare directly the relative efficacy and safety of glycerol rhizolysis with those of radiofrequency rhizolysis. In this study, however, seven patients were lost to follow-up, which must be considered when evaluating the overall efficacy of this procedure. In addition, meningitis, subarachnoid hemorrhage, and inadvertent intraparenchymal injection of glycerol are complications that can occur during glycerol injection.

In a recent observational study, 88% (15 of 17) of patients who underwent sectioning of the trigeminal sensory root at the level of the brainstem experienced complete or near-complete relief in the immediate postoperative period, and 76% went on to have long-term benefit (mean follow-up period 6.7 years).[79] Fifty-nine percent (10 of 17) of those patients did not require preventive medications after surgery and expressed satisfaction with the procedure. In another study, 57% (8 of 14) had complete or near-complete relief after only one trigeminal nerve section. Although 7 patients had to have a second surgery, 12 of 14 patients (85.7%) were able to live a normal life, with adequate pain control without medication (mean follow-up period 5.6 years). In both studies, complete sectioning of the nerve appeared to produce better results than partial sectioning. Stroke, death, weakness of the masticatory muscles, and painful facial dysesthesias or anasthesia dolorosa are potential adverse events.

Another potential complication with any surgical procedure is the development of contralateral cluster attacks, even in patients whose attacks have always been unilateral. Functional neuroimaging has provided recent evidence that the generator for cluster headache may reside in the periventricular hypothalamus.[80,81] Bilateral projections from each side of the hypothalamus to the caudal trigeminal nucleus and brainstem parasympathetic nuclei may explain why a unilateral lesion of the trigeminal sensory pathway does not exclude the possibility of contralateral trigeminal and parasympathetic pathways being recruited by a rostral diencephalic generator.

Trigeminal ablative procedures may therefore be an effective treatment with acceptable morbidity and complication rates for carefully selected patients with CCH who prove to be truly resistant to maximal medical therapy. Whether trigeminal root sectioning should be considered before a percutaneous ablative procedure, such as radiofrequency or glycerol trigeminal rhizolysis, will depend on the preferences of the treating physician and patient and the surgical expertise available. For most treating clinicians, sectioning of the sensory trigeminal nerve root will usually be considered as a last resort and may be considered only after a failed percutaneous procedure. Destructive procedures may always have the disadvantage of causing significant and permanent neurologic morbidity, and patients must be aware of these complications, but until newer therapies are proven more effective and safe, these procedures may offer relief from one of the most severe and disabling primary headache disorders.

## Deep Brain Stimulation

Based on the clinical benefit achieved with deep brain stimulation of relevant targets in movement disorders, two independent teams of investigators have demonstrated promising results using deep brain stimulation in patients with CCH.[82,83] With the demonstration, using PET, that the ipsilateral posterior inferior hypothalamic gray matter is central to the pathogenesis of cluster headache, these investigators stereotactically implanted stimulating electrodes into this region in 19 patients with medically refractory CCH. Thus far, the procedure appears to be effective in the majority of patients, durable, and well tolerated. One patient unfortunately expired fron an iatrogenic intracerebral hemorrhage during a procedure, reminding clinicians of the potential for serious morbidity and mortality associated with this procedure. Futher experience and longer follow-up are necessary, but the procedure offers hope to those who seem destined to live with CCH with a very poor quality of life. Consensus criteria were developed by a group of investigators to consider before subjecting a patient to deep brain stimulation.[84] These criteria should be strongly considered to maintain standardization so that outcome data can be compared across investigator sites (Table 6–6).

## Occipital Nerve Stimulation

Based on the convergent anatomy of the trigeminal cervical complex and the observations that occipital pain often occurs during cluster headache and occipital nerve blockade is effective for the acute relief of cluster headache, occipital nerve stimulation has been reported as an effective treatment in two patients with CCH.[85] Occipital nerve stimulation has also been reported to be effective in a group of patients with chronic migraine and chronic daily headache.[86,87] The mechanism of action is unclear, but stimulation may alter nociceptive processing with the trigeminal cervical complex and/or mobilize central pain-modulating networks. Further study of this procedure in patients with refractory CCH is certainly warranted because the procedure is minimally surgically invasive, with a much lower potential for the neurologic morbidity and mor-

**Table 6–6  Criteria for Electrode Implants in Intractable Chronic Cluster Headache**

CCH diagnosed according to IHS criteria; in addition, both of the following:

> CCH for at least 24 mo
>
> Attacks should normally occur on daily basis

Attacks must have always been strictly unilateral

Patients must be hospitalized to witness attacks and document their characteristics

All state-of-the-art drugs for CH prophylaxis must have been tried in sufficient dosages (unless they are contraindicated or have unacceptable side effects, etc), alone and in combination, where applicable. These include verapamil, lithium carbonate, methysergide, valproate, topiramate, gabapentin, melatonin, pizotifen, indomethacin, and corticosteroids.

Efficacy of placebo as abortive agent for the acute CH attacks must be tested (see text for full explanation)

Normal psychological profile

No medical/neurologic conditions contraindicating DBS, including

> Recent myocardial infarction
>
> Cardiac arrhythmia
>
> Cardiac malformation
>
> Epilepsy
>
> Stroke
>
> Deep brain stimulation for another reason
>
> Degenerative disorder of central nervous system
>
> Arterial hypertension or hypotension, not controlled by drugs
>
> Autonomic nervous system disorder
>
> Endocrinologic condition
>
> Major disturbance in electrolyte balance (eg, owing to renal insufficiency or hyperaldosteronism)

Normal neurologic examination except for symptoms characteristic of CH (eg, persistent Horner's syndrome)

Normal CT scan (base of the skull window). Normal cerebral MRI, including craniocervical transition and MRI arterial and venous angiography.

Neurosurgical team experienced at performing stereotactic implant of electrodes

Patient not pregnant

Ethics committee and institutional review board approval

Patient informed and gives written consent

CCH = chronic cluster headache; CH = cluster headache; CT = computed tomographic; DBS = deep brain stimulation; IHS = International Headache Society; MRI = magnetic resonance imaging.

tality associated with destructive trigeminal rhizotomies or deep brain stimulation.

## REFERENCES

1. Leandri M, Luzzani M, Cruccu G, Gottlieb A. Drug-resistant cluster headache responding to gabapentin: a pilot study. Cephalalgia 2001;21:744–6.

2. Headache Classification Subcommittee, International Headache Society. The international classification of headache disorders, 2nd edition. Cephalalgia 2004;24 Suppl 1:1–160.

3. Pearce JM. Natural history of cluster headache. Headache 1993;33:253–6.

4. Manzoni GC, Micieli G, Granella F, et al. Cluster headache—course over ten years in 189 patients. Cephalalgia 1991;11:169–74.

5. Kudrow L. Natural history of cluster headache. Part 1. Outcome of drop-out patients. Headache 1982;22:203–6.

6. Torelli, P, Cologno D, Cademartiri C, Manzoni GC. Possible predictive factors in the evolution of episodic to chronic cluster headache. Headache 2000;40:798–803.

7. Manzoni GC, Terzano MG, Bono G, et al. Cluster headache—clinical findings in 180 patients. Cephalalgia 1983;3:21–30.

8. Pearce JMS. Chronic migrainous neuralgia: a variant of cluster headache. Brain 1980;103:149–59.

9. Ekbom K. A clinical comparison of cluster headache and migraine. Acta Neurol Scand 1970;46 Suppl 41:1–44.

10. Kudrow L. Cluster headache. Mechanism and management. New York: Oxford University Press; 1980.

11. Kudrow L. Physical and personality characteristics in cluster headache. Headache 1974;13:197–202.

12. Levi R, Edman GV, Ekbom K, Waldenlind E. Episodic cluster headache. II: high tobacco and alcohol consumption in males. Headache 1992;32:184–7.

13. Graham JR, Rogado AZ, Rahman M, Gramer IV. Some physical, physiological, and psychological characteristics of patients with cluster headache. In: Cochrane AL, editor. Background to migraine. London: Heinemann; 1970. p. 38–51.

14. Hannerz J. Symptoms and diseases and smoking habits in female episodic cluster headache and migraine patients. Cephalalgia 1997;17:499–500.

15. Kudrow L. Cluster headache: diagnosis and management. Headache 1979;19:142–50.

16. Friedman AP, Mikropoulos HE. Cluster headaches. Neurology 1958;8:653–63.

17. Symonds C. A particular variety of headache. Brain 1956;79:217–32.

18. Bahra A, May A, Goadsby PJ. Cluster headache: a prospective study with diagnostic implications. Neurology 2002;58:354–61.

19. Dodick DW, Rozen TD, Goadsby PJ, Silberstein SD. Cluster headache. Cephalalgia 2000;20:787–803.

20. Goadsby PJ, Lipton RB. A review of paroxysmal hemicranias, SUNCT syndrome and other short-lasting headaches with autonomic features, including new cases. Brain 1997;120:193–209.

21. Boes CJ, Dodick DW. Refining the clinical spectrum of chronic paroxysmal hemicrania: a review of 74 patients. Headache 2002;42:699–708.

22. Dodick DW. Indomethacin-responsive headache syndromes. Curr Pain Headache Rep 2004;8:19–26.

23. Goadsby PJ, Edvinsson L. Human in vivo evidence for trigeminovascular activation in cluster headache. Brain 1994;117:427–34.

24. Goadsby PJ, Edvinsson L. Neuropeptide changes in a case of chronic paroxysmal hemicrania—evidence for trigemino-parasympathetic activation. Cephalalgia 1996;16:448–50.

25. Leone M, Bussone G. A review of hormonal findings in cluster headache. Evidence for hypothalamic involvement. Cephalalgia 1993;13:309–17.

26. Brzezinski A. Melatonin in humans. N Engl J Med 1997;336:186–95.

27. Leone M, Lucini V, D'Amico D, et al. Twenty-four hour melatonin and cortisol plasma levels in relation to timing of cluster headache. Cephalalgia 1995;15:224–9.

28. May A, Bahra A, Buchel C, et al. Hypothalamic activation in cluster headache attacks. Lancet 1998;352:275–8.

29. May A, Bahra A, Buchel C, et al. Functional magnetic resonance imaging in spontaneous attacks of SUNCT: short-lasting neuralgiform headache with conjunctival injection and tearing. Ann Neurol 1999;46:787–90.

30. May A, Kaube H, Buchel C, et al. Experimental cranial pain elicited by capsaicin: a PET study. Pain 1998;74:61–6.

31. May A, Ashburner J, Buchel C, et al. Correlation between structural and functional changes in brain in an idiopathic headache syndrome. Nat Med 1999;5:836–8.

32. Fogan L. Treatment of cluster headache. A double-blind comparison of oxygen air inhalation. Arch Neurol 1985;42:362–3.

33. Nilsson Remahl AIM, Ansjön R, Lind F, Waldenlind E. Hyperbaric oxygen treatment of active cluster headache: a double-blind placebo-controlled cross-over study. Cephalalgia 2002;22:730–9.

34. Ekbom K. Treatment of acute cluster headache with sumatriptan. N Engl J Med 1991;325:322–6.

35. Ekbom K, Krabbe A, Micieli G, et al. Sumatriptan Long Term Study Group. Cluster headache attacks treated for up to three months with subcutaneous sumatriptan (6 mg). Cephalalgia 1995;15:230–6.

36. Gobel H, Lindner V, Heinze A, et al. Acute therapy for cluster headache with sumatriptan: findings of a one-year long-term study. Neurology 1998;51:908–11.

37. van Vliet JA, Bahra A, Martin V, et al. Intranasal sumatriptan in cluster headache: randomized placebo-controlled double-blind study. Neurology 2003;60:630–3.

38. Sicuteri F, Geppetti P, Marabini S, Lembeck F. Pain relief by somatostatin in attacks of cluster headache. Pain 1984;18:359–65.

39. Geppetti P, Brocchi A, Caleri D, et al. Somatostatin for cluster headache attack. In: Pfaffenrath V, Lundberg PO, Sjaastad O, editors. Updating in headache. Berlin:Spring-Verlag; 1985. p. 302–5.

40. Matharu MS, Levy MJ, Meeran K, Goadsby PJ. Subcutaneous octreotide in cluster headache: randomized placebo-controlled double-blind crossover study. Ann Neurol 2004;56:488–94.

41. Andersson PG, Jespersen LT. Dihydroergotamine nasal spray in the treatment of attacks of cluster headache. Cephalalgia 1996;6:51–4.

42. Bahra A, Becker WJ, Blau JN. Efficacy of oral zolmitriptan in the acute treatment of cluster headache [abstract]. Cephalalgia 1999;19:457.

43. Yates R, Nairn K, Dixon R, et al. Preliminary studies of the pharmacokinetics and tolerability of zolmitriptan nasal spray in healthy volunteers. J Clin Pharmacol 2002;42:1237–43.

44. Uemura N, Charlesworth B, Onishi T, et al. Zolmitriptan is detectable in plasma 2 to 5 minutes after administration by nasal spray. Headache 2003;43:S159.

45. Bergström M, Wall A, Kågedal M, et al. An open label positron emission tomography study to investigate the distribution of intranasally administered [11C] zolmitriptan into the CNS. Neurology 2004;62 7 Suppl 5:A80–1.

46. Kågedal M, Duvauchelle T, Hovsepian L, et al. Zolmitriptan demonstrates good pharmacokinetic consistency between and within individuals following intranasal administration. Br J Clin Pharmacol 2004;57:679–80.

47. Zingmark P-H, Yates R, Hedlund C, et al. True nasopharyngeal absorption of zolmitriptan following administration of zolmitriptan nasal spray. Eur J Neurol 2003;10 Suppl 1:76.

48. Mathew NT, Kailasam J, Seifer T, Bouton T. Zolmitriptan (Zomig) nasal spray in cluster headache attacks; a single-blind observation—a preliminary report. Headache 2004;44:483.

49. Magnoux E, Zlotnik G. Outpatient intravenous dihydroergotamine for refractory cluster headache. Headache 2004;44:249–55.

50. Kudrow L. Cluster headache: mechanisms and management. London: Oxford University Press; 1980.

51. Ambrosini A, Vandenheede M, Rossi P, et al. Suboocipital (GON) injection with long-acting steroids in cluster headache: a double-blind placebo-controlled study. Cephalalgia 2003;23:734.

52. Leone M, D'Amico D, Attanasio A, et al. Verapamil is an effective prophylactic for cluster headache: results of a double-blind multicenter study versus placebo. In: Olesen J, Goadsby PJ, editors. Cluster headache and related conditions. Oxford (UK): Oxford University Press; 1999. p. 296–9.

53. Ekbom K. Lithium for cluster headache: review of the literature and preliminary results of long-term treatment. Headache 1981;21:132–9.

54. Bussone G, Leone M, Peccarisi C. Double blind comparison of lithium and verapamil in cluster headache prophylaxis. Headache 1990;30:411–7.

55. Stiener TJ, Hering R, Couturier EGM, et al. Double-blind placebo-controlled trial of lithium in episodic cluster headache. Cephalalgia 1997;17:673–5.

56. Krabbe A. Limited efficacy of methysergide in cluster headache. A clinical experience. Cephalalgia 1989;9:404–5.

57. Mueller L, Gallagher RM, Ciervo CA. Methylergonovine maleate as a cluster headache prophylactic: a study and review. Headache 1997;37:437–42.

58. Hering R, Kuritzky A. Sodium valproate in the treatment of cluster headache: an open trial. Cephalalgia 1989;9:195–8.

59. El Amrani M, Massiou H, Bousser MG. A negative trial of sodium valproate in cluster headache: methodological issues. Cephalalgia 2002;22:205–8.

60. Wheeler S, Carrazana EJ. Topiramate-treated cluster headache. Neurology 1999;53:234–6.

61. Láinez MJA, Pascual J, Pascual AM, et al. Topiramate in the prophylactic treatment of cluster headache. Cephalalgia 2003;43:784–9.

62. Leone M, Dodick D, Rigamonti A, et al. Topiramate in cluster headache prophylaxis: an open trial. Cephalalgia 2003;23:1001–2.

63. Ahmed F. Chronic cluster headache responding to gabapentin: a case report. Cephalalgia 2000;20:252–3.

64. Tay BA, Ngan Kee WD, Chung DC. Gabapentin for the treatment and prophylaxis of cluster headache. Reg Anesth Pain Med 2001;26:373–5.

65. Leone M, D'Amico D, Moschiano F, et al. Melatonin versus placebo in the prophylaxis of cluster headache: a double-blind pilot study with parallel groups. Cephalalgia 1996;16:494–6.

66. Pringsheim T, Magnoux E, Dobson CF, et al. Melatonin as adjunctive therapy in the prophylaxis of cluster headache: a pilot study.

67. Speight TM, Avery GS. Pizotifen (BC-105): a review of its pharmacological properties and its therapeutic efficacy in vascular headaches. Drugs 1972;3:159–203.

68. Ekbom K. Prophylactic treatment of cluster headache with a new serotonin antagonist, BC-105. Acta Neurol Scand 1969;45:601–10.

69. Antonaci F, Costa A, Ghirmai S, et al. Parenteral indomethacin (the INDOTEST) in cluster headache. Cephalalgia 2003;23:193–6.

70. Tfelt-Hansen P. Prophylactic pharmacotherapy of cluster headache. In: Oleson H, Goadsby PJ, editors. Cluster headache and related conditions.Oxford (UK): Oxford University Press; 1999. p. 257–63.

71. Rozen TD. Interventional treatment for cluster headache: a review of the options. Curr Pain Headache Rep 2002;6:57–64.

72. Meyer JS, Binns PM, Ericsson AS, et al. Sphenopalatine ganglionectomy for cluster headache. Arch Otolaryngol 1970;92:475–84.

73. Rowed DW. Chronic cluster headache managed by nervus intermedius section. Headache 1990;30:401–6.

74. Onofrio BM, Campbell JK. Surgical treatment of chronic cluster headache. Mayo Clin Proc 1986;61:537–44.

75. Kirkpatrick PJ, O'Brien MD, MacCabe JJ. Trigeminal nerve section for chronic migrainous neuralgia. Br J Neurosurg 1993;7:483–90.

76. Taha JM, Tew JM. Long-term results of radiofrequency rhizotomy in the treatment of cluster headache. Headache 1995;35:193–6.

77. Lovely TJ, Kotsiakis X, Jannetta PJ. The surgical management of chronic cluster headache. Headache 1998;38:590–4.

78. Pieper DR, Dickerson JBS, Hassenbusch SJ. Percutaneous retrogasserian glycerol rhizolysis for treatment of chronic intractable cluster headaches: long-term results. Neurosurgery 2000;46:363–70.

79. Jarrar R, Black D, Dodick DW, Davis D. Outcome of trigeminal nerve section in the treatment of chronic cluster headache. Neurology 2003;60:1360–2.

80. May A, Ashburner J, Buchel C, et al. Correlation between structural and functional changes in brain in an idiopathic headache syndrome. Nat Med 1999;5:836–8.

81. Goadsby PJ, May A. PET demonstration of hypothalamic activation in cluster headache. Neurology 1999;52:1522.

82. Leone M, Franzini A, D'Amico D, et al. Long-term follow-up of hypothalamic stimulation to relieve intractable chronic cluster headache [abstract]. Neurology 2004;62 Suppl 5:A355–6.

83. Vandenheede M, Maertens de Noordhout AS, Remacle JM, et al. Deep brain stimulation of posterior hypothalamus in chronic cluster headache [abstract]. Neurology 2004;29 Suppl 5:A356.

84. Leone M, May A, Franzini A, et al. Deep brain stimulation for intractable chronic cluster headache: proposals for patient selection. Cephalalgia 2004;24:934–7.

85. Dodick DW, Trentman T, Zimmerman R, Eross EJ. Occipital nerve stimulation for intractable chronic primary headache disorders. Cephalalgia 2003;23:701.

86. Popeney CA, Alo KM. Peripheral neurostimulation for the treatment of chronic, disabling transformed migraine. Headache 2003;43:369–75.

87. Matharu MS, Bartsch T, Ward N, et al. Central neuromodulation in chronic migraine patients with suboccipital stimulators: a PET study. Brain 2004;127:220–30.

# CHAPTER 7

# Chronic Paroxysmal Hemicrania

Christopher J. Boes, MD, and Juan A. Pareja, MD, PhD

Sjaastad and Dale reported a new treatable headache entity in 1974, and in 1976, they named the entity "chronic paroxysmal hemicrania" (CPH).[1,2] The first case seen by Sjaastad was described in detail in his book, *Cluster Headache Syndrome*, and it is quoted extensively here because of its importance:

> The first case of chronic paroxysmal hemicrania (CPH), a female aged 44 years with a 9-year history of headache, was brought to our cognizance in 1961, with a diagnosis of "typical cluster headache." However, the patient was a female (which, of course, may be consistent with a diagnosis of ordinary cluster headache, although females are admittedly rarely affected). There was another trait that, upon scrutiny, did not seem to be quite typical: there was a *multitude* of attacks per 24h, i.e. up to 24 or more per day. Another remarkable feature was the intractability of the headache… Over the course of the following years, every feasible drug was tried on her. Prior to each admission, she had discontinued her usual drug (mainly acetylsalicylic acid) which kept the attacks at a reasonable level. Each drug trial ended either with an absolutely negative response, or—more usually—with an adverse reaction. The latter response pattern was so typical that for almost every new drug that was tried she was brought from a stage of moderate or weak attacks to a stage of incapacitating and excruciatingly severe attacks… But she would not give up the hope that there was a solution to her problem. And she was the one who motivated us to try new approaches, not the other way around… To make matters even worse, she was diagnosed as being an hysterical person… despite the unilaterality of the pain, lacrimation, rhinorrhoea, etc…

> [T]he patient felt that everything centred on the eye… [W]e had arrived at a point where we were running out of arguments when trying to reject the patient's contention that an enucleation of the right (symptomatic side) eye would perhaps solve her pain problem.

> Fortunately, the following developments took place simultaneously. The patient had from the start claimed that salicylates seemed to give her some relief, not to the extent that the pain disappeared, but at times when they were not maximal the paroxysms could be modified by salicylates. Perhaps the paroxysms became even more rare during such medication. We thought that a lot of drugs would be more promising than salicylates as potential therapeutic agents. The anti-inflammatory agents were therefore put rather far down on our list of potentially effective drugs worthy of trial… When in late 1972 we finally arrived at indomethacin on our list, the response was no less than miraculous.[3]

A remitting form of the disease was subsequently recognized and termed "episodic paroxysmal hemicrania" (EPH).[4] The International Headache Society (IHS) gave diagnostic criteria for CPH in 1988,[5] and in 2004, the IHS classified CPH and EPH as subtypes of paroxysmal hemicrania (Table 7–1).[6]

## EPIDEMIOLOGY

The prevalence of CPH is unknown, but the relationship to cluster headache is reported to be approximately 1 to 3%.[7] Given that the prevalence of cluster headache is approximately 1 in 1,000, the prevalence of paroxysmal hemicrania would be approximately 1 in 50,000.[8] The reported female to male ratio ranges from

**Table 7–1** 2004 International Headache Society Diagnostic Criteria for Paroxysmal Hemicrania

Paroxysmal hemicrania has 2 subtypes:

Chronic: attacks occur for more than 1 yr without remission or with remissions lasting less than 1 mo

Episodic: attacks occur in periods lasting 7 d to 1 yr separated by pain-free periods lasting 1 mo or more; at least 2 attack periods required

Diagnostic criteria:

A.  At least 20 attacks fulfilling criteria B–D

B.  Attacks of severe unilateral orbital, supraorbital, or temporal pain lasting 2–30 min

C.  Headache is accompanied by at least 1 of the following:

  1.  Ipsilateral conjunctival injection and/or lacrimation

  2.  Ipsilateral nasal congestion and/or rhinorrhea

  3.  Ipsilateral eyelid edema

  4.  Ipsilateral forehead and facial sweating

  5.  Ipsilateral miosis and/or ptosis

D.  Attacks have a frequency above 5 per day for more than half of the time, although periods with lower frequency may occur

E.  Attacks are prevented completely by therapeutic doses of indomethacin*

F.  Not attributed to another disorder

Adapted from Headache Classification Subcommittee, International Headache Society.[6]

*To rule out an incomplete response, indomethacin should be used in a dose of ≥ 150 mg daily orally or rectally or ≥ 100 mg by injection, but for maintenance, smaller doses are often sufficient.

1.6 to 1[9] to 2.36 to 1.[7] CPH can begin at any age, but the mean age at onset is in the thirties.[7]

## CLINICAL FEATURES

Patients with CPH typically have unilateral, brief, severe attacks of pain associated with cranial autonomic features that recur several times per day. The pain is most often in a V1 distribution, but it can be extratrigeminal. In Antonaci and Sjaastad's retrospective review of 84 CPH patients, the maximal pain was most often in the ocular, temporal, maxillary, or forehead areas.[7] It was less often in the neck and shoulder, retro-ocular, or occipital regions. The quality of pain is usually claw-like or throbbing, but it can sometimes be described as dental, boring, or pressing.[7] The pain has an abrupt onset and cessation. Roughly 50% of patients prefer to sit or curl up in bed during attacks.[7] Photophobia (21%), nausea (14%), and vomiting (2%) may be present.[7] Twenty-seven of 31 patients noted at least one migrainous feature of photophobia, nausea, or vomiting during an attack.[9]

Ipsilateral autonomic features typically occur during attacks of pain. The most common symptoms are lacrimation and nasal congestion, but conjunctival injection, rhinorrhea, forehead and facial sweating, eyelid edema, ptosis, and miosis can also occur.[7] Bilateral autonomic symptoms can occur.[7] A dissociation between pain and autonomic features can be seen.[10]

The headache usually lasts 10 to 30 minutes (mean 20.9 minutes), with a range from 2 to 120 minutes.[7] The frequency ranges from 1 to 40 attacks per day, with a mean of 11 attacks per day.[7] In a review of 74 patients seen at the Mayo Clinic, the mean usual duration was 26 minutes and the mean usual attack frequency was six.[9] In a prospective study of 105 attacks in five patients, the mean duration was 13.3 minutes and the mean frequency was 14 per day.[11] Attacks seem to occur regularly throughout the 24-hour period, without the preponderance of nocturnal attacks typically seen in cluster headache. Nocturnal attacks associated with rapid eye movement (REM) sleep have been reported.[12] Interictal discomfort or pain is present in up to one-third of patients.[7]

Most attacks are spontaneous, but 10% of patients can trigger attacks with neck movement.[7] Alcohol ingestion triggers attacks in approximately 7% of patients.[7]

Paroxysmal hemicrania has chronic and episodic patterns, similar to cluster headache. In contradiction to cluster headache, however, the chronic form of paroxysmal hemicrania is more common than the episodic form, occurring in 80% of patients.[7] Around 20% of patients with paroxysmal hemicrania have clear intervals between bouts of attacks (EPH). The duration of the headache phase in EPH ranges from 2 weeks to 4.5 months.[13] Remissions in EPH range from 1 to 36 months.[13] EPH has been reported to stay episodic for up to 35 years.[7] The natural history of CPH is largely unknown. In a review of all reported cases in 1989, the mean duration of illness was 13.3 ± 12.2 years.[7] It seems to be a lifelong condition, although EPH can transform into CPH and vice versa.

CPH has been observed in association with other primary headache disorders, including trigeminal neuralgia (paroxysmal hemicrania–tic syndrome),[14,15] cluster headache,[16] migraine,[17] primary stabbing headache (PSH),[18] and primary cough headache.[19] Typically, each type of headache requires a separate treatment (except when CPH is associated with primary cough headache or PSH).

Unusual clinical features have been reported, including side-alternating attacks,[10,20,21] bilateral pain,[22] and an absence of autonomic features.[20,23,24] Cases presenting with primarily ear pain and a sensation of external acoustic meatus obstruction have been reported, and a case of CPH associated with red ear syndrome has been described.[24] Aura is rarely associated with attacks of CPH.[25]

## PATHOGENESIS

The pathogenesis of CPH is unknown. Any pathophysiologic explanation must account for the trigeminal location of the pain and the cranial autonomic features. Calcitonin gene–related peptide (CGRP) is elevated during attacks of CPH, reflecting trigeminovascular activation.[26] Vasoactive intestinal polypeptide (VIP) is also elevated during attacks, reflecting cranial parasympathetic activation.[26] The trigeminal autonomic reflex has been proposed to account for many of the features of CPH.[27] This reflex consists of a brainstem connection between the trigeminal nerve and the facial nerve parasympathetic outflow. Extratrigeminal pain in CPH could be explained by the caudal extension of the trigeminal nucleus caudalis to C1–2.[27]

A lesion in the ipsilateral cavernous sinus has been proposed to account for the features of CPH.[3] Orbital phlebography has been abnormal in CPH, as it has been in cluster headache and Tolosa-Hunt syndrome.[27] The findings on this test are felt to be neither specific nor pathophysiologically relevant.[27] A lesion in the pericarotid area in the cavernous sinus would not seem to explain the paroxysmal nature of CPH attacks.[28]

Goadsby and Lipton emphasize the pathophysiologic importance of the central nervous system in CPH:

There is little to suggest a fundamental neurobiological separation between CPH and cluster headache in regard to the final common pathways activated. The shorter attack duration, greater attack frequency and different effect of indomethacin perhaps point to differences in the generation thus central nervous system mechanisms of these disorders.[27]

Functional neuroimaging studies have not been reported in CPH. However, in the other two trigeminal autonomic cephalalgias (cluster headache and SUNCT syndrome [short-lasting, unilateral, neuralgiform headache attacks with conjunctival injection and tearing, functional neuroimaging has shown ipsilateral hypothalamic activation.[29,30] Hypothalamic activation is not seen in migraine or capsaicin-induced trigeminal pain.[8] The hypothalamus is known to have a modulatory role on the nociceptive and autonomic pathways, and there are direct hypothalamic-trigeminal connections.[8] It is possible that a similar hypothalamic process may be active in CPH, given its clinical similarities to the two other trigeminal autonomic cephalalgias.

The etiology of the exquisite responsiveness of CPH to indomethacin is unknown. It appears to be independent of its effect on prostaglandin synthesis because other nonsteroidal anti-inflammatory drugs (NSAIDs) are not usually efficacious.[31] Unlike other NSAIDs, indomethacin can decrease intracranial pressure,[31] but that seems unlikely to be important in CPH given that intracranial pressure was not elevated when measured during an attack of CPH.[32] This latter study was reported in 1970 as being done on a patient with cluster headache,[32] but this patient was eventually diagnosed with CPH after having a complete indomethacin response.[3] One patient with CPH and a cerebrospinal fluid opening pressure of 30 cm $H_2O$ has been reported, but that case was unusual in that the patient had side-alternating attacks that required indomethacin doses of 275 mg/d to control, and no comment was made about the presence or absence of papilledema.[21] Indomethacin inhibits the production of nitric oxide (NO), which is significant given that glycerol trinitrate (a NO donor) can trigger neurovascular headaches, such as cluster headache and migraine.[31] NO likely activates CGRP release from trigeminal fibers.[33,34] NO is colocalized with VIP within neurons and nerve fibers of the cranial parasympathetic system.[31] The elevated CGRP and VIP levels seen during attacks of CPH return to normal after treatment with indomethacin.[26] Thus, indomethacin may exert its effect on CPH by antagonizing one or more steps in the NO pathway, given that CPH is a disorder characterized by activation of the cranial parasympathetic system.[31]

## DIAGNOSIS

In CPH, as in any other primary headache disorder, there are no available biologic markers. Therefore, diagnosis relies on the clinical features and differentiation from other similar headaches (Table 7–2). Several secondary CPH cases have been reported (Table 7–3), highlighting the importance of neuroimaging with magnetic resonance imaging. Data obtained with sensitive instrumental methods should be considered as complementary and of relative help.

The diagnosis of CPH is based on the presence of strictly unilateral paroxysmal attacks centered on the orbital or periorbital area that are accompanied by a variable assortment of oculofacial autonomic features and that are absolutely responsive to indomethacin (see Table 7–1). The pharmacologic response to indomethacin should be considered diagnostic only when the test has been conducted in an optimal way.

### Testing Indomethacin Response

The appropriate test dosage should be 25 mg three times daily for 3 days. If that dose is not effective, another 3-

**Table 7–2** Clinical Features of the Trigeminal Autonomic Cephalalgias and Hemicrania Continua

| Feature | Cluster Headache | Paroxysmal Hemicrania | SUNCT Syndrome | Hemicrania Continua |
|---|---|---|---|---|
| Sex F:M | 1:2.5–7 | 1.6–2.36:1 | 1:1.3 | 2:1 |
| Pain | | | | |
|   Type | Stabbing, boring | Throbbing, boring, stabbing | Burning, stabbing, sharp | Background dull ache; throbbing/stabbing exacerbations |
|   Severity | Excruciating | Excruciating | Severe | Moderate background pain; severe exacerbations |
|   Site | Orbit, temple | Orbit, temple | Periorbital | Orbit, temple |
| Attack frequency | 1/alternate day to 8/d | 1–40/day (> 5/d for more than half the time) | 3–200/d | Continuous |
| Duration of attack | 15–180 min | 2–30 min | 5–240 s | Continuous background pain; exacerbations variable, lasting minutes to days |
| Autonomic features | Yes | Yes | Yes (prominent conjunctival injection and lacrimation) | Yes, mainly with exacerbations; less prominent than in other TACs |
| Migrainous features* | Yes (photophobia may be lateralized to pain side) | Yes (photophobia may be lateralized to pain side) | Very rarely (photophobia may be lateralized to pain side) | Yes, during exacerbations |
| Alcohol trigger | Yes | Occasional | No | Rare |
| Indomethacin effect | – | ++ | – | ++ |
| Abortive treatment | Sumatriptan injection Oxygen | Nil | Nil | Nil |
| Prophylactic treatment | Verapamil Methysergide Lithium | Indomethacin | Lamotrigine | Indomethacin |

Adapted from Matharu MS et al.[8]

SUNCT = short-lasting, unilateral, neuralgiform headache attacks with conjunctival injection and tearing; TAC = trigeminal autonomic cephalalgia; ++ = absolute response to indomethacin.

*Nausea, photophobia, or phonophobia.

**Table 7–3** Causes of Secondary Paroxysmal Hemicrania

*Vascular*

    Circle of Willis aneurysms

    Occipital, middle cerebral artery territory infarcts

    Parietal arteriovenous malformation

*Neoplastic*

    Malignant frontal tumor

    Cavernous sinus meningioma

    Petrous ridge meningioma

    Gangliocytoma sella turcica

    Pituitary adenoma

    Parotid epidermoid cerebral metastases

    Pancoast tumor

*Miscellaneous*

    Collagen vascular disease

    Intracranial hypertension

    Maxillary cyst

    Ophthalmic herpes zoster

    Essential thrombocythemia

Adapted from Matharu MS et al[8] and Boes CJ and Dodick DW.[9]

day course with a 150 mg daily dosage divided into six doses should be tried. The vast majority (if not all) of patients will respond within 24 hours. Many will respond within 8 hours with a standard oral dose of 75 to 150 mg daily.[35] The procedure may take up to 6 days or even more because an incomplete but substantial (60–80% improvement) response may indicate that the dosage needs to be increased. In chronic cases, this "delay" does not represent a diagnostic problem, but in remitting forms (especially in rarely occurring very short symptomatic periods), the delay in response becomes critical, and in such cases, high initial doses, even administered parenterally, are recommended.

The response to oral indomethacin may vary when the dose is titrated. With administration of 50 mg of indomethacin intramuscularly, a clear-cut response will be obtained within 1 to 1.5 hours.[36] This trial (the indotest) seems to be the ideal one in the diagnostically problematic case, chiefly because of the quick and clear response. Unfortunately, intramuscular indomethacin is not available in the United States.

When assessing the response to indomethacin diagnostically in remitting cases, the medication should be continued for several months (depending on the previous length and frequency of symptomatic periods) to avoid the possible confusion of a pharmacologic response with a spontaneous remission. Repeated trials, dosage reductions, and even drug discontinuation should also be carried out in doubtful cases to ascertain the diagnosis.

The diagnostic implications of a negative response to indomethacin are obvious, and this is another important reason for carefully testing the response to such a drug.

*Problem of Distinguishing Cluster Headache and CPH*
At this stage of development, the response to indomethacin should be a compulsory diagnostic criterion of CPH. Skipping such a pharmacologic criterion may bring about an unsolvable differentiation between cluster headache and CPH. Unilaterality and localization of attacks, excruciating severity of pain, and autonomic accompaniments are similar in cluster headache and CPH. According to the IHS classification, cluster headache attacks last for 15 to 180 minutes, whereas CPH attacks last for 2 to 30 minutes.[6] This means that in a given patient with attacks lasting 15 to 30 minutes, the distinction of both disorders is impossible unless the indomethacin response criterion is used. Alternatively, sophisticated instrumental examinations, such as evaporimetry, pupillometry, and dynamic tonometry, can provide similarities and differences between both disorders.[3] However, such investigations render information only during attacks or interictally and are not frequently available to most physicians.

## DIFFERENTIAL DIAGNOSIS

Some of the cardinal features of CPH may be present in other headache syndromes (see Table 7–2). CPH should be considered mainly when encountering a strictly unilateral, orbital or periorbital pain with prominent, ipsilateral, autonomic accompaniments and/or when the orbital pain paroxysms are short-lasting. The differential diagnostic possibilities seem to be limited and mainly consist of cluster headache, SUNCT syndrome, first division trigeminal neuralgia (V1 neuralgia), and PSH. Among long-lasting, unilateral headaches, only hemicrania continua (the other headache absolutely responsive to indomethacin) should be included in the diagnostic work-up.

Differential diagnosis of CPH versus the abovementioned headaches is relatively straightforward because complete relief from indomethacin is mandatory by definition in CPH,[6] and this drug has been shown to have no effect on the other short-lasting headaches (aside from PSH). Nevertheless, other distinguishing features are to be considered, thus strengthening the differences.

## Cluster Headache

As mentioned above, the indomethacin response is a factor that crucially distinguishes cluster headache from CPH. Nevertheless, there are important differences between the disorders: the differing sex preponderance, the prevalent temporal pattern, and the lack of effect of "cluster headache drugs" in CPH. Moreover, CPH attacks are briefer and more frequent compared with cluster headache and have a uniform distribution throughout the day and night. Almost as important may be the demonstration of a Horner-like syndrome and an abnormal sweating pattern in the central part of the forehead on the symptomatic side in cluster headache, which is not present in CPH.[3]

## SUNCT Syndrome

CPH differs from SUNCT syndrome as regards attack duration, temporal distribution of attacks, precipitating mechanisms, and sex preponderance.[7,37] SUNCT attacks typically last about 1 minute, with a duration exceeding 120 seconds being only rarely found.[38] Only exceptional attacks of CPH last less than 3 minutes, and the mean duration of attacks in CPH has been estimated at 13 minutes.[11] In SUNCT syndrome, nocturnal attacks are seldom reported, whereas CPH is characterized by a number of nocturnal attacks in addition to daytime attacks.

Most SUNCT attacks are precipitated by mechanisms acting on trigeminal and extratrigeminal innervated areas, such as the neck. Only a minority (~ 15%) of CPH patients exhibit precipitated attacks (with a latency of 5 seconds to 1 minute or more) after spontaneous neck movements or after prolonged external pressure over certain sensitive areas.[18]

## V1 Trigeminal Neuralgia

V1 neuralgia attacks last for 5 to 10 seconds, with durations longer than 30 seconds being very rare.[39] The response to carbamazepine is good. Otherwise, the attacks are never accompanied by conjunctival injection, although slight lacrimation may infrequently be noted.[40] V1 neuralgia attacks are typically precipitated by trivial stimuli on the trigeminal territory, whereas only some CPH patients exhibit precipitation mechanisms strictly acting on the nuchal or cervical areas. Trigeminal trigger zones do not exist in CPH.

## Primary Stabbing Headache

Topographically speaking, there is a strong difference between CPH and PSH, with the former being unilateral and the latter exhibiting a multidirectional, chaotic localization, with attacks changing localization in either the same or the opposite hemicranium. Rarely, PSH attacks recur in the same area, and in such cases, the orbit is frequently involved.[41,42] Even in such cases, the differentia-

tion from CPH is easy because most PSH attacks last 1 to 3 seconds (total range 1 to 10 seconds) and typically lack autonomic accompaniments. Stabs may (or may not) respond to standard oral doses of indomethacin.[42]

## Hemicrania Continua

Hemicrania continua is so far the only other headache absolutely responsive to indomethacin,[43] a fact that, along with both strict unilaterality and clear female preponderance, is similar to CPH. It should be emphasized that both headaches also exhibit remitting and nonremitting clinical forms. The two headaches clearly differ in the duration and intensity of pain (continuous/moderate in hemicrania continua and atrocious/shortlasting in CPH) and also as regards the extent of oculofacial autonomic involvement (modest/inconstant in hemicrania continua and dramatic/systematic in CPH).

## TREATMENT

Indomethacin is the treatment of choice for CPH and probably the only absolutely effective remedy. Indomethacin provides a remission, not a cure. Patients get rid of pain while on treatment. Withdrawal of indomethacin typically leads to resumption of symptoms after a variable (usually short) period of time. Therefore, the drug should be given continously in patients with the chronic form, as well as in the long-lasting or frequent episodic forms. In patients with infrequent symptomatic periods, the drug may be administered from the initial phase to the end of every symptomatic period, the reason being that the latency between administration and response is so short.

Indomethacin should be given orally in a dose of 75 to 150 mg daily divided in three to six doses. Patients are expected to absolutely respond within 24 hours.[35] Once the patient has improved, the dose should be titrated to the minimum necessary. The dosage requirement of indomethacin may fluctuate in parallel with the intensity of the symptoms but generally can be easily titrated by the patients themselves. In fact, the dose tends to be reduced with time.[44] Overall, the effective dose may range from 25 to 250 mg daily, with the usual dose being 75 to 100 mg/d. The need for a high dosage is exceptional and may indicate a symptomatic form,[45] requiring closer follow-up.

Virtually all NSAIDs have been tried in CPH, and in equipotent doses, none show the extraordinary effect provided by indomethacin.[3] Other drugs that have been reported as effective include aspirin,[1,46] piroxicam,[47] naproxen,[48] celecoxib,[49] rofecoxib,[50] flunarizine,[51] verapamil,[52] acetazolamide,[53] and corticosteroids.[54] These drugs are therapeutic alternatives in patients with intolerance to indomethacin.

# REFERENCES

1. Sjaastad O, Dale I. Evidence for a new (?), treatable headache entity. Headache 1974;14:105–8.

2. Sjaastad O, Dale I. A new (?) clinical headache entity "chronic paroxysmal hemicrania" 2. Acta Neurol Scand 1976;54:140–59.

3. Sjaastad O. Cluster headache syndrome. Major problems in neurology series. Vol 23. London: WB Saunders; 1992.

4. Kudrow L, Esperanca P, Vijayan N. Episodic paroxysmal hemicrania? Cephalalgia 1987;7:197–201.

5. Headache Classification Committee, International Headache Society. Classification and diagnostic criteria for headache disorders, cranial neuralgias and facial pain. Cephalalgia 1988;8 Suppl 7:1–96.

6. Headache Classification Subcommittee, International Headache Society. The international classification of headache disorders. 2nd edition. Cephalalgia 2004;24 Suppl 1:1–160.

7. Antonaci F, Sjaastad O. Chronic paroxysmal hemicrania (CPH): a review of the clinical manifestations. Headache 1989;29:648–56.

8. Matharu MS, Boes CJ, Goadsby PJ. Management of trigeminal autonomic cephalgias and hemicrania continua. Drugs 2003;63:1637–77.

9. Boes CJ, Dodick DW. Refining the clinical spectrum of chronic paroxysmal hemicrania: a review of 74 patients. Headache 2002;42:699–708.

10. Pareja JA. Chronic paroxysmal hemicrania: dissociation of the pain and autonomic features. Headache 1995;35:111–3.

11. Russell D. Chronic paroxysmal hemicrania: severity, duration and time of occurrence of attacks. Cephalalgia 1984;4:53–6.

12. Kayed K, Godtlibsen OB, Sjaastad O. Chronic paroxysmal hemicrania IV: "REM sleep locked" nocturnal headache attacks. Sleep 1978;1:91–5.

13. Newman LC, Lipton RB. Paroxysmal hemicranias. In: Goadsby PJ, Silberstein SD, editors. Headache. Boston: Butterworth-Heinemann; 1997. p. 243–50.

14. Caminero AB, Pareja JA, Dobato JL. Chronic paroxysmal hemicrania-tic syndrome. Cephalalgia 1998;18:159–61.

15. Boes CJ, Matharu MS, Goadsby PJ. The paroxysmal hemicrania-tic syndrome. Cephalalgia 2003;23:24–8.

16. Centonze V, Bassi A, Causarano V, et al. Simultaneous occurrence of ipsilateral cluster headache and chronic paroxysmal hemicrania: a case report. Headache 2000;40:54–6.

17. Pareja J, Pareja J. Chronic paroxysmal hemicrania coexisting with migraine. Differential response to pharmacological treatment. Headache 1992;32:77–8.

18. Sjaastad O, Egge K, Horven I, et al. Chronic paroxysmal hemicranial: mechanical precipitation of attacks. Headache 1979;19:31–6.

19. Mateo I, Pascual J. Coexistence of chronic paroxysmal hemicrania and benign cough headache. Headache 1999;39:437–8.

20. Pelz M, Merskey H. A case of pre-chronic paroxysmal hemicrania. Cephalalgia 1982;2:47–50.

21. Hannerz J, Jogestrand T. Intracranial hypertension and sumatriptan efficacy in a case of chronic paroxysmal hemicrania which became bilateral. (The mechanism of indomethacin in CPH.) Headache 1993;33:320–3.

22. Pollmann W, Pfaffenrath V. Chronic paroxysmal hemicrania: the first possible bilateral case. Cephalalgia 1986;6:55–7.

23. Bogucki A, Szymanska R, Braciak W. Chronic paroxysmal hemicrania: lack of pre-chronic stage. Cephalalgia 1984;4:187–9.

24. Boes CJ, Swanson JW, Dodick DW. Chronic paroxysmal hemicrania presenting as otalgia with a sensation of external acoustic meatus obstruction: two cases and a pathophysiologic hypothesis. Headache 1998;38:787–91.

25. Matharu MS, Goadsby PJ. Post-traumatic chronic paroxysmal hemicrania (CPH) with aura. Neurology 2001;56:273–5.

26. Goadsby PJ, Edvinsson L. Neuropeptide changes in a case of chronic paroxysmal hemicrania—evidence for trigemino-parasympathetic activation. Cephalalgia 1996;16:448–50.

27. Goadsby PJ, Lipton RB. A review of paroxysmal hemicranias, SUNCT syndrome and other short-lasting headaches with autonomic feature, including new cases. Brain 1997;120:193–209.

28. Goadsby PJ. Paroxysmal hemicrania. In: Gilman S, editor. MedLink neurology. San Diego (CA): MedLink Corporation. Available at: www.medlink.com (accessed Feb 2004).

29. May A, Bahra A, Buchel C, et al. Functional magnetic resonance imaging in spontaneous attacks of SUNCT: short-lasting neuralgiform headache with conjunctival injection and tearing. Ann Neurol 1999;46:791–4.

30. May A, Bahra A, Buchel C, et al. PET and MRA findings in cluster headache and MRA in experimental pain. Neurology 2000;55:1328–35.

31. Dodick DW. Indomethacin-responsive headache syndromes. In: Noseworthy J, editor. Neurological therapeu-

tics: principles and practices. London: Martin Dunitz; 2003. p. 142–50.

32. Broch A, Horven I, Nornes H, et al. Studies on cerebral and ocular circulation in a patient with cluster headache. Headache 1970;10:1–8.

33. Akerman S, Williamson DJ, Kaube H, Goadsby PJ. Nitric oxide synthase inhibitors can antagonize neurogenic and calcitonin gene-related peptide induced dilation of dural meningeal vessels. Br J Pharmacol 2002;137:62–8.

34. Pardutz A, Multon S, Malgrange B, et al. Effect of systemic nitroglycerin on CGRP and 5-HT afferents to rat caudal spinal trigeminal nucleus and its modulation by estrogen. Eur J Neurosci 2002;15:1803–9.

35. Pareja J, Sjaastad O. Chronic paroxysmal hemicrania and hemicrania continua. Interval between indomethacin administration and response. Headache 1996;36:20–3.

36. Antonaci F, Pareja JA, Caminero AB, Sjaastad O. Chronic paroxysmal hemicrania and hemicrania continua. Parenteral indomethacin: the "indotest." Headache 1998;38:122–8.

37. Pareja JA, Sjaastad O. SUNCT syndrome. A clinical review. Headache 1997;37:195–202.

38. Pareja JA, Shen JM, Kruszewski P, et al. SUNCT syndrome: duration, frequency, and temporal distribution of attacks. Headache 1996;36:161–5.

39. Sjaastad O, Pareja JA, Zukerman E, et al. Trigeminal neuralgia. Clinical manifestations of first division involvement. Headache 1997;37:346–57.

40. Pareja JA, Barón M, Gili P, et al. Objective assessment of autonomic signs during triggered first division trigeminal neuralgia. Cephalalgia 2002;22:251–5.

41. Lansche RK. Ophthalmodynia periodica. Headache 1964;4:247–9.

42. Pareja JA, Ruiz J, de Isla C, et al. Idiophathic stabbing headache (jabs and jolts syndrome). Cephalalgia 1996;16:93–6.

43. Sjaastad O, Spierings EL. "Hemicrania continua": another headache absolutely responsive to indomethacin. Cephalalgia 1984;4:65–70.

44. Pareja JA, Caminero AB, Franco E, et al. Dose, efficacy and tolerability of long-term indomethacin treatment of chronic paroxysmal hemicrania and hemicrania continua. Cephalalgia 2001;21:906–10.

45. Sjaastad O, Stovner LJ, Stolt-Nielsen A, et al. CPH and hemicrania continua: requirements of high indomethacin dosages—an ominous sign? Headache 1995;35:363–7.

46. Kudrow DB, Kudrow L. Successful aspirin prophylaxis in a child with chronic paroxysmal hemicrania. Headache 1989;29:280–1.

47. Sjaastad O, Antonaci F. A piroxicam derivative partly effective in chronic paroxysmal hemicrania and hemicrania continua. Headache 1995;35:549–50.

48. Durko A, Klimek A. Naproxen in the treatment of chronic paroxysmal hemicrania. Cephalalgia 1987;7:361–2.

49. Mathew NT, Kailasam J, Fisher A. Responsiveness to celecoxib in chronic paroxysmal hemicrania. Neurology 2000;55:316.

50. Lisotto C, Maggioni F, Mainardi F, Zanchin G. Rofecoxib for the treatment of chronic paroxysmal hemicrania. Cephalalgia 2003;23:318–20.

51. Coria F, Clavería LE, Jiménez-Jiménez FJ, de Seijas EV. Episodic paroxysmal hemicrania responsive to calcium channel blockers. J Neurol Neurosurg Psychiatry 1992;55:166.

52. Shabbir N, McAbee G. Adolescent chronic paroxysmal hemicrania responsive to verapamil monotherapy. Headache 1994;34:209–10.

53. Warner JS, Wamil AW, McLean MJ. Acetazolamide for the treatment of chronic paroxysmal hemicrania. Headache 1994;34:597–9.

54. Hannerz J, Ericson K, Bergstrand G. Chronic paroxysmal hemicrania: orbital phlebography and steroid treatment. A case report. Cephalalgia 1987;7:189–92.

# Short-Lasting, Unilateral, Neuralgiform Headache Attacks with Conjunctival Injection and Tearing (SUNCT) Syndrome

Manjit S. Matharu, MRCP, and Peter J. Goadsby, MD, PhD, DSc, FRACP, FRCP

Short-lasting, unilateral, neuralgiform headache attacks with conjunctival injection and tearing (SUNCT) syndrome, as its name implies, is a disorder characterized by strictly unilateral, severe, neuralgiform attacks centered on the ophthalmic trigeminal distribution that are brief in duration and occur in association with conjunctival injection and lacrimation. SUNCT syndrome was described only relatively recently in 1978[1] and more fully characterized in 1989.[2] Goadsby and Lipton proposed diagnostic criteria for SUNCT syndrome in 1997.[3] The syndrome is now sufficiently validated, and the second edition of the International Headache Society (IHS) classification criteria recognizes SUNCT syndrome as a subgroup of trigeminal autonomic cephalgias (TACs) (Table 8–1).[4] A review of 21 patients (19 primary and 2 secondary cases) was initially published in 1997.[5] More recently, a comprehensive review of 63 SUNCT patients was published.[6] This chapter provides a review of 82 SUNCT (64 primary and 18 secondary cases) patients reported in the English-language literature to date.

## EPIDEMIOLOGY

The prevalence or incidence of primary (idiopathic) SUNCT syndrome is not known, although the extremely low number of reported cases suggests that it is a very rare syndrome. The disorder has a male predominance (35 males, 29 females) with a male to female ratio of 1.2:1. In an earlier review of SUNCT syndrome, the male preponderance among primary cases was greater than that reported here, with a male to female ratio of 3.75 (15 males, 4 females).[5] The trend toward increasing the female to male ratio over time probably reflects an ascertainment issue. The typical age at onset is between 35 and 65 years (69% of primary SUNCT

cases), although it ranges from 10 to 77 years (mean 50 ± 15 years). The mean duration of the disorder at reporting was 7 ± 8 years (range 6 months to 48 years).

## CLINICAL FEATURES

### Site of Pain

The pain is usually maximal in the ophthalmic distribution of the trigeminal nerve, especially the orbital or retro-orbital regions (91%), forehead (50%), and temple (31%). It may radiate to the other ipsilateral trigeminal divisions (cheek, 14%; nose, 6%; lip, 3%; palate, 2%; gums, 2%; upper teeth, 2%) and, rarely, even to extratrigeminal regions such as the ear[5,7] and occiput.[8,9] There is one report of a case purported to be extratrigeminal SUNCT syndrome with pain centered on the throat without trigeminal involvement; although the authors raise the possibility that it may represent glossopharyngeal neuralgia, it is noteworthy that the clinical phenotype, including the temporal profile of the

**Table 8–1**  Diagnostic Features of Short-Lasting, Unilateral, Neuralgiform Headache Attacks with Conjunctival Injection and Tearing (SUNCT)

A. At least 20 attacks fulfilling criteria B–E

B. Attacks of unilateral orbital, supraorbital, or temporal stabbing or pulsating pain lasting from 5–240 s

C. Attack frequency from 3–200/d

D. Pain is accompanied by ipsilateral conjunctival injection and lacrimation

E. Not attributed to another disorder

Adapted from Headache Classification Committee, International Headache Society.[4]

pain and the intense cranial autonomic symptoms, was otherwise typical for SUNCT syndrome.[10]

## Laterality of Attack

Attacks are typically strictly unilateral and side-locked (89%); however, in four patients (6%), the pain was simultaneously experienced on the opposite side,[5,11] whereas three patients (5%) reported strictly unilateral but side-alternating attacks.[8,12,13]

The pain is present more frequently on the right side (47%) than the left (40%) in primary SUNCT patients (right-sided attacks, 26 patients; left-sided attacks, 22 patients; bilateral attacks, 3 patients; side-alternating attacks, 4 patients; data not available on 9 patients).

## Severity of Pain

The intensity of the pain is generally severe. In the 64 primary SUNCT cases reviewed, the usual pain intensity was described as moderate in 6 patients (14%), severe or intense in 27 patients (63%), and very severe or excruciating in 10 patients (23%). Five of the 27 patients with severe pain were reported to have a pain intensity ranging from moderate to severe. In 21 patients, data on the intensity of the pain were not available. The intensity of pain in SUNCT syndrome has generally been described as moderate to severe.[5] However, our data suggest that the intensity of pain is severe in the majority of patients and moderate in a small minority only. This is in line with our own clinical experience in that the SUNCT patients we have managed describe the severity of their pain as ranging between severe and excruciating.

## Character of Pain

The pain had a neuralgic character in the majority of patients (46 patients; 85%), usually being described as stabbing, sharp, burning, pricking, piercing, shooting, lancinating, or electric shock–like. The character of pain was described as pulsatile or throbbing in 3 patients (6%), steady in 2 patients (4%), spasmodic in 1 patient (2%), staccato in 1 patient (2%) and pressing in 1 patient (2%). No description of character of pain was given in 10 cases.

## Duration of the Individual Attack

Three different types of pain have been described in SUNCT syndrome: relatively short-lasting attacks, long-lasting attacks, and a continuous or intermittent background ache.

The individual short-lasting attacks are very brief, lasting between 5 and 120 seconds in the majority of patients (51 patients, 84%). The attacks were described as lasting less than 5 seconds in 5 patients (8%) and more than 120 seconds in 5 patients (8%). No data were available on 3 patients. The median duration of the usual attack was 40 seconds. The range of the usual attack

duration was between 2 seconds and 20 minutes.[8,13,14] In a study that objectively measured the duration of 348 attacks in 11 patients, the range of duration was 5 to 250 seconds, and the mean duration was 49 seconds.[15]

There are four reported cases of SUNCT syndrome in whom prolonged attacks, lasting 1 to 2 hours, are described.[16–18] In all of these patients, the majority of the attacks were short-lasting and were otherwise typical for SUNCT syndrome; the relatively long-lasting attacks were phenotypically similar to the short-lasting attacks except for the duration of the attack.

Most patients are completely pain free between attacks, although there are seven case reports of a dull interictal ipsilateral discomfort over the same site; the interictal discomfort has been reported to be continuous in five cases[5,11,13,14] and intermittent in the other two.[19,20] There is also one case report of a bilateral continuous interictal discomfort over the forehead.[13] In addition, a burning sensation lasting 2 hours following the attacks has also been reported.[21]

## Temporal Profile of the Individual Attack

The short-lasting paroxysms begin abruptly, reaching the maximum intensity within 2 to 3 seconds.[5] In the majority of patients, the pain is maintained at the maximum intensity before abating rapidly. However, several temporal patterns for the individual attack, besides the plateau-like pattern, have been described, including a repetitive pattern of spike-like paroxysms; a sawtooth pattern, in which repetitive spike-like paroxysms occur without reaching the pain-free baseline between the individual spikes; and plateau-like plus exacerbations pattern, in which a plateau-like attack had superimposed, random, ultrashort exacerbations of 1 to 2 seconds.[22]

## Frequency and Periodicity of Attacks

In the majority of patients, SUNCT syndrome presents in an episodic manner; the temporal pattern is quite variable, with the symptomatic periods alternating with remissions in an erratic manner. Symptomatic periods generally last from a few days to several months and occur once or twice annually, although a maximum of 22 bouts per annum have been reported.[5] Remissions typically last a few months, although they can range from 1 week to 8.5 years.[23] Symptomatic periods appear to increase in frequency and duration over time.[5] Circannual periodicity is not typically a feature of SUNCT.

Earlier reviews noted that the chronic form of SUNCT was not sufficiently validated.[24] However, there are now 18 case reports in which the disorder was clearly chronic, with the symptomatic period lasting more than 1 year. In these cases, the mean duration of the chronic phase was 5.3 ± 5.0 years (range 1 to 17 years). In 13 of these cases, the disorder was chronic from onset.[3,13,17,20,25–31] In 5 patients, the disorder was episodic at onset before transforming into the chronic form.[11,13,18,32,33] In addition, there are several case reports of SUNCT syndrome in which the chronic phase alternates with the episodic phase.[2,28,34,35] These data indicate that the chronic form of SUNCT is now sufficiently validated; therefore, the subclassification of SUNCT syndrome should include episodic and chronic forms, thereby bringing it in line with that of cluster headache and paroxysmal hemicrania.

The attack frequency during the symptomatic phase varies immensely between sufferers and within an individual sufferer. Attacks may be as infrequent as once a day or less to more than 60 per hour.[36] Objective assessment of the frequency of attacks in four patients demonstrated a mean of 16 attacks daily, with a range of 1 to 86 attacks daily.[15] There are six case reports of a SUNCT-like status, when patients experience severe exacerbations with frequent, easily triggered, high-intensity pain attacks in a repetitive and overlapping fashion for several hours or days at a time.[5,28,36]

SUNCT attacks occur either exclusively or predominantly during the daytime. Exclusively diurnal attacks were reported in 5 (17%) patients. Nocturnal attacks were reported to occur occasionally in 20 (66%) patients and frequently in 5 (17%) patients. However, these results need to be interpreted cautiously because no data were available in over half of the reported cases (34 patients; 53%). Objective assessment of the timing of 585 attacks in 4 patients demonstrated that a bimodal distribution occurs with morning and afternoon or evening predominance, with only 1.2% occurring at night; however, given the small number of patients studied, these data need to be interpreted cautiously.[15] Although we agree that the attacks are predominantly diurnal in SUNCT, we feel that this is overstated because we have seen several cases in whom frequent nocturnal attacks occur. The timing of the attacks needs to be studied objectively in a larger and more representative group.

## Associated Features

Acute headache episodes in SUNCT syndrome are accompanied by a variety of associated symptoms. The attacks are virtually always accompanied by both ipsilateral conjunctival injection (64 patients; 100%) and lacrimation (61 patients; 95%). Ipsilateral rhinorrhea (35 patients; 55%), nasal congestion (28 patients; 44%), eyelid edema (19 patients; 30%), ptosis (12 patients; 19%), miosis (4 patients; 6%), and facial redness (4 patients; 6%) or sweating (2 patients; 3%) are less commonly reported. These cranial autonomic symptoms, particularly conjunctival injection and lacrimation, are typically very prominent in SUNCT syndrome. The associated conjunctival injection and tearing usually begin 1 to 2 seconds after onset of the pain and may outlast the pain by a few seconds. Rhinorrhea, when present, is delayed, occurring relatively late in the course of

the headache.[5] Unlike in cluster headache, restlessness is not a prominent feature of SUNCT syndrome and has been described only in four patients.[13,20]

Nausea (one patient; 2%), vomiting, photophobia (three patients; 5%), phonophobia (one patient; 2%), osmophobia, and worsening of pain with movement (two patients; 3%) are not normally associated with SUNCT syndrome. A migrainous aura in association with SUNCT was reported in two patients. There is a report of tingling sensation over the ipsilateral temple in association with the attacks[36] and another report of ipsilateral facial tingling lasting 5 to 10 minutes and occurring 5 to 15 minutes prior to the SUNCT attacks.[13]

## Triggers

Most SUNCT patients have both spontaneous and triggered attacks (48 patients), whereas a minority seem to exhibit exclusively spontaneous attacks (9 patients). No patients had exclusively triggered attacks, and data were not available on 7 patients.

Data on the triggers were available in 40 of the 48 patients with triggerable attacks. The most commonly reported triggers were touching certain trigger zones within trigeminal innervated distribution and, occasionally, even from an extratrigeminal territory (29 patients; 73%), mastication (27 patients; 68%), and head or neck movements (15 patients; 38%). Less common triggers included talking (8 patients; 20%), brushing teeth (7 patients; 18%), blowing the nose (7 patients; 18%), air blowing on the face (7 patients; 18%), swallowing (6 patients; 15%), rapid eye movements (6 patients; 15%), coughing (5 patients; 13%), sneezing (5 patients; 13%), bright lights (5 patients; 13%), yawning (4 patients; 10%), touching the palate with the tongue (3 patients; 8%), squeezing the eyes (3 patients; 8%), making sudden or jerking movements (2 patients; 5%), emotional stress (2 patients; 5%), walking (2 patients; 5%), putting ice in the mouth (2 patients; 5%), laughing (1 patient; 3%), loud noises (1 patient; 3%), mental concentration (1 patient; 3%), physical exertion (1 patient; 3%), and bending forward (1 patient; 3%). Some patients could lessen or abort the attacks by continuously rotating their neck.[2,5]

## Refractory Period

It has been suggested that, unlike in trigeminal neuralgia, most SUNCT patients have no refractory period.[5] Indeed, 11 case reports either explicitly state or implicitly suggest that there is a lack of a refractory period.[9,13,14,22,32,36–38] In contrast, there are two case reports of an absolute refractory period in SUNCT syndrome.[39,40] In addition, there is a report of a patient with both short- and long-lasting attacks who demonstrated the presence of an absolute refractory period after the prolonged attacks in the absence of even a relative refractory period after the shorter attacks.[18] However, these data need to be interpreted with caution because 50 case reports make no mention of a refractory period. This may be due to a lack of awareness of this feature; consequently, refractoriness in SUNCT syndrome may be underreported.

## Comorbidity

Two patients reported a history of migraine with aura.[5,18] There are three case reports of the headaches starting as trigeminal neuralgia before "transformation" to SUNCT.[19,28,41] This led to the suggestion that trigeminal neuralgia and SUNCT represent different spectrums of the same disorder.[19,41] Conversely, the differences in the clinical phenotypes and treatment response overwhelmingly suggest that they are distinct syndromes (Table 8–2).[42–44] What, then, is the explanation for the purported "transformation" from trigeminal neuralgia to SUNCT in these cases? One possibility is that they represent the co-occurrence of two distinct headache syndromes. An alternative possibility is that a headache syndrome may express different clinical phenotypes, for example, migraine patients often also have tension-type headaches, the biologic basis of which is probably different from pure tension-type headaches.[45]

Comorbidity with other diseases or disorders was noted in a number of patients. The most frequently reported condition was arterial hypertension in eight patients. Glaucoma and otitis media were reported in three and two patients, respectively. The following conditions and surgical procedures were reported in one patient each: diabetes mellitus, hypercholesterolemia, atrial fibrillation, supraventricular tachycardia, hypothyroidism, stroke, chemical meningitis after

exposure to a bacterioside, postconcussional anosmia, essential tremor, sinusitis, bacterial pneumonia, infectious mononucleosis, chicken pox, herpes zoster infection affecting trigeminal mandibular distribution, postviral fatigue syndrome, ambylopia, laryngeal cancer, prostatic cancer, immunoglobulin G lambda monoclonal gammopathy, adrenal adenoma, multinodular goiter, renal cysts, prostatic hypertrophy, chronic active hepatitis, duodenal ulcer, hiatus hernia, post-traumatic stress disorder, chronic anxiety, depression, periodontitis, thrombophlebitis, osteoarthritis, Caldwell-Luc procedure, hysterectomy, inguinal hernia repair, surgery for calcaneal spur, cholecystectomy, and cholelithiasis. No pattern of association of a disease or disorder with SUNCT could be noted.

### Physical Examination

The physical examination is normal in the vast majority of patients. Slight allodynia or hyperesthesia over the ophthalmic and mandibular trigeminal divisions has been reported in seven patients.[5,7,11,21,29] Trigeminal hypoesthesia has been reported in four patients,[5,13,14] although two of these patients had previously had invasive surgical procedures of the trigeminal nerve.[13,14] Horner's syndrome was previously thought not to be a feature of SUNCT. However, there have been two recent descriptions of persistent Horner's syndrome in association with SUNCT.[31,38] Persistent ipsilateral ptosis[20] and eyelid edema[19,31] were reported in one and two patients, respectively. One patient was described as having transient ipsilateral miosis without ptosis that lasted one bout only.[2]

## SECONDARY SUNCT

There are 18 case reports of secondary SUNCT syndrome in the medical literature. A close scrutiny of these cases reveals that the pathologic lesions occurred at two main sites: the posterior fossa and the pituitary gland.

There are eight case reports of SUNCT syndrome secondary to a posterior fossa abnormality, including homolateral cerebellopontine angle arteriovenous malformations in two patients,[46,47] a brainstem cavernous hemangioma,[48] a posterior fossa lesion in a patient with human immunodeficiency virus/acquired immune deficiency syndrome (HIV/AIDS),[3] severe basilar impression causing pontomedullary compression in a patient with osteogenesis imperfecta,[49] craniosynostosis resulting in a foreshortened posterior fossa,[50] ischemic brainstem infarction,[51] and a homolateral pontocerebellar astrocytoma.[52] In addition, there is a case report of SUNCT in association with two intracranial lesions, suggestive of meningiomas, at the homolateral cerebellopontine angle and frontal lobe.[53]

There are five case reports of SUNCT syndrome secondary to pituitary adenomas in the medical litera-

**Table 8–2** Differentiating Features of SUNCT Syndrome and Trigeminal Neuralgia

| Feature | SUNCT | Trigeminal Neuralgia |
|---|---|---|
| Gender ratio, male:female | 1.2:1 | 1:2 |
| Site of pain | V1 | V2/3 |
| Severity of pain | Severe | Very severe |
| Duration, s | 5–240 | < 5 |
| Autonomic features | Prominent | Sparse or none |
| Refractory period | Absent | Present |
| Response to carbamazepine | Partial | Complete |

SUNCT = short-lasting, unilateral, neuralgiform headache with conjunctival injection and tearing.

ture. Before the acronym SUNCT was proposed, a patient with a nonfunctioning pituitary macroadenoma and trigeminal neuralgia-like attacks, compatible with a diagnosis of SUNCT syndrome, was described.[54] The differential diagnosis between trigeminal neuralgia and SUNCT can be difficult. Subsequently, Massiou and colleagues described two patients with SUNCT syndrome and prolactinomas; one of the patients had a microprolactinoma, whereas the other had a macroprolactinoma with cavernous sinus invasion.[55] Recently, we described two additional patients with SUNCT syndrome and prolactinomas; one of the patients had a microprolactinoma,[56] whereas the other had a macroprolactinoma with cavernous sinus invasion.[57] The significance of these cases is further underlined by the findings that headache was the initial presentation in all cases of prolactinoma reported hitherto and that there can be a considerable time lag before the onset of pituitary-related symptoms. Hence, all patients presenting with suspected SUNCT syndrome should be questioned for symptoms associated with pituitary neoplasms either due to a hormonal imbalance or a mass effect.

There are four other case reports of secondary SUNCT syndrome. There is a report of SUNCT in association with a cavernous sinus leiomyosarcoma[58] and another in association with an orbital cyst.[59] A case of SUNCT in an HIV-positive patient, in whom there were no opportunistic infections and brain imaging was normal, was reported; the authors raised the possibility of a causal relationship between the two conditions,[60] although an alternative explanation is a coincidental occurrence of the two conditions. A patient with episodic SUNCT in whom magnetic resonance imaging (MRI) demonstrated compression of the ipsilateral trigeminal nerve by the superior cerebellar artery was reported.[61] This sole case of vascular compression of the trigeminal nerve in SUNCT contrasts with trigeminal neuralgia, in which it is reported in 47 to 77% of the patients.[62–65]

## DIFFERENTIAL DIAGNOSIS

The differential diagnosis of very brief headaches includes SUNCT (primary and secondary forms), trigeminal neuralgia, primary stabbing headache, and paroxysmal hemicrania.

Differentiating SUNCT from trigeminal neuralgia can be challenging in some cases because there is a considerable overlap in the clinical phenotypes of the two syndromes. Both headaches are short-lasting, can have a high frequency of attacks, and display clustering of attacks. Both are principally unilateral headaches, and the trigger zones behave similarly. The usual onset is during middle or old age in both. However, there are a number of striking differences between these two

syndromes (see Table 8–2), awareness of which can aid in their differentiation.[42]

Primary stabbing headache (also known as idiopathic stabbing headache) refers to brief, sharp, or jabbing pain in the head that occurs either as a single episode or in brief repeated volleys. The pain is usually over the ophthalmic trigeminal distribution, whereas the face is generally spared. The pain usually lasts a fraction of a second but can persist for up to 1 minute, thereby overlapping with the phenotype of SUNCT, and recurs at irregular intervals (hours to days). These headaches are generally easily distinguishable clinically because they differ in several respects: in primary stabbing headache, there is a female preponderance; the site and radiation of pain often vary between attacks; the majority of the attacks tend to be spontaneous; cranial autonomic features are absent; and the attacks commonly subside with the administration of indomethacin.[66]

SUNCT syndrome also has to be differentiated from short-lasting paroxysmal hemicrania. Paroxysmal hemicrania prevails in females, the attacks have a uniform distribution through day and night, the triggers differ from those in SUNCT, and the attacks are exquisitely responsive to indomethacin. If there is any diagnostic uncertainty, then a trial of indomethacin is warranted.

## INVESTIGATIONS

The association of secondary SUNCT syndrome with pituitary and posterior fossa abnormalities emphasizes the absolute need for cranial MRI, including an adequate view of the pituitary. In addition, these patients should have a screen for basal hormone measurements, including prolactin, thyroid-stimulating hormone, free thyroxine, cortisol, adrenocorticotrophic hormone, luteinizing hormone, follicle-stimulating hormone, estrogen, testosterone, and growth hormone. We routinely perform a therapeutic trial of indomethacin to exclude an indomethacin-responsive headache.

## TREATMENT

### Drug Therapies

Several categories of drugs used in headache and other pain syndromes have been tried in SUNCT. Most of these drugs have been reported to be ineffectual, and, until recently, SUNCT was thought to be highly refractory to treatment. The drug therapies that have been tried in SUNCT are reviewed below.

## Nonsteroidal Anti-Inflammatory Drugs and Cyclooxygenase 2 Inhibitors

Nonsteroidal anti-inflammatory drugs (NSAIDs), including aspirin, diclofenac, ibuprofen, ketoprofen, mefenamic acid, naproxen, and piroxicam, are ineffective in SUNCT.[12,13,26,27,67] Indomethacin (administered orally at 100 to 300 mg daily in 36 patients and 100 mg intramuscular injection in 4 patients) has generally been found to be ineffective[3,7,8,11–14,18,20,21,26–31,33,34,36,38,41,67–70]; only 1 patient reported a partial benefit, with oral indomethacin 150 mg daily reducing the severity but not the frequency of attacks.[25]

The cyclooxygenase 2 inhibitors nimesulide and celecoxib have been tried in SUNCT. Nimesulide was reported to be ineffective in one patient.[12] Celecoxib was partially effective in one patient but had to be discontinued because of significant side effects, whereas it was ineffective in another patient.[13,70]

## Analgesics

Simple analgesics (acetaminophen [paracetamol], aspirin, metamizole)[7,8,12,27,31,67] and opiates (tramadol, buprenorphine, codeine, dihydrocodeine, hydrocodone, meperidine, morphine)[13,28,67,71] have been tried without benefit, except in one patient treated with hydrocodone 10 mg and acetaminophen 500 mg who experienced a slight reduction in the intensity of the pain.[14]

## Oxygen

Inhalation of oxygen as abortive treatment has been tried in nine patients without benefit.[11,13,18,19,22,34,37,70] We have tried high-dose and flow-rate oxygen (100% at 7 to 12 L/min) in several patients without any beneficial response (AS Cohen et al, unpublished observations).

## Serotoninergic Agonists and Antagonists

Sumatriptan has been tested, either orally (100 to 300 mg daily) or subcutaneously (6 mg), in 15 patients. One patient who received the oral formulation had a slight improvement, whereas 4 patients who received the subcutaneous formulation were reported to have a positive response, with no spontaneous attacks occurring for 3 to 5 hours following administration[28,34,67]; 10 patients failed to respond.[3,7,11,13,14,18,36,67] No trials of the other triptans have been reported. There is one case report of a poor response to "triptans" but the authors did not state which triptans were tried.[70] In contrast to the occasional response reported with sumatriptan, ergot derivatives have been universally ineffective. Oral or intravenous ergotamine and intravenous dihydroergotamine were ineffectual in 12 patients.[3,7,14,28,34,67,72] It is interesting to note that one patient who responded to sumatriptan failed to respond to ergotamine.[28]

Methysergide has been tried in eight patients.[3,14,28,34,67,70] It was ineffective in six patients, led to a worsening in one patient, and was partially effective in one patient but had to be discontinued because of significant side effects. Pizotifen was ineffective in the two patients treated with this agent.[3,13]

## Adrenoreceptor Agonists and Antagonists

The β-blockers propranolol and timolol have been tested in SUNCT. Oral propranolol has been tried in three patients, without any benefit.[2,3] Timolol eyedrops were reported to be ineffective in two patients.[67] Guanethidine eyedrops, which act at the sympathetic neuroeffector junction by inhibiting or interfering with the release and distribution of catecholamines, were ineffective in one patient.[67] Clonidine, a central α-adrenoreceptor agonist, did not produce a beneficial response in one patient.[14] Similarly, doxazosin, an $\alpha_1$-adrenoreceptor blocker, was ineffective in two patients.[67]

## Histamine Desensitization and Antagonist

Histamine desensitization has been attempted in one patient without benefit.[67] Cyproheptadine, an antihistaminic and antiserotoninergic agent, was reported to produce a transient initial improvement before becoming ineffective in one patient.[34]

## Calcium Channel Antagonists

The therapeutic response of various calcium channel antagonists, including verapamil, nifedipine, amlodipine, flunarizine, and diltiazem, has been examined in SUNCT syndrome. Verapamil has been tried in 18 patients.[3,7,11,14,18–21,23,27–29,67,70] In 17 patients, it was tried alone; in 2 of these patients, it was also tried in combination with other medications.[11,14] In one patient, it was tried only in combination with other medications.[18] When verapamil was administered solely, it was ineffective in all patients; in fact, five patients reported a worsening of the attacks with verapamil.[3,23,67] Of the three patients in whom it was used in combination with other agents, a beneficial response was reported in two of them; in one patient, verapamil was highly effective when used in combination with carbamazepine,[18] whereas it was partially effective when used in combination with carbamazepine, naloxone, and lithium in the other patient.[11] A trial of verapamil as a pharmacologic precipitant of attacks was advocated in SUNCT syndrome.[23] This approach is likely to be fraught with difficulties given that verapamil induces a worsening in only about one-third of patients, there is a marked spontaneous variability in the attack frequency of SUNCT syndrome, the placebo and nocebo response rates are unknown, and there is an ethical concern of administering a drug that worsens a pain syndrome in the absence of a rapidly effective abortive or preventive agent.

Nifedipine has been tried in one patient in whom it reduced the frequency of attacks and the intensity of pain by approximately 50%.[2] Amlodipine has been reported to worsen the attacks in the sole patient to whom it was administered.[23] Flunarizine and diltiazem have been tried in two and one patient, respectively, without any benefit.[36,67,73]

### γ-Aminobutyric Acid Agonists

Baclofen is a structural analog of the inhibitory neurotransmitter γ-aminobutyric acid (GABA) and exerts its effects by stimulation of the GABA$_B$ receptor. It has been tried in eight patients with SUNCT syndrome, without any benefit.[13,14,20,28,35,41,67,68]

The benzodiazepines are agonists at the GABA$_A$ receptor. They increase channel opening frequency at the GABA$_A$ receptor, resulting in an enhanced chloride uptake into the neuron and neuronal hyperpolarization. The three benzodiazepines that have been tried in SUNCT syndrome, namely, diazepam,[11] clonazepam,[13,14,41,68] and lorazepam,[19] were ineffective in one, four, and one patient, respectively.

### Tricyclic Antidepressants

The main mechanism of action of the tricyclic antidepressants is the inhibition of neural uptake of serotonin and noradrenaline, although they possess antagonistic properties at a variety of neurotransmitter receptors, including muscarinic cholinergic receptors, $\alpha_1$-adrenoreceptors, and H$_1$-histamine receptors. The tricyclic antidepressants that have been tried in SUNCT include amitriptyline, nortriptyline, lofepramine, imipramine, and desipramine. Amitriptyline has been used in 13 patients[3,13,14,21,26–29,34,41,67,68]; it was ineffective in all except one patient, in whom it reduced the frequency of attacks and the intensity of pain by approximately 50%.[41] There is one case report of a patient who transiently improved on nortriptyline when used in combination with valproate and prednisone.[19] Lofepramine, imipramine, and desipramine were reported to be ineffective in one patient each.[2,13]

### Selective Serotonin Reuptake Inhibitors

Fluoxetine was reported to be ineffective in one patient.[13] One case report states that selective serotonin reuptake inhibitors were tried without any beneficial response in a patient, although the agents used were not stated.[73]

### Lithium

Lithium is thought to act, at least in part, on second-messenger systems, including the adenylate cyclases, phosphoinositol turnover, and calcium influx, via various mechanisms.[74] It has been tried in seven patients with SUNCT syndrome, without any beneficial effect.[3,14,19,28,67] On the other hand, lithium used in com-bination with verapamil, carbamazepine, and naloxone was reported to be partially effective in one patient.[11]

### Corticosteroids and Azathioprine

The response to corticosteroids has been reported in 18 patients. Eleven patients were administered prednisone,[7,19,29,34,67] and five patients were administered prednisolone or methylprednisolone.[11,13,14,21,36] In two patients, it was stated that corticosteroids were tried, but the agent used was not stated.[3,26] Four of the 11 patients taking prednisone reported a beneficial response: 2 reported a partial effect,[2,34] 1 reported a complete response,[7] and 1, who used prednisone in combination with valproate and nortriptyline, improved transiently.[19] Two of the five patients taking prednisolone or methylprednisolone also reported a beneficial response: one patient treated with prednisolone and carbamazepine reported a complete response,[21] whereas the other treated with intravenous methylprednisolone, in combination with carbamazepine and followed by oral prednisolone, was seemingly rendered pain free on three occasions for a variable period of time.[36]

Azathioprine was claimed to be beneficial in a patient who demonstrated a partial response to prednisone.[34]

### Anticonvulsants

Several anticonvulsants, including carbamazepine, phenytoin, valproic acid, lamotrigine, gabapentin, and topiramate, have been tried in SUNCT syndrome. The therapeutic response of these agents in SUNCT is reviewed below.

Carbamazepine acts via blockade of use- and frequency-dependent sodium channels, although a blockade of the *N*-methyl-D-aspartate receptor–activated sodium and calcium influx and the effects on the purine, monoamine, and acetylcholine receptors have also been proposed. The therapeutic response to car-bamazepine was reported in 45 cases. In 30 of these cases, there was no beneficial response with the sole use of carbamazepine.[3,7,11,13,14,19,20,26–31,33,36,41,67–71] However, two of these nonresponders demonstrated a partial or good response when carbamazepine was used in com-bination with other agents: a partial response was reported with a combination of carbamazepine, naloxone, verapamil, and lithium in one patient,[11] whereas the other patient treated with carbamazepine, in combination with intravenous methylprednisolone and followed by oral prednisolone, was seemingly rendered pain free on three occasions for a variable period of time.[36] In 11 of the 45 cases, a partial response was reported,[8,9,13,21,38,67] although in some patients, this was variable[28] or transient.[14,35] A complete or almost complete response was noted in four patients. One of these patients responded completely and consistently for 2 years to carbamazepine alone but thereafter required a combination of carbamazepine and verapamil to render him pain free.[18] Another patient had substantial relief on carbamazepine and prednisolone.[21] The third patient had complete relief with some courses of treatment, but this effect was inconsistent.[34] The fourth patient responded consistently and almost completely over 10 years.[31]

Phenytoin acts largely by blocking ionic movements in the sodium channel during the depolarization process. It may also modulate GABA receptors and inhibit neurotransmitter release by reducing calcium-dependent phosphorylation of membrane proteins. Phenytoin was tried in 13 patients and was reported to be ineffective in all except 2 patients.[13,14,20,28,31,34,67,70,71] A possible slight improvement was noted in one patient,[67] whereas a single intravenous injection of phenytoin 250 mg was reported to have reduced the attack frequency and severity for 2 hours in another patient.[31]

Valproic acid is thought to act via multiple mechanisms, which include the inhibition of excitatory amino acids (glutamate, aspartate, $\gamma$-hydroxybutyrate) and the reduction of the excitability of neuronal membranes through its influence on sodium and potassium channels. Valproic acid was tried in 11 patients with SUNCT syndrome. It was ineffective in nine patients and produced a possible slight improvement in one patient.[3,13,14,20,67,70] There is one case report of a patient who responded completely but transiently on a combination of valproate, nortriptyline, and prednisone.[19]

Lamotrigine acts mainly by blockade of voltage-dependent sodium channel conductance, although antifolate, antiglutamate, and antiaspartate actions have been suggested. Recently, lamotrigine was reported to be highly efficacious in 12 SUNCT patients.[8,27,30,33,69–71] Lamotrigine, given in an open manner at 100 to 400 mg daily, induced a complete remission in nine patients and produced about an 80% improvement in the other three patients. Conversely, it was reported to be ineffective in three patients,[13,14] although the maximum dose of lamotrigine that was tried in one of these patients was only 50 mg daily. In addition, one patient had to discontinue lamotrigine after a few days of initiation of treatment owing to development of Stevens-Johnson syndrome.[29]

Gabapentin is thought to act via blockade of voltage-gated calcium channels and may be a $GABA_B$ agonist, although the precise knowledge of its mechanism of action remains elusive. Gabapentin was tried in 13 SUNCT patients. It was highly effective in three patients, completely suppressing the attacks when used at 800 to 2,700 mg daily.[7,25,75] However, it was reported to be completely ineffective in 10 patients.[13,14,18,26,28,31,36,71]

Topiramate has multiple mechanisms of action. It exerts its action through blockade of the voltage-gated sodium channels, enhancement of GABA-mediated chloride influx involving the $GABA_A$ receptor, and antagonism of the glutamate kainate/$\alpha$-amino-3-hydroxy-5-methyl-4-isoxazoleproprionic acid (AMPA) receptor. The effect of topiramate in SUNCT was reported in eight cases. Topiramate was ineffective in three patients,[14,30] whereas five patients responded completely to topiramate at 50 to 300 mg daily.[13,29,76]

### Lidocaine

Lidocaine mediates its effect through blockade of sodium channels. An intravenous lidocaine 100 mg bolus followed by 4 mg/min over 48 hours was reported to be ineffective when administered to two patients with SUNCT syndrome.[67] In contrast, intravenous lidocaine 1.3 to 3.3 mg/kg/h was highly effective at completely suppressing the headaches in four SUNCT patients.[13]

Intranasal lidocaine was reported to be ineffective in six cases.[13,18,67] In addition, intranasal local anesthetic was stated to be ineffective in one case, although the agent used was not stated.[35] Lidocaine mouthwash was reported to produce a possible, slight improvement in two of five patients.[67]

### Miscellaneous Drugs

Other agents reported to be ineffective in SUNCT syndrome include neuroleptics (pimozide, levomepromazine), central nervous system stimulants (methylphenidate, pemoline), somatostatin, angiotensin-converting enzyme inhibitors (captopril, enalapril), aprotinin, tranexamic acid, omeprazole, vitamin $B_{12}$, and acyclovir.[11,34,36,67]

### Conclusion

Open-label studies and case reports clearly play an important role in the generation and testing of hypotheses. In SUNCT syndrome, several groups of pharmacologic strategies have been excluded and a partial or complete effectiveness suggested with the use of sumatriptan, corticosteroids, lamotrigine, topiramate, gabapentin, carbamazepine, and intravenous lidocaine. However, the ultimate confirmation of the effectiveness of any agent in the treatment of this syndrome should come from randomized, double-blind, placebo-controlled clinical trials because open studies are difficult to judge for various reasons, including the following: there is probably a publication bias involved in that positive results are more likely to be published than negative ones; in some case reports, measures of efficacy are not adequately described; the highly variable frequency of attacks in SUNCT syndrome makes it difficult to determine whether an agent is truly potent; and it is difficult to distinguish a true response from a placebo effect. It has been suggested that controlled trials are not required in TACs because these conditions do not demonstrate a placebo effect[67,77]; in fact, this has now been demonstrated to be an erroneous supposition, at least in cluster headache, in which the reported placebo response rate is 7 to 62%.[78,79] No controlled studies have been published in paroxysmal hemicrania and SUNCT syndrome.

On the basis of the data available in the literature and our clinical experience, we have outlined our approach to the management of SUNCT syndrome. Lamotrigine is the treatment of choice, whereas topiramate and, perhaps, gabapentin are reasonable second-line agents in patients who fail a trial of lamotrigine. It should be remembered that some patients have a useful response to carbamazepine, and its use can be considered if the other agents are ineffective. When patients with SUNCT syndrome experience severe exacerbations with frequent, easily triggered, high-intensity pain attacks, acute interventions are needed because the patients are severely affected. They may not be able to eat or drink because these actions trigger attacks. In that situation, intravenous lidocaine can be used to temporarily ameliorate the attacks while conventional therapy is being optimized. Corticosteroids can also be considered in this situation, although they need to be used with caution because of the potential for serious side effects, especially with prolonged courses. Given the short-lasting transient effect of sumatriptan, it has no role in the management of SUNCT syndrome.

It is interesting to note that the common mechanism of action in lamotrigine, topiramate, lidocaine, and carbamazepine is blockade of sodium channels. This raises the possibility that the therapeutic response of effective agents is mediated via sodium channel blockade. However, some sodium channel blockers, such as valproic acid and phenytoin, do not appear to be beneficial in SUNCT syndrome. Advances in the delineation of the pathophysiologic basis of SUNCT syndrome and characterization of the mechanism of action of the pharmacologic agents are likely to lead to better treatments for this condition.

## Surgery

Several surgical approaches have been tried in SUNCT syndrome. The approaches attempted can be subdivided into two main groups: local blockades and invasive procedures involving the trigeminal nerve.

### Local Blockades

Local blockades of pericranial nerves with anesthetics, alcohol, phenol, or opioids have generally been reported to be ineffectual.

Supraorbital blockades were reported in 10 patients; the blockades were performed with lidocaine in 7 patients, bupivacaine in 1 patient, bupivacaine and corticosteroids in 1 patient, and alcohol in 1 patient.[28,67,70] The blockades were ineffective at suppressing spontaneous attacks in all patients, although it was more difficult to precipitate attacks by touching the anesthetized area in some patients. Infraorbital blockades were performed in nine patients; the blockades were performed with lidocaine in six patients, alcohol in one patient, bupivacaine and phenol (at different times) in one patient, and an unnamed local anesthetic in one patient.[28,67] These blockades were ineffective in all patients except one who received phenol, in whom a variable benefit lasting 1 to 12 months was reported. Lidocaine blockades of the greater occipital nerve, lacrimal nerve, orbicularis oculi muscles, and retrobulbar region were performed in three, one, two, and one patient, respectively, without any beneficial responses.[67] Similarly, greater occipital nerve blockade with bupivacaine and corticosteroid was reported to be ineffective in one patient.[70]

One patient has had a stellate ganglion blockade with bupivacaine without benefit.[67] Sphenopalatine ganglion blockade with phenol produced a variable benefit lasting 1 to 12 months in one patient.[28] There is one report of a partial response with local opioid blockade of the superior cervical ganglion.[11]

### Invasive Surgical Procedures Involving the Trigeminal Nerve

There are nine case reports of either apparently successful treatment or temporary relief of SUNCT syndrome with surgical procedures. The procedures that have been used include the Jannetta procedure, percutaneous trigeminal ganglion compression, trigeminal ganglion thermocoagulation, retrogasserian glycerol rhizolysis, and trigeminal nerve balloon compression.

Three patients were treated with the Jannetta procedure.[31,72,80] In two of these patients, there was no recurrence of attacks after a follow-up period of 3 and 18 months, respectively. In the third patient, the attacks recurred after 2 years. One patient had percutaneous trigeminal ganglion compression,[26] which rendered the patient asymptomatic during the 18-month follow-up period. Two patients had trigeminal ganglion thermocoagulation, which rendered the patients pain free for 2 years before the attacks recurred.[13,70] Three patients were treated with retrogasserian glycerol rhizolysis, two of whom were treated twice. All five treatments provided complete pain relief, although the duration of the benefit ranged from 7 months to 4.5 years. One of these patients went on to have trigeminal nerve balloon compression with a good result.[28]

Given that the follow-up period in some of these patients was limited to less than 18 months, it is difficult to assess the actual effectiveness of the procedures given the variable nature of attack frequency in this syndrome. Nonetheless, it is worth noting that the benefit was temporary in all reported cases with prolonged follow-up.

Black and Dodick reported on two SUNCT cases refractory to various surgical procedures.[14] The first patient underwent a glycerol rhizotomy, gamma-knife radiosurgery, and microvascular decompression of the trigeminal nerve, whereas the second patient underwent gamma-knife radiosurgery of the trigeminal root exit zone and two microvascular decompressions of the trigeminal nerve. Neither patient benefited from these procedures. In addition, the first patient suffered from anesthesia dolorosa and the second patient from unilateral deafness, chronic vertigo, and disequilibrium as a result of surgery. Hannerz and Linderoth made a brief reference to a patient who had not benefited from trigeminal vascular decompression and two gamma-knife radiosurgeries of the trigeminal root.[28] There is one case report of a patient who underwent trigeminal microvascular decompression, following which, the attacks worsened.[13]

Given the uncertain efficacy of trigeminal procedures, together with the potential for complications, surgery should be considered only as a last resort and only when the pharmacologic options have been exploited to the fullest.

## NATURAL HISTORY

The natural history of SUNCT syndrome is poorly understood. The average duration of symptoms at reporting was $7 \pm 8$ years. In 20 of these patients, the duration of SUNCT exceeded 10 years. The longest reported duration of SUNCT is 48 years.[5] It appears to be a lifelong disorder once it starts, although more prospective data are needed. The syndrome itself is not fatal and does not cause any long-term neurologic sequelae.

## CLASSIFICATION AND DIAGNOSTIC CRITERIA

The TACs are a group of primary headache disorders characterized by unilateral trigeminal distribution pain that occurs in association with ipsilateral cranial autonomic features.[3] The group comprises SUNCT syndrome, paroxysmal hemicrania, and cluster headache. The revised IHS classification criteria recognize SUNCT syndrome as a subgroup of TACs.[4]

The IHS classification criteria of SUNCT have some notable problems. First, the name of the syndrome and the proposed classification criteria imply that all patients must have both conjunctival injection and tearing. Our clinical experience and the data from this review suggest that this is not invariably the case. Indeed, cases of SUNCT without either conjunctival injection or tearing may have been erroneously mislabeled as other syndromes and hence underreported in the medical literature. It has been proposed that a more appropriate term for the syndrome may be short-lasting, unilateral, neuralgiform headache attacks with cranial autonomic symptoms (SUNA).[4,6] Second, the attack frequency of SUNCT is rather unhelpful given its breadth. Because the attacks are usually daily, changing the frequency requirement may be helpful. Third, the pain attacks can be difficult to differentiate from ophthalmic division trigeminal neuralgia. The main differentiating features in the proposed criteria are the duration of the attack and the presence of autonomic features. However, there can be a considerable overlap in the duration of the attack, and autonomic features can occur with trigeminal neuralgia but are generally not prominent. One possibility is to propose the requirement of prominent cranial autonomic feature(s), but this would introduce subjectivity into the criteria unless what constitutes "prominent" autonomic symptoms is clearly defined. Another suggestion might be to introduce the absence of a refractory period to cutaneous stimulation as a criterion, although the drawback is that this feature is not adequately validated in this syndrome. Fourth, both episodic and chronic forms are now adequately validated. These subdivisions should be incorporated into the classification system, thereby bringing it in line with that of cluster headache and paroxysmal hemicrania. Some of these problems were addressed in the proposed criteria for SUNA and require validation (Table 8–3).[4]

## PATHOPHYSIOLOGY

Any pathophysiologic construct for TACs must account for the two major clinical features characteristic of the various conditions that comprise this group: trigeminal distribution pain and ipsilateral autonomic features. The pain-producing innervation of the cranium projects through branches of the trigeminal and upper cervical nerves to the trigeminocervical complex, from whence nociceptive pathways project to higher centers. This implies an integral role for the ipsilateral trigeminal nociceptive pathways in TACs. The ipsilateral autonomic features suggest cranial parasympathetic activation and sympathetic hypofunction. Goadsby and Lipton suggested that the pathophysiology of the TACs revolves around the trigeminal-autonomic reflex.[3] There is considerable experimental animal literature to document that stimulation of trigeminal efferents can result in cranial autonomic outflow, the trigeminal-autonomic reflex.[81] In fact, some degree of cranial autonomic symptomatology is a normal physiologic response to cranial nociceptive input,[82,83] and patients with other headache syndromes may report these symptoms.[84–86] The distinction between the TACs and other headache syndromes is the degree of cranial autonomic activation.[43]

The cranial autonomic symptoms may be prominent in the TACs owing to a central disinhibition of the trigeminal-autonomic reflex.[43] Supporting evidence is emerging from functional imaging studies: a functional MRI study in SUNCT syndrome[17] and a positron emission tomography study in cluster headache[87] have both demonstrated ipsilateral hypothalamic activation. Hypothalamic activation is specific to these syndromes and is not seen in migraine[88,89] or experimental ophthalmic trigeminal distribution head pain.[90] There are direct hypothalamic-trigeminal connections,[91] and the hypothalamus is known to have a modulatory role on the nociceptive[92,93] and autonomic pathways.[94] Hence, SUNCT syndrome is possibly due to an abnormality in the hypothalamus with subsequent trigeminovascular and cranial autonomic activation.

Several studies have demonstrated the diverse parasympathetic manifestations of SUNCT syndrome. Forehead sweating is usually increased during bouts,[95] unlike paroxysmal hemicrania, in which it is normal. Pupillary studies using pupillometry and pharmacologic approaches have revealed no abnormalities.[96] Given that conjunctival injection occurs during SUNCT syndrome, it is not surprising that intraocular pressure and corneal temperatures are elevated during attacks,[97] most likely reflecting local vasodilatation consequent to the marked parasympathetic activation. Similarly, a report of bradycardia in association with attacks of SUNCT syndrome indicates increased parasympathetic outflow.[98] Systolic blood pressure is sometimes elevated, although ventilatory function is normal.[99]

Conversely, orbital phlebography is reported to be abnormal in SUNCT syndrome, with a narrowed superior ophthalmic vein and the cavernous sinus homolateral to the pain.[100] This finding leads to the suggestion that SUNCT syndrome may be a form of orbital venous vasculitis,[34] although there are similar reports in cluster headache, Tolosa-Hunt syndrome, and paroxysmal hemicrania.[3] However, transcranial Doppler ultrasonography and single-photon emission computed tomography studies have not demonstrated convincing change in the vasomotor activity[101] or cerebral blood flow during attacks of pain.[102] Similarly, no intracranial vessel activation was apparent in a functional MRI study.[17] The hypothalamic activation and the diverse parasympathetic manifestations, taken together with the paucity of evidence for vascular changes, favor a central pathogenesis for SUNCT rather than a peripheral vasculitic cause.

## SUMMARY

SUNCT syndrome is a rare condition that predominates slightly in males. The mean age at onset is 50 years. It is characterized by strictly unilateral attacks centered on the orbital or periorbital regions, forehead, and temple. The pain is generally severe and neuralgic in character. The usual duration ranges from 5 to 120 seconds, although the reported range of duration is 2 seconds to 20 minutes. Both ipsilateral conjunctival injection and lacrimation are present in most, but not all, patients. Attacks can be triggered mainly from within the trigeminal innervated areas but also from the extratrigeminal areas. Most patients have both spontaneous and triggered attacks, although a minority have exclusively spontaneous attacks. Most patients are thought to have no refractory periods, although refractoriness may be underreported. Both episodic and chronic forms of SUNCT exist. The disorder is chronic in 28% of patients. In episodic SUNCT, an irregular temporal pattern occurs, with symptomatic periods alternating with remissions in a highly variable fashion. The attack frequency varies from less than one

---

**Table 8–3** Proposed Classification Criteria for Short-Lasting, Unilateral, Neuralgiform Headache Attacks with Cranial Autonomic Symptoms (SUNA)[4]

A. At least 20 attacks fulfilling criteria B–F

B. Attacks of unilateral orbital, supraorbital, or temporal stabbing or pulsating quality of pain lasting from 2 s to 10 min

C. Attacks occur with a frequency of ≥ 1/d for more than half of the time

D. Pain is accompanied by 1 of

    1. Conjunctival injection and/or lacrimation

    2. Nasal congestion and/or rhinorrhea

    3. Eyelid edema

E. No refractory period follows attacks triggered from trigger areas

F. Not attributed to another disorder

*Episodic SUNA:* At least 2 periods of attacks lasting (untreated patients) from 7 d to 1 yr and separated by remissions of at least 1 month.
*Chronic SUNA:* Absence of remission phases for 1 yr or more or with remissions lasting less than 1 mo.
Adapted from Headache Classification Committee, International Headache Society.[4]

attack daily to more than 60 attacks per hour. The attacks are predominantly diurnal, although frequent nocturnal attacks can occur in some patients. A functional MRI study in SUNCT syndrome has demonstrated ipsilateral hypothalamic activation. SUNCT was thought to be highly refractory to treatment. However, recent open-label trials of lamotrigine, topiramate, gabapentin, corticosteroids, and intravenous lidocaine have produced beneficial therapeutic responses. These results offer the promise of better treatments for this syndrome, although they require validation in controlled trials. Several invasive trigeminal procedures have been attempted with uncertain results; these procedures are best avoided until the drug therapies have been exhausted.

## REFERENCES

1. Sjaastad O, Russell D, Horven I, Bunaes U. Multiple neuralgiform, unilateral headache attacks associated with conjunctival injection and appearing in clusters. A nosological problem. Proc Scand Migraine Soc 1978;31.

2. Sjaastad O, Saunte C, Salvesen R, et al. Shortlasting unilateral neuralgiform headache attacks with conjunctival injection, tearing, sweating, and rhinorrhea. Cephalalgia 1989;9:147–56.

3. Goadsby PJ, Lipton RB. A review of paroxysmal hemicranias, SUNCT syndrome and other short-lasting headaches with autonomic feature, including new cases. Brain 1997;120:193–209.

4. Headache Classification Committee, International Headache Society. The international classification of headache disorders (second edition). Cephalalgia 2004;24:1–195.

5. Pareja JA, Sjaastad O. SUNCT syndrome. A clinical review. Headache 1997;37:195–202.

6. Matharu MS, Cohen AS, Boes CJ, Goadsby PJ. Short-lasting unilateral neuralgiform headache with conjunctival injection and tearing syndrome: a review. Curr Pain Headache Rep 2003;7:308–18.

7. Graff-Radford SB. SUNCT syndrome responsive to gabapentin. Cephalalgia 2000;20:515–7.

8. D'Andrea G, Granella F, Ghiotto N, Nappi G. Lamotrigine in the treatment of SUNCT syndrome. Neurology 2001;57:1723–5.

9. Cohen A, Matharu M, Goadsby P. SUNCT syndrome in the elderly. Cephalalgia 2004;24:508–9.

10. Wingerchuk, Nyquist PA, Rodriguez M, Dodick DW. Extratrigeminal short-lasting unilateral neuralgiform headache with conjunctival injection and tearing (SUNCT): new pathophysiologic entity or variation on a theme? Cephalalgia 2000;20:127–9.

11. Sabatowski R, Huber M, Meuser T, Radbruch L. SUNCT syndrome: a treatment option with local opioid blockade of the superior cervical ganglion? A case report. Cephalalgia 2001;21:154–6.

12. D'Andrea G, Granella F. SUNCT syndrome: the first case in childhood. Cephalalgia 2001;21:701–2.

13. Matharu MS, Cohen AS, Goadsby PJ. SUNCT syndrome responsive to intravenous lidocaine. Cephalalgia 2004;24:985–92.

14. Black DF, Dodick DW. Two cases of medically and surgically intractable SUNCT: a reason for caution and an argument for a central mechanism. Cephalalgia 2002;22:201–4.

15. Pareja JA, Shen JM, Kruszewski P, et al. SUNCT syndrome: duration, frequency, and temporal distribution of attacks. Headache 1996;36:161–5.

16. Pareja JA, Joubert J, Sjaastad O. SUNCT syndrome. Atypical temporal patterns. Headache 1996;36:108–10.

17. May A, Bahra A, Buchel C, et al. Functional magnetic resonance imaging in spontaneous attacks of SUNCT: short-lasting neuralgiform headache with conjunctival injection and tearing. Ann Neurol 1999;46:791–4.

18. Matharu MS, Boes CJ, Goadsby PJ. SUNCT syndrome: prolonged attacks, refractoriness and response to topiramate. Neurology 2002;58:1307.

19. Sesso RM. SUNCT syndrome or trigeminal neuralgia with lacrimation and conjunctival injection? Cephalalgia 2001;21:151–3.

20. van Vliet JA, Ferrari MD, Haan J. SUNCT syndrome resolving after contralateral hemispheric ischaemic stroke. Cephalalgia 2003;23:235–7.

21. Raimondi E, Gardella L. SUNCT syndrome. Two cases in Argentina. Headache 1998;38:369–71.

22. Pareja JA, Sjaastad O. SUNCT syndrome in the female. Headache 1994;34:217–20.

23. Jimenez-Huete A, Franch O, Pareja JA. SUNCT syndrome: priming of symptomatic periods and worsening of symptoms by treatment with calcium channel blockers. Cephalalgia 2002;22:812–4.

24. Pareja JA. SUNCT syndrome: the clinical picture. In: Olesen J, Goadsby PJ, editors. Cluster headache and related conditions. Oxford (UK): Oxford University Press; 1999. p. 71–7.

25. Hunt CH, Dodick DW, Bosch EP. SUNCT responsive to gabapentin. Headache 2002;42:525–6.

26. Morales-Asin F, Espada F, Lopez-Obarrio LA, et al. A SUNCT case with response to surgical treatment. Cephalalgia 2000;20:67–8.

27. Gutierrez-Garcia JM. SUNCT syndrome responsive to lamotrigine. Headache 2002;42:823–5.

28. Hannerz J, Linderoth B. Neurosurgical treatment of short-lasting, unilateral, neuralgiform hemicrania with conjunctival injection and tearing. Br J Neurosurg 2002;16:55–8.

29. Rossi P, Cesarino F, Faroni J, et al. SUNCT syndrome successfully treated with topiramate: case reports. Cephalalgia 2003;23:998–1000.

30. Chakravarty A, Mukherjee A. SUNCT syndrome responsive to lamotrigine: documentation of the first Indian case. Cephalalgia 2003;23:474–5.

31. Schwaag S, Frese A, Husstedt IW, Evers S. SUNCT syndrome: the first German case series. Cephalalgia 2003;23:398–400.

32. Lain AH, Caminero AB, Pareja JA. SUNCT syndrome; absence of refractory periods and modulation of attack duration by lengthening of the trigger stimuli. Cephalalgia 2000;20:671–3.

33. Leone M, Rigamonte A, Usai S, et al. Two new SUNCT cases responsive to lamotrigine. Cephalalgia 2000;20:845–7.

34. Hannerz J, Greitz D, Hansson P, Ericson K. SUNCT may be another manifestation of orbital venous vasculitis. Headache 1992;32:384–9.

35. Becser N, Berky M. SUNCT syndrome: a Hungarian case. Headache 1995;35:158–60.

36. Montes E, Alberca R, Lozano P, et al. Statuslike SUNCT in two young women. Headache 2001;41:826–9.

37. Pareja JA, Pareja J, Palomo T, et al. SUNCT syndrome: repetitive and overlapping attacks. Headache 1994;34:114–6.

38. Prakash KM, Lo YL. SUNCT syndrome in association with persistent Horner syndrome in a Chinese patient. Headache 2004;44:256–8.

39. Sjaastad O, Zhao JM, Kruszewski P, Stovner LJ. Short-lasting unilateral neuralgiform headache attacks with conjunctival injection, tearing, etc. (SUNCT): III. Another Norwegian case. Headache 1991;31:175–7.

40. Wober C, Wober-Bingol C, Wessely P. [SUNCT syndrome—case report and review of the literature]. Fortschr Neurol Psychiatr 1993;61:378–82.

41. Bouhassira D, Attal N, Esteve M, Chauvin M. "SUNCT" syndrome. A case of transformation from trigeminal neuralgia? Cephalalgia 1994;14:168–70.

42. Sjaastad O, Kruszewski P. Trigeminal neuralgia and "SUNCT" syndrome: similarities and differences in the clinical pictures. An overview. Funct Neurol 1992;7:103–7.

43. Goadsby PJ, Matharu MS, Boes CJ. SUNCT syndrome or trigeminal neuralgia with lacrimation. Cephalalgia 2001;21:82–3.

44. Pareja JA, Caminero AB, Sjaastad O. SUNCT syndrome: diagnosis and treatment. CNS Drugs 2002;16:373–83.

45. Lipton RB, Stewart WF, Cady R, et al. Sumatriptan for the range of headaches in migraine sufferers: results of the spectrum study. Headache 2000;40:783–91.

46. Bussone G, Leone M, Dalla Volta G, et al. Short-lasting unilateral neuralgiform headache attacks with tearing and conjunctival injection: the first "symptomatic" case? Cephalalgia 1991;11:123–7.

47. Morales F, Mostacero E, Marta J, Sanchez S. Vascular malformation of the cerebellopontine angle associated with "SUNCT" syndrome. Cephalalgia 1994;14:301–2.

48. De Benedittis G. SUNCT syndrome associated with cavernous angioma of the brain stem. Cephalalgia 1996;16:503–6.

49. ter Berg JW, Goadsby PJ. Significance of atypical presentation of symptomatic SUNCT: a case report. J Neurol Neurosurg Psychiatry 2001;70:244–6.

50. Moris G, Ribacoba R, Solar DN, Vidal JA. SUNCT syndrome and seborrheic dermatitis associated with craniosynostosis. Cephalalgia 2001;21:157–9.

51. Penart A, Firth M, Bowen JR. Short-lasting unilateral neuralgiform headache with conjunctival injection and tearing (SUNCT) following presumed dorsolateral brainstem infarction. Cephalalgia 2001;21:236–9.

52. Blattler T, Capone Mori A, Boltshauser E, Bassetti C. Symptomatic SUNCT in an eleven-year-old girl. Neurology 2003;60:2012–3.

53. Ramirez-Moreno J, Fernandez-Portales I, Garcia-Castanon I, et al. SUNCT syndrome and neoplasms in the central nervous system. A new association. Neurologia 2004;19:326–30.

54. Ferrari MD, Haan J, van Seters AP. Bromocriptine-induced trigeminal neuralgia attacks in a patient with a pituitary tumor. Neurology 1988;38:1482–4.

55. Massiou H, Launay JM, Levy C, et al. SUNCT syndrome in two patients with prolactinomas and bromocriptine-induced attacks. Neurology 2002;58:1698–9.

56. Levy MJ, Matharu MS, Goadsby PJ. Prolactinomas, dopamine agonists and headache: two case reports. Eur J Neurol 2003;10:169–73.

57. Matharu MS, Levy MJ, Merry RT, Goadsby PJ. SUNCT syndrome secondary to prolactinoma. J Neurol Neurosurg Psychiatry 2003;74:1590–2.

58. Kaphan E, Eusebio A, Donnet A, et al. Shortlasting, unilateral, neuralgiform headache attacks with conjunctival injection and tearing (SUNCT syndrome) and tumour of the cavernous sinus. Cephalalgia 2003;23:395–7.

59. Lim EC, Teoh HL. Headache—it's more than meets the eye: orbital lesion masquerading as SUNCT. Cephalalgia 2003;23:558–60.

60. Barea LM, Forcelini CM. Onset of short-lasting, unilateral, neuralgiform headache with conjunctival injection and tearing (SUNCT) after acquired human immunodeficiency virus (HIV): more than a coincidence? Cephalalgia 2001;21:518.

61. Ertsey C, Bozsik G, Afra J, Jelencsik I. A case of SUNCT syndrome with neurovascular decompression. Cephalalgia 2000;20:325.

62. Majoie CB, Hulsmans FJ, Verbeeten B Jr, et al. Trigeminal neuralgia: comparison of two MR imaging techniques in the demonstration of neurovascular contact. Radiology 1997;204:455–60.

63. Kuroiwa T, Matsumoto S, Kato A, et al. MR imaging of idiopathic trigeminal neuralgia: correlation with non-surgical therapy. Radiat Med 1996;14:235–9.

64. Yang J, Simonson TM, Ruprecht A, et al. Magnetic resonance imaging used to assess patients with trigeminal neuralgia. Oral Surg Oral Med Oral Pathol Oral Radiol Endod 1996;81:343–50.

65. Baldwin NG, Sahni KS, Jensen ME, et al. Association of vascular compression in trigeminal neuralgia versus other "facial pain syndromes" by magnetic resonance imaging. Surg Neurol 1991;36:447–52.

66. Pareja JA, Kruszewski P, Caminero AB. SUNCT syndrome versus idiopathic stabbing headache (jabs and jolts syndrome). Cephalalgia 1999;19:46–8.

67. Pareja JA, Kruszewski P, Sjaastad O. SUNCT syndrome: trials of drugs and anesthetic blockades. Headache 1995;35:138–42.

68. Benoliel R, Sharav Y. SUNCT syndrome: case report and literature review. Oral Surg Oral Med Oral Pathol Oral Radiol Endod 1998;85:158–61.

69. D'Andrea G, Granella F, Cadaldini M. Possible usefulness of lamotrigine in the treatment of SUNCT syndrome. Neurology 1999;53:1609.

70. Piovesan EJ, Siow C, Kowacs PA, Werneck LC. Influence of lamotrigine over the SUNCT syndrome: one patient follow-up for two years. Arq Neuropsiquiatr 2003;61:691–4.

71. Malik K, Rizvi S, Vaillancourt PD. The SUNCT syndrome: successfully treated with lamotrigine. Pain Med 2002;3:167–8.

72. Gardella L, Viruega A, Rojas H, Nagel J. A case of a patient with SUNCT syndrome treated with Jannetta procedure. Cephalalgia 2001;21:996–9.

73. Porta-Etessam J, Martinez-Salio A, Berbel A, Benito-Leon J. Gabapentin (neurontin) in the treatment of SUNCT syndrome. Cephalalgia 2002;22:249.

74. Post RM. Comparative pharmacology of bipolar disorder and schizophrenia. Schizophr Res 1999;39:153–8; discussion 163.

75. Porta-Etessam J, Benito-Leon J, Martinez-Salio A, Berbel A. Gabapentin in the treatment of SUNCT syndrome. Headache 2002;42:523–4.

76. Matharu MS, Goadsby PJ. Persistence of attacks of cluster headache after trigeminal nerve root section. Brain 2002;125:976–84.

77. Antonaci F, Costa A, Ghirmai S, et al. Parenteral indomethacin (the Indotest) in cluster headache. Cephalalgia 2003;23:193–6.

78. Fogan L. Treatment of cluster headache. A double-blind comparison of oxygen v air inhalation. Arch Neurol 1985;42:362–3.

79. El Amrani M, Massiou H, Bousser M. A negative trial of sodium valproate in cluster headache: methodological issues. Cephalalgia 2002;22:205–8.

80. Lenaerts M, Diederich N, Phuce K. A patient with SUNCT cured by the Jannetta procedure. Cephalalgia 1997;17:461.

81. May A, Goadsby PJ. The trigeminovascular system in humans: pathophysiologic implications for primary headache syndromes of the neural influences on the cerebral circulation. J Cereb Blood Flow Metab 1999;19:115–27.

82. May A, Buchel C, Turner R, Goadsby PJ. Magnetic resonance angiography in facial and other pain: neurovascular mechanisms of trigeminal sensation. J Cereb Blood Flow Metab 2001;21:1171–6.

83. Frese A, Evers S, May A. Autonomic activation in experimental trigeminal pain. Cephalalgia 2003;23:67–8.

84. Avnon Y, Nitzan M, Sprecher E, et al. Different patterns of parasympathetic activation in uni- and bilateral migraineurs. Brain 2003;126:1660–70.

85. Barbanti P, Fabbrini G, Pesare M, et al. Unilateral cranial autonomic symptoms in migraine. Cephalalgia 2002;22:256–9.

86. Benoliel R, Sharav Y. Trigeminal neuralgia with lacrimation or SUNCT syndrome? Cephalalgia 1998;18:85–90.

87. May A, Bahra A, Buchel C, et al. Hypothalamic activation in cluster headache attacks. Lancet 1998;352:275–8.

88. Weiller C, May A, Limmroth V, et al. Brain stem activation in spontaneous human migraine attacks. Nat Med 1995;1:658–60.

89. Bahra A, Matharu MS, Buchel C, et al. Brainstem activation specific to migraine headache. Lancet 2001;357:1016–7.

90. May A, Kaube H, Buchel C, et al. Experimental cranial pain elicited by capsaicin: a PET study. Pain 1998;74:61–6.

91. Malick A, Burstein R. Cells of origin of the trigemino-hypothalamic tract in the rat. J Comp Neurol 1998;400:125–44.

92. Wang Q, Mao LM, Han JS. Naloxone-reversible analgesia produced by microstimulation of the arcuate nucleus of the hypothalamus in pentobarbital-anesthetized rats. Exp Brain Res 1990;80:201–4.

93. Dafny N, Dong WQ, Prieto-Gomez C, et al. Lateral hypothalamus: site involved in pain modulation. Neuroscience 1996;70:449–60.

94. Lumb BM, Lovick TA. The rostral hypothalamus: an area for the integration of autonomic and sensory responsiveness. J Neurophysiol 1993;70:1570–7.

95. Kruszewski P, Zhao JM, Shen JM, Sjaastad O. SUNCT syndrome: forehead sweating pattern. Cephalalgia 1993;13:108–13.

96. Zhao JM, Sjaastad O. SUNCT syndrome: VIII. Pupillary reaction and corneal sensitivity. Funct Neurol 1993;8:409–14.

97. Sjaastad O. Cluster headache syndrome. Major problems in neurology series. Vol 23. London: WB Saunders; 1992.

98. Kruszewski P, Sand T, Shen JM, Sjaastad O. Short-lasting, unilateral, neuralgiform headache attacks with conjunctival injection and tearing (SUNCT syndrome): IV. Respiratory sinus arrhythmia during and outside paroxysms. Headache 1992;32:377–83.

99. Kruszewski P, Fasano ML, Brubakk AO, et al. Shortlasting, unilateral, neuralgiform headache attacks with conjunctival injection, tearing, and subclinical forehead sweating ("SUNCT" syndrome): II. Changes in heart rate and arterial blood pressure during pain paroxysms. Headache 1991;31:399–405.

100. Kruszewski P. Shortlasting, unilateral, neuralgiform headache attacks with conjunctival injection and tearing (SUNCT syndrome): V. Orbital phlebography. Cephalalgia 1992;12:387–9.

101. Shen JM, Johnsen HJ. SUNCT syndrome: estimation of cerebral blood flow velocity with transcranial Doppler ultrasonography. Headache 1994;34:25–31.

102. Poughias L, Aasly J. SUNCT syndrome: cerebral SPECT images during attacks. Headache 1995;35:143–5.

# CHAPTER 9

# Hemicrania Continua

Mario F. P. Peres, MD, PhD

Hemicrania continua (HC) is one of the primary chronic daily headache (CDH) disorders. It is characterized by a continuous, unilateral, moderately severe headache; exacerbations of severe pain associated with migrainous and autonomic features (tearing, conjunctival injection, ptosis); and complete responsiveness to indomethacin.

HC was once thought to be a rare headache disorder, but many cases have been reported. It is an under-recognized headache syndrome. The earliest recognition of a headache syndrome involving one side of the head is attributed to Aretaeus of Cappadocia (2nd century AD). However, Egyptian descriptions appear in papyri dating from 1500 BC.[1] Galen (131–201 AD) introduced the term "hemicrania" for unilateral headache. It was later transformed into the old English *megrim* and the French *migraine*. We now accept the term "migraine," derived from hemicrania. It differs from HC in its episodic nature.

Medina and Diamond probably were the first authors to describe HC in a subset of 54 patients who had cluster headache variants, as well as strictly unilateral, continuous headaches that were responsive to indomethacin.[2]

The term "hemicrania continua" was coined by Sjaastad and Spierings in 1984.[3] They reported two patients, a woman aged 63 years and a man aged 53 years, who developed a strictly unilateral headache that was continuous from onset and absolutely responsive to indomethacin. In 1983, Boghen and Desaulniers described a patient with a similar headache that they called "background vascular headache responsive to indomethacin."[4]

HC is not that uncommon in clinical practice and should not be that rare in the general population. The prevalence of primary CDH in the general population is 4%. Epidemiologic studies never found HC in the population because the indomethacin trial has never been applied to the suspected cases. However, unilateral headache was found in 42% of chronic tension-type headache and 61% of chronic migraine patients.[5] HC has been reported in different countries and races. The first Japanese case was reported in 2002.[6] Wheeler also reported HC in African Americans.[7]

HC exists in continuous and remitting forms. The continuous variety can be subclassified into (1) an evolutive, unremitting form that arises from the remitting form and (2) an unremitting form characterized by continuous headache from the onset.

Ninety-seven patients had available descriptions of their temporal pattern; 83 (85%) were reported to be the continuous form and 14 (15%) the remitting form. Of patients who had the continuous form, 64% had it since the beginning and 36% of patients had the continuous form evolved from the remitting form.

A wide range of gender distribution has been reported. Bordini and colleagues reported a female preponderance (5:1) in the first 18 cases reported.[8] Newman and colleagues found less female preponderance (1.8:1),[9] and Espada and colleagues presented a slight male preponderance (1.25:1).[10] Wheeler reported the highest female preponderance (29:1).[11] Peres and colleagues found a 2.4:1 female to male ratio.[12] Summarizing all of the cases for which gender data are available, the female to male ratio is 2.6:1.

One of the essential features of HC is unilateral headache; however, some bilateral[13] or alternating side[14,15] cases have been reported. Ekbom reported side alternation in 10% of patients with episodic cluster headache.[16] Bilateral cases have been reported in the literature in chronic paroxysmal hemicrania[17] and in cluster headache, and a mechanism of failed contralateral suppression was proposed by Young and Rozen.[18]

Bilateral HC may be underdiagnosed because one would not consider HC in a patient presenting with bilateral CDH. Hannerz reported an indomethacin test performed in a population of CDH patients with bilateral headaches who met diagnostic criteria for tension-type headache.[19] An absolute response was found in three patients. There may be a subgroup of patients with bilateral chronic headache who respond to indomethacin in the group of patients otherwise diagnosed as having chronic tension-type headache or even new daily persistent headache and chronic (transformed) migraine.

Associated symptoms present in HC can be divided into three main categories: autonomic symptoms, "jabs and jolts" (stabbing headaches) and migrainous features. Autonomic symptoms consist of conjunctival injection, tearing, rhinorrhea, nasal stuffiness, eyelid edema, and forehead sweating. These symptoms are not as prominent in HC as they are in cluster headache and chronic paroxysmal hemicrania. Symptoms of ocular discomfort, at times premonitory, have been described by patients with HC. Some patients report a feeling of sand in the eye, which may be specific for HC.[20] Peres and colleagues found autonomic symptoms to be more common in the exacerbation period compared with the baseline in HC.[12] At least one autonomic symptom was found in 75% of patients.

Jabs and jolts syndrome is described as sharp pain that lasts less than 1 minute; it occurs in patients with tension-type, migraine, and cluster headache or in headache-free individuals and responds to indomethacin. Jabs and jolts pain occurs in HC, more frequently in the exacerbation periods. Jabs and jolts syndrome is described in 26% of HC cases reported in the literature. Peres and colleagues found it in 41% of cases.[12] Its prevalence in the general population is 30%. Because of its low sensitivity and specificity, it should not be part of the diagnostic criteria for HC.

Migrainous features (nausea, vomiting, photophobia, or phonophobia) are common in HC, particularly in the exacerbation period.[21] The association between HC and visual auras was recently described.[22] Evers and colleagues reported a patient with HC and attacks of hemiparesis with a familial history of hemiplegic migraines.[23] Pasquier and colleagues reported a patient with unilateral paresthesias.[13] Little is known about the natural history of HC during pregnancy and reproductive life events. Hemicrania postpartum, a new HC variant, was recently reported.[24]

The pathophysiology of HC is unknown. It has been speculated that HC might be a migraine variant because many patients have headaches that have migrainous features. HC has been reported to be coexistent with familial hemiplegic migraine,[23] and HC with aura was recently described.[22] The mechanisms of indomethacin response are still unknown. Theories have included decreased cerebral blood flow, reduced cerebrovascular permeability, decreased cerebrospinal fluid pressure, an effect on melatonin secretion, and an antagonist effect on nitric oxide.[25]

Neuroimaging findings have improved our understanding of HC etiology. Matharu and colleagues studied seven patients with HC in two sessions.[26] In one session,

patients were pain free after receiving indomethacin 100 mg intramuscularly. In the other session, patients were scanned with functional magnetic resonance imaging during baseline pain and when still in pain after receiving intramuscular placebo. The control group included seven age- and sex-matched nonheadache subjects. Scans revealed significant activation of the contralateral posterior hypothalamus and ipsilateral dorsal rostral pons, as well as activation of the ipsilateral ventrolateral midbrain, which extended over the red nucleus, the substantia nigra, and the bilateral pontomedullary junction. The scan exposed no obvious intracranial vessel dilation. This study demonstrated activation of various subcortical structures, in particular the posterior hypothalamus and the dorsal rostral pons. If posterior hypothalamic and brainstem activation are considered markers of trigeminal autonomic cephalgias and migrainous syndromes, then the activation pattern demonstrated in HC mirrors the overlapping clinical phenotype. However, the activation was opposite to that seen in trigeminal autonomic cephalgias and migrainous syndromes. In migraine, the brainstem is activated contralateral to the side of headache, but in HC, it is ipsilateral. In cluster headache, the hypothalamus is activated ipsilateral to the side of headache but contralateral in HC.

The management of HC is basically centered on indomethacin. Indomethacin is a nonsteroidal anti-inflammatory drug that is often poorly tolerated. Drugs other than indomethacin that are helpful in HC include ibuprofen, piroxicam β-cyclodextrin, and rofecoxib. Kumar and Bordiuk reported a complete response to ibuprofen 800 mg two times daily.[27] In 1992, Antonaci and Sjaastad found that four of six patients responded to piroxicam β-cyclodextrin 20 to 40 mg/d.[28] One patient had a moderate response, and one had no response.[28] Peres and Zukerman reported a case that was responsive to rofecoxib.[29] Other classes of drugs have not been successful in controlling HC. Antonaci and colleagues reported the lack of efficacy of sumatriptan in seven patients.[30] All analgesics were reported to be of no benefit. The dose for indomethacin response ranges from 50 to 300 mg/d. Kuritzky reported four cases that were unresponsive to 100 mg of indomethacin, but higher doses were not attempted.[31] Pascual reported other cases that were unresponsive to 225 mg.[32]

An outpatient test of indomethacin starts with administering 25 mg of the drug three times a day for the first 2 days and subsequently increasing the dose to 250 mg/d if necessary. An alternative to the indomethacin trial is the so-called "indotest." Twelve patients with HC were given 50 mg of intramuscular indomethacin, and some of them were given 100 mg on a second day. The time between indomethacin injection and complete pain relief was 66 to 73 minutes with the 50 mg injection and 56 to 61 minutes with the 100 mg injection. The pain-free period was 8 to 13 hours after the 50 mg injection and 10 to 13 hours after the 100 mg injection. The authors suggest a standard dose of 50 mg of intramuscular indomethacin with observation for up to 3 hours because relief occurred in all patients by 2 hours.[33]

Rozen recently reported that melatonin 6 to 12 mg at bedtime was an effective therapy for indomethacin-responsive headaches for one patient with HC and two patients with idiopathic stabbing headache.[34] Melatonin may be an alternative treatment for the indomethacin-responsive headaches; its molecular structure is similar to that of indomethacin,[35] and it tends to be more tolerable.

The differential diagnosis of HC includes other CDHs that can also be strictly unilateral. The continuous form of HC should be differentiated from the other primary CDH disorders (transformed migraine, chronic tension-type headache, and new daily persistent headache) by an indomethacin test. All patients who have strictly unilateral headaches should undergo an indomethacin trial to rule out a diagnosis of HC.

Chronic paroxysmal hemicrania does not have the continuous baseline headache found in HC; headache duration is shorter (2 to 45 minutes), and frequency is usually more than five a day. It is precipitated by neck movement, a feature that is not found in HC. Autonomic symptoms are more prominent in chronic paroxysmal hemicrania and cluster headache than in HC.

Three secondary cases have been reported. One patient had a mesenchymal tumor,[23] one had human immunodeficiency virus (HIV),[36] and one had a 2.5 cm adenocarcinoma lung mass.[37] HC can be aggravated by a C7 root irritation owing to a disk herniation.[38]

Bigal and colleagues compared two different diagnostic criteria for HC and found Goadsby and Lipton's to be more clinically useful.[39] The new classification in the International Headache Society's classification system includes diagnostic criteria for HC (Table 9–1).[40]

Espada and colleagues studied prognosis in five men and four women who had HC (eight continuous, one remitting).[10] All nine patients had initial relief with indomethacin (mean daily dose 94.4 mg; range 50 to 150 mg). Follow-up was possible in eight patients. Indomethacin could be discontinued after 3, 7, and 15 months, respectively, and patients remained pain free. Three patients discontinued treatment because of side effects and had headache recurrence; two had relief with aspirin. Two other patients continued to take indomethacin with partial relief. Pareja and colleagues reported a patient who began in the continuous stage but 5 years later, after discontinuing indomethacin, remained pain-free.[41] This may have represented a continuous stage turning into a remitting course or a spontaneous remission. Pareja and colleagues studied HC and chronic paroxysmal hemicrania patients and found that 42% of patients experienced a decrease of up to 60% in the dose of indomethacin required to maintain a pain-free state; 23% of patients reported gastrointestinal complaints that were relieved with ranitidine.[42] Direct complications from the disease are not seen, but side effects from indomethacin (bleeding, renal failure, neuropathy) should be monitored.

**Table 9–1** Diagnostic Criteria for Hemicrania Continua According to the International Classification of Headache Disorders, Second Edition[40]

A. Headache for > 3 mo fulfilling criteria B–D

B. All of the following characteristics:

    1.    Unilateral pain without side-shift

    2.    Daily and continuous without pain-free periods

    3.    Moderate intensity but with exacerbation of severe pain

C. At least one of the autonomic features occurs during exacerbation, ipsilateral to the side of pain:

    1. Conjuctival lacrimation and/or lacrimation

    2. Nasal congestion and/or rhinorrhea

    3. Ptosis and/or miosis

D. Complete response to therapeutic doses of indomethacin

E. Not attributed to another disorder

## REFERENCES

1. Borghouts J. The magical texts of papyrus Leiden I 348. Leiden: E.J. Brill; 1971.

2. Medina J, Diamond S. Cluster headache variant. Spectrum of a new headache syndrome. Arch Neurol 1981;38:705–9.

3. Sjaastad O, Spierings EL. "Hemicrania continua": another headache absolutely responsive to indomethacin. Cephalalgia 1984;4:65–70.

4. Boghen D, Desaulniers N. Background vascular headache: relief with indomethacin. Can J Neurol Sci 1983;10:270–1.

5. Scher AI, Stewart WF, Liberman J, Lipton RB. Prevalence of frequent headache in a population sample. Headache 1998;38:497–506.

6. Ishizaki K, Takeshima T, Ijiri T, et al. Hemicrania continua: the first Japanese case report. Rinsho Shinkeigaku 2002;42:754–6.

7. Wheeler SD. Hemicrania continua in African Americans. J Natl Med Assoc 2002;94:901–7.

8.  Bordini C, Antonaci F, Stovner LJ, et al. "Hemicrania continua": a clinical review. Headache 1991;31:20–6.

9.  Newman LC, Lipton RB, Solomon S. Hemicrania continua: ten new cases and a review of the literature. Neurology 1994;44:2111–4.

10. Espada F, Escalza I, Morales-Asin F, et al. Hemicrania continua: nine new cases. Cephalalgia 1999;19:442.

11. Wheeler SD. Clinical spectrum of hemicrania continua. San Diego (CA): American Academy of Neurology 52nd Annual Meeting; 2000.

12. Peres MF, Silberstein SD, Nahmias S, et al. Hemicrania continua is not that rare. Neurology 2001;57:948–51.

13. Pasquier F, Leys D, Petit H. "Hemicrania continua": the first bilateral case? Cephalalgia 1987;7:169–70.

14. Newman LC, Lipton RB, Russell M, Solomon S. Hemicrania continua: attacks may alternate sides. Headache 1992;32:237–8.

15. Peres MF, Young WB. Side-shifting hemicrania continua with aura or chronic migraine with autonomic symptoms responsive to indomethacin. Cephalalgia 2003;23:735–6.

16. Ekbom K. Clinical aspects of cluster headache. Headache 1974;13:176–80.

17. Pollmann W, Pfaffenrath V. Chronic paroxysmal hemicrania: the first possible bilateral case. Cephalalgia 1986;6:55–7.

18. Young WB, Rozen TD. Bilateral cluster headache: case report and a theory of (failed) contralateral suppression. Cephalalgia 1999;19:188–90.

19. Hannerz J. Chronic bilateral headache responding to indomethacin. Headache 2000;40:840–3.

20. Pareja JA. Hemicrania continua: ocular discomfort heralding painful attacks. Funct Neurol 1999;14:93–5.

21. Peres MF. Hemicrania continua: recent treatment strategies and diagnostic evaluation. Curr Neurol Neurosci Rep 2002;2:108–13.

22. Peres MF, Siow HC, Rozen TD. Hemicrania continua with aura. Cephalalgia 2002;22:246–8.

23. Evers S, Bahra A, Goadsby PJ. Coincidence of familial hemiplegic migraine and hemicrania continua? A case report. Cephalalgia 1999;19:533–5.

24. Spitz M, Peres MF. Hemicrania continua postpartum. Cephalalgia 2004;24:603–4.

25. Castellano AE, Micieli G, Bellantonio P, et al. Indomethacin increases the effect of isosorbide dinitrate on cerebral hemodynamic in migraine patients: pathogenetic and therapeutic implications. Cephalalgia 1998;18:622–30.

26. Matharu MS, Cohen AS, McGonigle DJ, et al. Posterior hypothalamic and brainstem activation in hemicrania continua [abstract]. Headache. 2004;44:462–3.

27. Kumar KL, Bordiuk JD. Hemicrania continua: a therapeutic dilemma. Headache 1991;31:345.

28. Antonaci F, Sjaastad O. Hemicrania continua: a possible symptomatic case, due to mesenchymal tumor. Funct Neurol 1992;7:471–4.

29. Peres MF, Zukerman E. Hemicrania continua responsive to rofecoxib. Cephalalgia 2000;20:130–1.

30. Antonaci F, Pareja JA, Caminero AB, Sjaastad O. Chronic paroxysmal hemicrania and hemicrania continua: lack of efficacy of sumatriptan. Headache 1998;38:197–200.

31. Kuritzky A. Indomethacin-resistant hemicrania continua. Cephalalgia 1992;12:57–9.

32. Pascual J. Hemicrania continua. Neurology 1995; 45:2302–3.

33. Antonaci F, Pareja JA, Caminero AB, Sjaastad O. Chronic paroxysmal hemicrania and hemicrania continua. Parenteral indomethacin: the 'indotest.' Headache 1998;38:122–8.

34. Rozen TD. Melatonin as a treatment for indomethacin-responsive headaches. Headache 2003;43:591.

35. Peres MF, Stiles MA, Oshinsky M, Rozen TD. Remitting form of hemicrania continua with seasonal pattern. Headache 2001;41:592–4.

36. Brilla R, Evers S, Soros P, Husstedt IW. Hemicrania continua in an HIV-infected outpatient. Cephalalgia 1998;18:287–8.

37. Eross EJ, Swanson JW. Hemicrania continua: an indomethacin-responsive case with an underlying malignant etiology. Philadelphia: American Academy of Neurology 53rd Annual Meeting; 2001.

38. Sjaastad O, Stovner LJ, Stolt-Nielsen A, et al. CPH and hemicrania continua: requirements of high indomethacin dosages—an ominous sign? Headache 1995;35:363–7.

39. Bigal ME, Tepper SJ, Rapoport AM, Sheftell FD. Hemicrania continua: comparison between two different classification systems. Cephalalgia 2002;22:242–5.

40. International Headache Society Classification Subcommittee. International classification of headache disorders. 2nd ed. Cephalalgia 2004;24 Suppl 1:1–160.

41. Pareja JA, Palomo T, Gorriti MA, et al. Hemicrania episodica—a new type of headache or pre-chronic stage of hemicrania continua. Headache 1990;30:344–6.

42. Pareja JA, Caminero AB, Franco E, et al. Dose, efficacy and tolerability of long-term indomethacin treatment of chronic paroxysmal hemicrania and hemicrania continua. Cephalalgia 2001;21:906–10.

# CHAPTER 10

# Hypnic Headache

Stefan Evers, MD, PhD, and David W. Dodick, MD, FRCPC, FACP

Hypnic headache is a rare headache syndrome first described by Raskin in 1988 and later termed "clockwise headache" or "alarm-clock headache."[1–3] Since then, more than 80 similar cases have been reported in the literature, and a recent systematic review of all published cases described the typical clinical picture of and treatment options for hypnic headache.[4] All authors thus far have assumed that hypnic headache is an idiopathic headache disorder, and diagnostic criteria were first proposed in 1997.[5] Hypnic headache has now been included in the revised version of the headache classification of the International Headache Society (IHS).[6] The actual diagnostic criteria for hypnic headache are presented in Table 10–1. In this chapter, the clinical picture and options for the management of hypnic headache are described, based on a recent review[4] and on the case series published since then.[7–10]

## CLINICAL FEATURES

Eighty-two published cases could be analyzed (for the original references, see Evers and Goadsby[4]). The data for these cases are described separately for the different clinical and pathophysiologic observations to give an impression of the clinical features and varieties of hypnic headache.

### Demographic Data

The mean age at onset of hypnic headache was 62 ± 11 years (range 36–84 years). There was a female preponderance (62%). The mean duration of disease before diagnosis was 5 ± 7 years (range 0.1–35 years), suggesting that this condition is poorly recognized and perhaps underdiagnosed. Only 14 patients experienced spontaneous remission of hypnic headache during the observation period. There was no case with a family history of hypnic headache.

The prevalence or incidence of hypnic headache cannot be calculated based on the literature. Hypnic headache was reported to be the main diagnosis in 0.07% of all patients in the Headache Division at the Mayo Clinic[3]; in another sample, hypnic headache could be diagnosed in about 0.1% of all headache patients in a German supraregional headache outpatient clinic.[11]

### Clinical Data

The average intensity of pain was mild in 4%, moderate in 60%, and severe in 37%. There were no relevant changes in the untreated intensity of headaches during the course of the disease. The most prominent charac-

---

**Table 10–1** Diagnostic Criteria of the International Headache Society for Hypnic Headache

Diagnostic criteria:

A. Dull headache fulfilling criteria B–D

B. Develops only during sleep and awakens patient

C. At least 2 of the following characteristics:

   1. Occurs > 15 times/mo

   2. Lasts ≥ 15 min after waking

   3. First occurs after age of 50 yr

D. No autonomic symptoms and no more than 1 of nausea, photophobia, or phonophobia

E. Not attributed to another disorder

*Note:* Intracranial disorders must be excluded. Distinction from one of the trigeminal autonomic cephalgias is necessary for effective management.
*Comment:* The pain of hypnic headache is usually mild to moderate, but severe pain is reported by approximately 20% of patients. Pain is bilateral in about two-thirds of cases. The attack usually lasts from 15 to 180 minutes, but longer durations have been described. Caffeine and lithium have been effective treatments in several reported cases.

ter of pain was dull in 57%, throbbing or pulsating in 39%, and sharp or stabbing in 4%.

The pain was bilateral in 60% of the cases and always one-sided in 40% (13% right, 16% left, 11% alternating sides). The localization of the typical headache was frontotemporal (including periorbital) in 45%, posterior in 3%, and diffuse in 52%.

The average duration of untreated attacks was 88 $\pm$ 95 minutes (range 15–500 minutes), whereas the maximum duration of a single attack for the total sample was 500 minutes in a patient whose average headache duration was 240 minutes. The frequency of attacks was 1.2 $\pm$ 0.8 per 24 hours (range one per week to six per night). The time of onset during the course of sleep was presented in the majority of published patients. In 4% of the patients, the onset of the first attack was within 30 to 60 minutes after falling asleep; in 9% of the patients, this onset was between 60 and 120 minutes after falling asleep. Most of the patients (75%) had the onset of their first attack between 120 and 480 minutes after falling asleep, and only 12% of the patients had the first attack later than 4 hours after sleep onset. In 60% of the patients, the onset of an attack occurred regularly within a time interval of 60 minutes, most often about 3 hours after falling asleep and between 1 and 3 am. However, the variability of the time interval with the attack onset was up to 4 hours.

Data on concomitant symptoms during the headache were described only by a minority of patients. In 8% of the patients, autonomic symptoms fulfilling the IHS criteria for cluster headache or chronic paroxysmal hemicrania could be recorded (lacrimation [four], in part with nasal congestion or rhinorrhea, and ptosis [two]). However, none of these patients fulfilled the complete IHS criteria for cluster headache or chronic paroxysmal hemicrania. Nausea was reported in 22% of the patients during the headache; none reported vomiting. Mild photophobia, phonophobia, or both were reported in 5% of the patients.

In seven patients, it was explicitly noted that the headache was worse when they remained supine. These patients experienced marked relief of the headache when they assumed an upright position. However, nearly all patients got up during the headache and were active, and there was no report of headache aggravation by physical activity. Four patients reported occurrence of headache even during daytime sleep, whereas three patients had consistently no headache during their daytime nap.

In three patients, alcohol was reported to be a trigger for hypnic headache attacks. However, it was noted that alcohol did not have an influence on the occurrence of attacks in 19 patients. Other triggers were not reported.

The main clinical and demographic features are presented in Table 10–2.

## Neurophysiologic and Neuroradiologic Findings

Magnetic resonance imaging (MRI) and computed tomography of the brain were performed in 46 and 56 cases, respectively. In 10 cases, no brain imaging was reported. There were no pathologic findings except nonspecific white matter lesions, including lacunar infarctions (six), meningioma (two), and mild atrophy

**Table 10–2** Demographic and Clinical Features of the Patients with Hypnic Headache Analyzed in This Review (N = 82)

| | |
|---|---|
| Sex, % | |
| Men | 38 |
| Women | 62 |
| Age at onset, yr | 62 $\pm$ 11 (36–84) |
| Duration of attacks, min | 88 $\pm$ 95 (15–500) |
| Frequency of attacks per 24 h | 1.2 $\pm$ 0.8 (1/wk–6) |
| Intensity of pain, % | |
| Mild | 4 |
| Moderate | 60 |
| Severe | 37 |
| Character of pain, % | |
| Dull | 57 |
| Throbbing/pulsating | 39 |
| Sharp/stabbing | 4 |
| Side of headache, % | |
| Unilateral | 40 (13 right, 16 left, 11 alternating) |
| Bilateral | 60 |
| Localization, % | |
| Frontotemporal | 45 |
| Posterior | 3 |
| Diffuse | 52 |
| Concomitant symptoms, % | |
| Nausea | 22 |
| Photo–/phonophobia | 5 |
| Lacrimation | 5 |
| Ptosis | 3 |

Data are given as a percentage or as an arithmetic mean with simple standard deviation (range in brackets). Data were not available from all patients for every aspect.

(two). All neurophysiologic examinations (electroencephalography, Doppler ultrasonography, evoked potentials) were reported to be normal. Data on blood analysis were given in a minority of patients. However, in none of these patients were abnormalities recorded that could not be explained by a concomitant disorder or disease independent from hypnic headache.

## Sleep Recordings

Polysomnography was performed in nine patients, with evidence for occurrence of the headache attacks always during the rapid eye movement (REM) sleep stage in five patients and during sleep stage 3 in one patient; the remaining three patients did not have a headache attack during polysomnography.[9,11–13] In all five patients with REM-associated hypnic headache, the attack occurred during the first REM stage. Two of these patients had multiple REM-associated attacks per night. Another seven patients reported onset of headache attacks during dreams, three of them during nightmares or vivid dreams.

Other measures of sleep quality were normal except a decreased sleep efficiency (ie, time of sleep during time in bed) of down to 60% in seven patients with polysomnography. Sleep apnea was recorded in one patient, and snoring was reported in 10 patients. Oxygen saturation was decreased mildly down to 90% in two patients and 70% in another two patients for several minutes. One patient showed periodic limb movement during a night with a hypnic headache, whereas seven did not. Interestingly, one patient had a remission of hypnic headache for 3 months after traveling across time zones.[14]

## Comorbidity

In 44 cases, the previous headache history was reported. Fifteen cases had migraine, three of them with aura in their prior history. In seven cases, episodic tension-type headache was reported. Two had chronic daily headache, one had unspecified hemicranial headache, and one had cervicogenic headache. In 18 cases, the absence of headache in the history was reported.

Comorbidity with other diseases or disorders was noted in a number of patients. The most frequently reported condition was arterial hypertension in 12 patients; in 27 patients, however, arterial hypertension was excluded. There were no reports of nocturnal hypertension. In 2 patients, smoking of at least 20 pack-years was described, but in the majority of patients, no information on smoking habits was given. The remaining conditions reported were atrial fibrillation, diabetes mellitus (2), depression or dysthymia (4), coronary heart disease, including myocardial infarction (4), malignant neoplasm (5), obstructive sleep apnea syndrome (2 without polysomnography), stroke, Meniere's disease, hiatus hernia, tuberculosis, essential tremor (2), epilepsy (2), cystic kidneys, human immunodeficiency virus (HIV) infection without acquired immune deficiency syndrome (AIDS), pituitary microadenoma, and Sjögren's syndrome. No pattern of diseases or disorders typically associated with hypnic headache could be noted.

## MANAGEMENT

In all case reports on hypnic headache, the efficacy of different drugs and treatment procedures tried in the patients were described. Acute medication in the attack was tested only in a few patients. Notably, sumatriptan administered subcutaneously and oxygen inhalation, the drugs of first choice for the treatment of cluster headache attacks, were not effective. Only acetylsalicylic acid demonstrated, on average, moderate efficacy for the acute relief of hypnic headache attacks.

From the standpoint of preventive medications reported, lithium was used most frequently and also showed the best average efficacy. It has been suggested to be the drug of first choice by several authors. Similar ratios of successful versus unsuccessful treatment could be obtained for indomethacin, flunarizine, and caffeine. The efficacy of indomethacin is of special interest because this drug is also effective in paroxysmal hemicrania and hemicrania continua.[5] It has been suggested that indomethacin may be helpful only in patients whose hypnic headache attacks are unilateral.[15] All other drugs did not provide benefit for the prevention of hypnic headache attacks better than an expected placebo rate of about one-third. In particular, antidepressant drugs and β-blockers were not useful. A list of all drugs applied in at least two patients and their efficacy, as reported by the respective authors, is presented in Table 10–3.

Nondrug therapy, such as sleep-behavior therapy or physiotherapy, was not reported. Continuous positive airway pressure (CPAP) was completely successful in one patient with obstructive sleep apnea, demonstrated by overnight polysomnography,[12] whereas continuous oxygen supply was tried in three patients without any benefit.

## PATHOPHYSIOLOGY

The pathophysiology of hypnic headache must remain speculative because there are no experimental studies on its nature. It has been debated whether hypnic headache is a particular subtype of cluster headache. However, only the nocturnal occurrence of hypnic headache supports this hypothesis. There is no strict unilaterality and no obligatory symptoms indicating paraympathetic activation in hypnic headache, as is

**Table 10–3**  Different Drug Treatments in the Case Reports on Hypnic Headache*

| Drug Name | Efficacy | | |
|---|---|---|---|
| | None | Moderate | Good |
| Acute drugs | | | |
| Acetylsalicylic acid (9) | 3 | 5 | 1 |
| Triptans, including subcutaneous formulation (8) | 6 | 1 | 1 |
| Ergotamine derivatives (6) | 3 | 2 | 1 |
| Acetaminophen (5) | 3 | 2 | — |
| Oxygen inhalation (4) | 4 | — | — |
| Nimesulide (2) | 1 | — | 1 |
| Prophylactic drugs | | | |
| Lithium (43) | 5 | 5 | 33 |
| Indomethacin (21) | 8 | 5 | 8 |
| Caffeine (21) | 9 | 4 | 8 |
| Tricyclic antidepressants (20) | 19 | 1 | — |
| β-Blockers (15) | 14 | — | 1 |
| NSAR (prophylactic) (11) | 7 | 4 | — |
| Verapamil (9) | 6 | 1 | 2 |
| Melatonin (9) | 4 | 2 | 3 |
| Flunarizine (7) | 3 | — | 4 |
| Anticonvulsants others than gabapentin (6) | 6 | — | — |
| Prednisone (6) | 3 | 1 | 2 |
| Antidepressants others than tricyclic (4) | 4 | — | — |
| Benzodiazepines (4) | 3 | — | 1 |
| Pizotifen (4) | 3 | — | 1 |
| Methysergide (3) | 3 | — | — |
| Gabapentin (3) | — | 2 | 1 |
| Clonidine (3) | 2 | 1 | — |
| Opiates (2) | 2 | — | — |
| Barbiturates (2) | 1 | — | 1 |

*Number of patient reports in brackets. Only the drugs tried in at least two patients are presented.
The efficacy is classified according to the statements of the respective authors.

usually observed for the trigeminal autonomic cephalgias. It has been assumed that hypnic headache is a spectrum disorder (eg, some patients with unilateral headache and some with autonomic symptoms), with an overlap with other primary headache disorders.[3] Interestingly, some cases of cluster headache would fulfill the criteria for hypnic headache, but not vice versa, if the absence of autonomic symptoms was omitted from the criteria.

More striking is the observation that the onset of hypnic headache attacks is associated with REM sleep, which was observed in all but one patient with polysomnography or sleep history. Although the number of cases is too small for any final conclusions, this observation suggests that pain-processing structures are activated during REM sleep. This might be a similar mechanism as, for example, in Schenck's syndrome, when the pyramidal motor system is active during REM sleep. Other authors have described headache owing to arterial hypertension, which might also occur during REM sleep,[16] and owing to low oxygenation during REM sleep.[12] The former condition has been called nocturnal headache-hypertension syndrome, and these headaches could be successfully treated by antihypertensive medication, which is adjusted to lower the nocturnal increase of blood pressure.[16]

It is known that the different types of sleep apnea coincide with morning or nocturnal headache.[17,18] However, in the case series with polysomnography in hypnic headache, no obstructive sleep apnea syndrome was found.[4,9] Only one patient improved after CPAP and oxygen supplementation,[12] whereas three patients did not.[4]

It was suggested that hypnic headache might be a REM sleep disorder owing to a disturbance of the sleep-related physiology of brainstem areas.[12] During REM sleep, the activity of the dorsal raphe and the locus cerulei nuclei is absent.[19] These areas are, together with the periaqueductal gray matter, essential parts of the human antinociceptive system, and it may be that in hypnic headache, this inactivity facilitates ascending transmission of trigeminal nociception in susceptible individuals.[12] Certainly, headaches occur frequently during sleep and, specifically during REM sleep, in headache-susceptible individuals (ie, migraine and cluster headache). This observation supports the concept that changes in the activity of aminergic nuclei during sleep are important for modulation of spontaneous activity and ascending transmission from the trigeminal nucleus caudalis.

Furthermore, hypnic headache might be a chronobiologic disturbance because many patients experience the headache attack always at the same time in the night (alarm-clock headache). The most important brain structure for the endogenous circadian rhythm is the suprachiasmatic nuclei (SCN). The SCN have afferent and efferent projections with the periaqueductal gray and aminergic nuclei, which are the most important brainstem structures for pain modulation. With advanced age, the function of the hypothalamic-pineal axis, and in particular of the SCN, is diminished, and melatonin secretion is impaired or absent after the age of 60 years. This phenomenon can also be observed in cluster headache.[20] There are several biologic functions of melatonin, which could explain how decreased levels of this hormone would lead to the development of headache.[3] The nature of hypnic headache as a chronobiologic disorder is also supported by the efficacy of

lithium, which has therapeutic value in other chronobiologic disorders, such as cluster headache and affective disorders. Lithium indirectly increases the level of melatonin[21–23] and may thus affect the pathophysiology of hypnic headache. In one patient with hypnic headache, the efficacy of melatonin has been shown.[12] In addition, lithium is able to affect serotonin metabolism by down-regulation of serotonin receptors and increased serotonin release.[24] Hence, it could be speculated that serotonin metabolism is also affected in patients with hypnic headache.

Structural lesions or metabolic dysfunction could not be detected in any of the cases reviewed. This suggests that hypnic headache is a primary headache disorder rather than a symptomatic or secondary headache. However, a symptomatic headache cannot be fully dismissed because there are no systematic studies on metabolic changes or other underlying sleep disorders. Furthermore, there is no evidence for a genetic disposition for hypnic headache, which would support the hypothesis of a primary headache disorder. Admittedly, the number of cases is too small to exclude genetic mechanisms, and the lack of a genetic influence is evident in other rare primary headache disorders, such as chronic paroxysmal hemicrania and SUNCT (short-lasting, unilateral, neuralgiform headache with conjunctival infection and tearing) sydrome. The variety of drugs reported to be effective in hypnic headache also underscores the possibility that the pathophysiology might be heterogeneous.

## SYMPTOMATIC CASES

According to the IHS criteria for hypnic headache, intracranial lesions must be excluded. This is certainly difficult because older patients frequently show nonnspecific intracranial abnormalities, such as microangiopathic leukoencephalopathy ($T_2$-weighted hyperintensities or asymptomatic lacunar infarctions) or brain atrophy, which cannot be regarded as the cause of hypnic headache. However, some symptomatic cases have been described in which the hypnic headache was linked to the onset of an intracranial lesion or disappeared after its removal. Peatfield and Mendoza presented the case of a 54-year-old female patient who suffered from typical hypnic headache and was diagnosed with posterior fossa meningioma.[25] After removal of the tumor, no further attacks of hypnic headache occurred. In addition, in a 72-year-old male patient with hypnic headache, attacks occurred after an ischemic stroke in the midrostral upper pons, which is the anatomic localization of the pontine reticular formation[26] and aminergic nuclei. In a 43-year-old black female patient, the diagnostic work-up of a typical hypnic headache revealed a nonspecific inflammatory meningeal lesion in the region of the foramen lacerum.[8] At this time, the patient was also diagnosed as having an HIV infection with involvement of several cranial nerves. Causation in this particular case cannot be certain, however.

## CONCLUSIONS

It can be concluded that hypnic headache is most likely a primary headache syndrome. Given that accompanying autonomic symptoms are lacking in the majority of cases and are very mild in the remaining, hypnic headache is appropriately not classified as a trigeminal autonomic cephalgia but must be classified as one of the miscellaneous headaches not associated with structural lesions (group 4 of the IHS classification). The diagnostic work-up of patients presenting with the typical clinical picture of hypnic headache should include MRI of the brain to exclude brainstem lesions. In some cases, overnight polysomnography may be helpful to distinguish hypnic headache from obstructive sleep apnea, REM sleep-behavior disorder, or other parasomnias. The most effective preventive agent for hypnic headache appears to be lithium carbonate and, to a lesser extent, indomethacin or caffeine given in the evening. Acute treatment of hypnic headache attacks is often not possible or necessary owing to the short duration and mild or moderate intensity of the attacks. The triptans and oxygen do not appear to provide significant pain relief, at least according to the limited evidence available. Because of the different treatment approaches, it is important for the clinician to distinguish hypnic headache from other primary headache disorders, especially cluster headache and paroxysmal hemicrania, both of which can also occur exclusively or predominantly during sleep. Patients should be reassured regarding the benign nature and favorable prognosis of the condition and the possibility for spontaneous remission, although long-term treatment appears to be necessary in most patients.

## REFERENCES

1. Raskin NH. The hypnic headache syndrome. Headache 1988;28:534–6.

2. Newman LC, Lipton RB, Solomon S. The hypnic headache syndrome: a benign headache disorder of the elderly. Neurology 1990;40:1904–5.

3. Dodick DW, Mosek AC, Campbell JK. The hypnic ("alarm clock") headache syndrome. Cephalalgia 1998;18:152–6.

4. Evers S, Goadsby PJ. Hypnic headache. Clinical features, pathophysiology, and treatment. Neurology 2003;60:905–10.

5. Goadsby PJ, Lipton RB. A review of paroxysmal hemicranias, SUNCT syndrome and other short-lasting headaches with autonomic feature, including new cases. Brain 1997;120:193–209.

6. Headache Classification Subcommittee, International Headache Society. The international classification of headache disorders. Cephalalgia 2004;24 Suppl 1:1–160.

7. Ghiotti N, Sances G, Di Lorenzo G, et al. Report of eight new cases of hypnic headache and mini-review of the literature. Funct Neurol 2002;211–9.

8. Vieira-Dias M, Esperance P. Cefaleas hipnicas: cuatro casos clinicos. Rev Neurol 2002;34:950–1.

9. Pinessi I, Rainero I, Cicolin A, et al. Hypnic headache syndrome: association of the attacks with REM sleep. Cephalalgia 2003;23:150–4.

10. Sibon I, Ghorayeb I, Henry P. Successful treatment of hypnic headache syndrome with acetazolamide. Neurology 2003;61:1157–8.

11. Evers S, Rahmann A, Schwaag S, et al. Hypnic headache—the first German cases including polysomnography. Cephalalgia 2003;23:20–3.

12. Dodick DW. Polysomnography in hypnic headache syndrome. Headache 2000;40:748–52.

13. Molina Arjona JA, Jimenez-Jimenez FJ, Vela-Bueno A, Tallon-Barranco A. Hypnic headache associated with stage 3 slow wave sleep. Headache 2000;40:753–4.

14. Martins IP, Gouveia IRG. Hypnic headache and travel across time zones: a case report. Cephalalgia 2001;21:928–31.

15. Dodick DW, Jones JM, Capobianco DJ. Hypnic headache: another indomethacin-responsive headache syndrome? Headache 2000;40:830–5.

16. Cugini P, Granata M, Strano S, et al. Nocturnal headache-hypertension syndrome: a chronobiologic disorder. Chronobiol Int 1992;9:310–3.

17. Aldrich MS, Chauncey JB. Are morning headaches part of obstructive sleep apnea syndrome? Arch Intern Med 1990;150:1265–7.

18. Loh NK, Dinner DS, Foldvary N, et al. Do patients with obstructive sleep apnea wake up with headaches? Arch Intern Med 1999;159:1765–8.

19. Somers VK, Dyken ME, Mark AL, Abboud FM. Sympathetic-nerve activity during sleep in normal subjects. N Engl J Med 1993;328:303–7.

20. Leone M, Lucini V, D'Amico D, et al. Twenty-four hour melatonin and cortisol plasma levels in relation to timing of cluster headache. Cephalalgia 1995;15:224–9.

21. Chazot G, Claustrat B, Brun J, Zaidan R. Effects of the patterns of melatonin and cortisol in cluster headache of a single administration of lithium at 7:00 p.m. daily

over one week: a preliminary report. Pharmacopsychiatry 1987;20:222–3.

22. Lewis AJ, Kerenyi NA, Feuer G. Neuropharmacology of pineal secretion. Drug Metab Drug Interact 1990;8:247–312.

23. Pablos MI, Santaolaya MJ, Agapito MT, Recio JM. Influence of lithium salts on chick pineal gland melatonin secretion. Neurosci Lett 1994;174:55–7.

24. Treiser SL, Cascio CS, O'Donohue TL, et al. Lithium increases serotonin release and decreases serotonin receptors in the hippocampus. Science 1981;213:1529–37.

25. Peatfield RC, Mendoza ND. Posterior fossa meningioma presenting as hypnic headache. Headache 2003;43:1007–8.

26. Moon HS, Chung CS, Kim HY, Kim DH. Hypnic headache syndrome: report of a symptomatic case. Cephalalgia 2003;23:673–4.

# Secondary Chronic
# Daily Headache

# CHAPTER 11

# Medication-Overuse Headache

Hans-Christoph Diener, MD, PhD, Volker Limmroth, MD, and Zaza Katsarava, MD

## INTERNATIONAL HEADACHE SOCIETY CLASSIFICATION AND DEFINITION

Frequent intake of analgesics leads to chronic headache. This was probably first observed in Switzerland, where workers in the pharmaceutical industry were given free samples of pain medication containing phenacetin at the workplace.[1] Peters and Horton observed the same phenomenon in patients with excessive use of ergotamine preparations and later described 52 patients who took ergotamine on a daily basis, developed daily headache, and significantly improved after ergotamine was withdrawn.[2,3] The literature up to 1988 is summarized by Diener and Wilkinson and up to 2004 by Diener and Limmroth.[4,5] Just 1 year after their introduction in 1993, it became evident that the triptans (5-hydroxytryptamine [5-HT]$_{1B/D}$ agonists), like all other drugs for the treatment of headache, would lead to medication-overuse headache (MOH) but might cause a "pure" increase in migraine frequency.[6,7]

Many terms have served to describe this entity, which was first defined under the name "drug-induced headache" by the International Headache Society (IHS) in 1988.[8] This term has been criticized because the single intake of several drugs, such as nitrates, may also lead to headache. To emphasize the regular intake of drugs as the basis of this headache form, the new term, "medication-overuse headache," has now been introduced with the new IHS classification from 2004.[9] The new classification further extends the definition according to different clinical symptoms caused by different drugs (Table 11–1).

## DRUGS THAT MAY CAUSE MOH

There is now substantial evidence that all drugs used for the treatment of headache may cause MOH in patients with primary headache disorders. The use of drugs that lead to chronic MOH varies considerably from country to country and is influenced by cultural factors. In many patients, it is difficult to identify a single "responsible" substance because 90% of patients take more than one compound at a time and because each component contained in antimigraine drugs can potentially induce headache. This has been shown even for substances such as acetylsalicylic acid and acetaminophen.[10]

Four studies investigating the frequency of the chemical compounds of various drugs have been performed.[11–14] Combination analgesics containing butalbital (short-acting barbiturate), caffeine, and aspirin with or without codeine were the leading candidates for MOH in an American study.[14] Until the mid-1990s, combination analgesics with codeine or caffeine or ergots combined with codeine were most frequently (mis)used in many European countries.[11–13] The introduction of triptans and the fact that ergots have recently been withdrawn from some markets (eg, in Germany) is now changing the picture. Sumatriptan-induced MOH was first observed in patients who abused ergotamine previously.[6,15] De novo cases, however, were later reported.[16–18] Studies involving patients who developed MOH from naratriptan, zolmitriptan, or rizatriptan usually were published 1 year after a drug had been approved.[7,19] Today, there is no doubt that all available triptans may cause MOH. Owing to the delay between frequent triptan intake and the development of MOH, similar cases will probably be observed in the future because other triptans (eletriptan, frovatriptan, almotriptan) have been approved. Headache patients who have a history of analgesic and/or ergotamine misuse are at a higher risk. It will be interesting to observe whether new treatment principles, such as calcitonin gene–related peptide antagonism,[20] will also lead to MOH once introduced into the treatment of migraine attacks.

**Table 11–1**   Diagnostic Criteria of Medication-Overuse Headache According to the Second Classification of Headache Disorders*

| Type of MOH | Diagnostic Criteria |
| --- | --- |
| Ergotamine-overuse headache (8.2.1, G44.411) | A: Headache present on ≥ 15 d/mo, with at least 1 of the following characteristics and fulfilling criteria C and D: |
| |    1. Bilateral |
| |    2. Pressing/tightening quality |
| |    3. Mild or moderate intensity |
| | B: Ergotamine intake on ≥ 10 d/mo on a regular basis for > 3 mo |
| | C: Headache has developed or markedly worsened during ergotamine overuse |
| | D: Headache resolves or reverts to its previous pattern within 2 mo after discontinuation of ergotamine |
| Triptan-overuse headache (8.2.2, G44.41) | A: Headache present on ≥ 15 d/mo |
| | B: Triptan intake (any formulation) on ≥ 10 d/mo on a regular basis for ≥ 3 mo |
| | C: Headache frequency has markedly increased during triptan overuse |
| | D: Headache reverts to its previous pattern within 2 mo after discontinuation of triptan |
| Analgesic-overuse headache (8.2.3, G44.410) | A: Headache present on ≥ 15 d/mo |
| | B: Intake of simple analgesics on ≥ 15 d/mo on a regular basis for > 3 mo |
| | C: Headache has developed or markedly worsened during analgesic overuse |
| | D: Headache resolves or reverts to its previous pattern within 2 mo after discontinuation of analgesics |
| Opioid-overuse headache (8.2.4, G44.83) | A: Headache present on ≥ 15 d/mo fulfilling criteria C and D: |
| | B: Opioid intake on ≥ 10 d/mo for > 3 mo |
| | C: Headache has developed or markedly worsened during opioid overuse |
| | D: Headache resolves or reverts to its previous pattern within 2 mo after discontinuation of opioids |
| Combination medication–overuse headache (8.2.5, G44.410) | A: Headache present on ≥ 15 d/mo |
| | B: Intake of simple analgesics on ≥ 10 d/mo on a regular basis for > 3 mo |
| | C: Headache has developed or markedly worsened during analgesic overuse |
| | D: Headache resolves or reverts to its previous pattern within 2 mo after discontinuation of combination medication |
| Probable medication-overuse headache (8.2.7, G44.41, or 44.83) | A: Headache fulfilling criteria A–C for any 1 of the subforms above |
| | B: One or other of the following: |
| |    1. Overuse medication has not yet been withdrawn |
| |    2. Medication overuse has ceased within the last 2 mo, but headache has not so far resolved or reverted to its previous pattern |

MOH = medication-overuse headache.

*International Classification of Headache Disorders II code 8.2; International Classification of Diseases 10 G44.4 or G44.83.

## CLINICAL MANIFESTATION

Despite the IHS classification[9] and the fact that the diagnosis of MOH does not require any additional examinations (only to exclude symptomatic forms of chronic headache) and is based on the patient's history and the clinical presentation only, MOH is frequently overlooked. Almost no experimental work has been done in this field, and the following is based mainly on clinical series describing patients presenting at headache clinics with this problem, with subsequent treatment and follow-up. Several clinical characteristics may help identify MOH in patients with primary headache disorders.[14] Table 11–2 summarizes important clinical characteristics.

A prospective study of 96 patients investigated the characteristics of MOH with regard to different substances.[19,21] In this study, conducted between 1999 and 2001, triptan overuse far outnumbered ergot overuse. This reflects the fact that, despite high costs, triptans have become widely used (and overused) and suggests that they are about to become the most important group to cause MOH. Unlike patients who suffer from MOH following ergot or analgesic overuse, migraine patients (but not tension-type headache patients) with triptan-induced headache did not describe the typical tension-type daily headache but rather a migraine-like daily headache (a unilateral, pulsating headache with autonomic disturbances) or a significant (and pure) increase in migraine attack frequency. Furthermore, the delay between the frequent medication intake and the development of daily headache was shortest for triptans (1.7 years), longer for ergots (2.7 years), and longest for analgesics (4.8 years). The intake frequency (single dosages per month) was lowest for triptans (18 single dosages per month), higher for ergots (37 single dosages per month), and highest for analgesics (114 single dosages per month). Hence, triptans not only cause a different spectrum of clinical features but are able to cause MOH faster and with lower dosages compared with other substance groups.

Diener and Dahlöf performed a meta-analysis summarizing 29 studies comprising a total of 2,612 patients with chronic MOH.[22] Sixty-five percent of the patients reported migraine as their primary headache, 27% reported tension-type headache as their primary headache, and 8% reported mixed or other headaches as their primary headache. Women were more prone to MOH than men (3.5:1; 1,533 women, 442 men). This ratio is slightly higher than would be expected from the gender differences in the frequency of migraine. The mean duration of primary headache was 20.4 years. The mean admitted time of frequent drug intake was 10.3 years, and the mean duration of daily headache was 5.9 years. The results from headache diaries show that the number of tablets or suppositories taken per day averages 4.9 (range 0.25–25). On average, patients take 2.5 to 5.8 different pharmacologic components simultaneously (range 1–14).[22] As seen in the recent study by Katsarava and colleagues, the number of doses per day is much smaller in patients who abuse triptans.[19]

**Table 11–2**  Clinical Characteristics of Medication-Overuse Headache

| | |
|---|---|
| General headache symptoms and observations | The headaches are refractory, daily, or near-daily. |
| | The headache itself varies in its severity, type, and location from time to time. |
| | Physical or intellectual effort may bring on headache. In other words, the threshold for head pain appears to be low. |
| | Withdrawal symptoms are observed when patients are taken off pain medication abruptly. |
| | Spontaneous improvement of headache occurs when the medications are discontinued after a few days. |
| | Concomitant prophylactic medications are (and are reported) to be ineffective while the patients are consuming excess amounts of immediate-relief medication. |
| Associated symptoms | Asthenia, nausea, gastrointestinal symptoms |
| | Irritability, anxiety, restlessness, depression |
| | Memory problems and difficulty in intellectual concentration |
| Special symptoms under ergot overuse | Cold extremities, tachycardia, paresthesias, "irritable bowl syndrome" |
| | Diminished pulse, hypertension, lightheadedness, muscle pain of the extremities, weakness of the legs |

## ETIOLOGY AND PATHOPHYSIOLOGY

The etiology of MOH is still widely unknown. Several mechanisms, however, appear to play an important role.

### Genetic Disposition

The association between analgesic overuse and headache has been studied in conditions other than primary headache disorders. Chronic overuse of analgesics does not cause increased headache in nonmigraineurs. For example, patients who were consuming fairly large amounts of analgesics regularly for arthritis did not show an increased incidence of headache.[23] In patients with cluster headache, who often consume large amounts of analgesics or triptans, MOH is not reported. In contrast, it has recently been shown that patients with migraine who are forced to take analgesics for the treatment of other pain conditions than headache are significantly more likely to develop MOH than nonmigraineurs.[24] The conclusion drawn from various clinical observations and studies is that MOH may be restricted to individuals who are already headache sufferers. The basis for this could either be genetic or the fact that migraine pain is more severe than, for example, joint pain.

### Receptor and Enzyme Physiology and Regulation

There is no doubt that the regular exposure to the same substance will induce significant changes regarding expression and sensitization of receptors, as well as changes for the threshold of receptor activation. The extent of these changes and the velocity in which these changes occur depend on the receptor type (eg, ion channels or G protein–coupled receptors) and the duration and concentration of drug exposure. Recently, it was shown in rats that regular (daily) exposure to 5-$HT_{1B/D}$ agonists (triptans), such as sumatriptan or zolmitriptan, causes a significant down-regulation of these receptors in various cortical regions, the extrapyramidal system, and the brainstem and influences the synthesis rate of serotonin.[25,26] Moreover, from *in vivo* studies, it is well known that down-regulation of 5-HT receptors may occur as early as 24 to 96 hours following chronic exposure.[27] Chronic or frequent exposure to 5-$HT_{1B/D}$ agonists may lead in humans to a down-regulation of 5-HT receptors and change central inhibitory pathways significantly. The same mechanisms account for the regulation of enzymes such as cyclooxygenase I and II, which are the main pharmacologic targets of analgesics, such as acetylsalicylic acid or ibuprofen. Enzyme regulation, however, is slower and needs a longer exposure time and a higher drug concentration.[28] These theoretical aspects, however, are well in line with clinical experience and a recently conducted trial on withdrawal symptoms showing that MOH will develop faster under triptans than under analgesic misuse but that the intensity and duration of withdrawal symptoms will be significantly milder and shorter when triptans have been misused.[29] Thus, it is tempting to hypothesize that the down-regulation of 5-HT receptors and/or prostaglandin-synthesizing enzymes within anatomic structures involved in the transmission or modulation of nociceptive signals such as the perioquaeductual gray (PAG) (which exhibits serotoninergic descending inhibitory pathways mainly to trigeminal nuclei) may lead to an impairment of antinociceptive activity and subsequently result in a permanent feeling of head pain.

### Psychological and Behavioral Mechanisms

Psychological factors include the reinforcing properties of pain relief by drug consumption, a very powerful component of positive conditioning. Many patients report that they take migraine drugs prophylactically because they are worried about missing work or an important social event or they fear an imminent headache. They are often instructed by physicians or by the instructions supplied with the medication to take the migraine drug as early as possible at the start of either the aura or the headache phase of a migraine attack. Early treatment also bears the danger that patients consume more medication than necessary and thereby steadily increases their intake frequency, even for headache attacks, which would not have been treated otherwise. This model behavior can be relevant in families because children may learn the early and low-threshold consumption of analgesic from their parents.

Withdrawal headache is an additional factor. When the patient tries to stop or reduce the medication, the preexisting headache worsens. Barbiturates that are contained in drugs used to treat tension-type headache have a high potency for addiction. The stimulating action of analgesics or migraine drugs and their psychotropic side effects, such as sedation or mild euphoria, may lead to drug dependency. Barbiturates, codeine, other opioids, and caffeine are most likely to have this effect. Caffeine increases vigilance, relieves fatigue, and improves performance and mood.[30,31] The typical symptoms of caffeine withdrawal, such as irritability, nervousness, restlessness, and, especially, "caffeine withdrawal headache,"[32,33] which may last for several days, encourage patients to continue their abuse.

### Physical Dependencies

Headache patients have been reported to develop physical dependency on codeine and other opioids.[34,35] Although some headache patients have been on codeine for as long as 10 years, no studies have investigated the effects of codeine intake over this time period.[36] It should be remembered that up to 10% of codeine is metabolized to morphine. Ergotamine and dihydroergotamine (DHE) may lead to physical dependency.[37] Many migraineurs take ergotamine as prophylactic treatment. The reason for the physical dependency on ergotamine remains obscure. One study found that the tyramine-induced mydriasis after ergotamine administration was increased during abuse but not after withdrawal of ergotamine, which would indicate a central inhibition of pupillary sympathetic activity during abuse.[38] Thus, a possible central nervous system (CNS) effect of ergotamine can be observed after chronic use but not after a single dose of the drug. Other studies investigating the effect of the chronic use of ergotamine on CNS regulation of the autonomic nervous system are needed.

## EPIDEMIOLOGY

Cross-sectional population-based epidemiologic studies indicate that chronic headache is common, with prevalence rates between 2 and 5%,[36–40] and a prevalence rate of chronic headache associated with medication overuse or probable MOH is seen in about 1%.[39–42] Unfortunately, there is growing evidence that the overuse of analgesics and subsequent MOH is not only prevalent in the Western world but a growing problem in Asian countries, such as China or Taiwan, as well,[40] with the same prevalence as observed in Europe. Furthermore, it seems that it completely escapes public attention that analgesic overuse and MOH are already a problem in early adolescence and even childhood.[43] A recent study on caffeine-induced headache in children revealed that MOH may occur in children as early as age 6 years. In this study, children suffered from MOH, on average, for over 12 months, indicating that the overuse was initiated at age 4 or 5 years.[44] Although precise data on the prevalence of MOH in children are not yet available, the first reports on MOH withdrawal therapy in children clearly demonstrate the magnitude of this rising problem.[45]

Most headache centers report that between 5 and 10% of the patients they see fulfill the criteria of MOH.[46] Micieli and colleagues observed an incidence of 4.3% in 3,000 consecutive headache patients.[12] A survey of family doctors showed that MOH was the third most common cause of headache.[47] In some specialized headache clinics in North America, medication overuse has been reported to be present in up to 70% of cases.[47]

A potential problem arises from the recent concept to recommend drug intake as early as possible.[48–51] Although the degree of drug efficacy (triptans in particular) may improve in migraine attacks, it enhances the likelihood that the patient will take medication more frequently than necessary and subsequently paves the way for the development of MOH. At least some of the early headaches may not develop into a migraine attack or may represent a phase of episodic tension-type headache that requires a different type of treatment. Therefore, the general recommendation to treat as early as possible should be given only to patients who have been told about this aspect, who are suffering from migraine only, or who are able to distinguish migraine attacks from episodic tension-type headache even in the early phases of the headache.

Taken together, these studies indicate that MOH is a major health problem all over the world. Considering the potential secondary effects of chronic medication overuse on other organ systems, which include chronic kidney failure (combination analgesics), gastrointestinal ulcers (nonsteroidal anti-inflammatory drugs [NSAIDs]), or ergotism,[52–54] education on MOH should be mandatory for medical students and all physicians who treat headache patients.

## DIAGNOSTIC WORK-UP

Unfortunately, there is no technical tool to prove the presence of MOH. Medical history, the course of the disorder, the history of drug intake, and intake frequency, ideally supported by a well-maintained headache diary, are the only available tools. Some patients may be reluctant to reveal their entire drug consumption. Hence, it is key to explain to patients the concept of MOH and the need to know these details.

Patients frequently take several different substances daily, despite the fact that their effect is negligible. This behavior is merely an attempt to avoid a disabling withdrawal headache. If not available, patients should record their present and previous use of prescription drugs and nonprescription compounds and caffeine intake. Many patients also abuse other substances, such as tranquilizers, opioids, decongestants, and laxatives. It is often helpful to have patients keep a diagnostic headache diary for 1 month to record headache pattern and drug use. The history and examination should also search for possible complications of regular drug intake, for example, recurrent gastric ulcers, bowel disease, anemia, hypertension, and signs of ergotism. A good indicator for MOH is the number of physicians the patient has consulted and the number of previous unsuccessful therapies. One study showed that headache patients had consulted an average of 5.5 physicians, who had prescribed 8.6 different therapies.[55]

The careful inquiry regarding the course of the headache and acute medication use may suggest chronic migraine when the transformation is gradual over a period of many months or years. An abrupt increase in medication consumption may be caused by a spontaneous increase in the frequency of migraine or tension-type headache. Concomitant medical problems, stress, sleep disturbance, hormonal factors, depression, and certain nonheadache medications can cause an increase in headache frequency. If there is no obvious nonorganic cause for the change in headache pattern, clinical reevaluation is advisable. If clinical reevaluation suggests the possibility of serious medical or neurologic illness, appropriate diagnostic testing, including imaging, is indicated.

## DIFFERENTIAL DIAGNOSIS

All conditions leading to more than 15 headache days per month must be considered in the differential diagnosis of MOH. The high frequency of drug intake, however, does not necessarily mean that MOH is present, but may reflect the fact that patients suffer from another chronic headache disorder or that the patient is in the transition phase to MOH but the biologic transformation to MOH has not yet occurred.[51] A diagnostic diary is often helpful to monitor the precise drug intake and to reveal the extent of overuse. The important differential diagnoses that have to be considered are shown in Table 11–3.

With the new IHS classification,[9] the term "chronic migraine" (similar but not identical to "transformed migraine" [see Chapter 4, "Chronic Migraine"]) has been introduced and defined. The diagnosis requires that patients have a history of episodic migraine attacks, which increased in frequency over time, and that the diagnostic criteria of migraine are fulfilled on more than 15 days per month. In some cases, the differentiation between MOH and chronic migraine may be impossible by clinical criteria alone and will require withdrawal therapy. According to the new classification, these cases can be classified as "probable chronic migraine" (International Classification of Headache Disorders [ICHD]-II 1.6.5; International Classification of Disorders [ICD]-10NA G43.83) or as "probable MOH" (ICHD-II 8.2.7; ICD-10NA G44.41/G44.83).

### Table 11–3    Important Differential Diagnoses to Medication-Overuse Headache

Primary headache disorders

   Chronic migraine

   Chronic tension-type headache

   Hemicrania continua

   New daily persistent  headache

Secondary headache disorders

   Cerebral venous and sinus thrombosis

   Giant cell arteritis

Chronic tension-type headache (CTTH) is a diffuse, dull, nonlocalized headache with or without minimal autonomic features. Headache intensity is lower than that of migraine. Patients find it difficult to describe the character of the pain. Sometimes it is described as a feeling of a metal band around the head or a feeling of increased pressure. Many patients with CTTH complain of mild autonomic disturbances, such as nausea, photophobia, or phonophobia. The IHS definition of CTTH requires head pain on at least 15 days per month for at least 6 months. CTTH has a prevalence of 2 to 3%.[42,56] When patients take an analgesic on more than 15 days per month or combined analgesics on more than 10 days per month, CTTH with medication overuse can be differentiated from CTTH without medication overuse only after drug withdrawal or a drug holiday. If the headache persists, the intake of analgesics was not responsible for the chronic headache. Until the withdrawal therapy is completed, these patients can be coded as "probable CTTH" (ICHD-II 2.4.3; ICD-10NA G44.28) or as "probable MOH" (ICHD-II 8.2.7; ICD-10NA G44.41/G44.83).

Sometimes it is impossible to separate migraine from tension-type headache. In these cases, treating at least three headache days with a triptan is recommended. If the headache responds to the triptan, headache prophylaxis is performed as if a migraine exists.[57–59] The other patients are treated for CTTH.

Patients who have hemicrania continua suffer from daily headache of moderate intensity. Superimposed exacerbation of severe headache with ipsilateral autonomic features, such as ptosis, miosis, tearing, and sweating,[60,61] may occur. Some patients have photo- and phonophobia or nausea. In some cases, the head pain may alternate sides. Hemicrania continua is differentiated from cluster headache and chronic paroxysmal hemicrania by its continuous pain character; furthermore, the autonomic symptoms during acute pain exacerbations are less pronounced compared with cluster headache or chronic paroxysmal hemicrania. Both forms can be successfully treated with indomethacin.

Patients with new daily persistent headache abruptly develop chronic headache without remission. Many patients remember the exact day the headache started. These patients did not have a previous history of migraine or episodic tension-type headache. In some patients, a viral infection was suspected to cause this form of headache.[62] The headache usually does not respond to ergots, triptans, or simple analgesics.

Among several secondary headaches, at least two differential diagnoses should be excluded. Thrombosis of the venous sinus may occur acutely or chronically (over weeks/month). Because the clinical presentation encompasses a variety of symptoms, such as headache, seizures, focal neurologic deficits, and more, the diagnosis can be a challenge. Still, the most frequently reported symptom is a holocranial headache in 70 to 90% of all cases. Typically, the headache is resistant to classic antiheadache medication and tends to increase with time. Giant cell arteritis is a segmental granulomatous inflammation of medium-sized arteries and the most common vasculitic syndrome, with a high prevalence in elderly patients. The clinical presentation may vary, but the majority of patients complain about a unilateral headache without a significant response to classic antiheadache medication. Other associated symptoms, such as painful jaw claudication, induration, and decreased pulse of the temporal artery, together with a marked elevation of the erythrocyte sedimentation rate, should facilitate the differential diagnosis.

## MANAGEMENT

Abrupt drug withdrawal is the treatment of choice for MOH (Table 11–4). However, no prospective and randomized trials on the natural course of MOH or the tapering of the offending drugs are available. A survey of 22 studies dealing with therapy of drug-induced headache showed that most centers use drug withdrawal as the primary therapy.[22] Clinical experience indicates that medical and behavioral headache treatment fails as long as the patient continues to take symptomatic drugs daily. No study until today, however, has prospectively treated MOH patients de novo with a migraine prophylactic drug to investigate whether headache frequency and intake of medication for treating acute headache can be influenced. Such a study is under way with topiramate.

The typical withdrawal symptoms last for 2 to 10 days (average 3.5 days) and include withdrawal headache, nausea, vomiting, arterial hypotension, tachycardia, sleep disturbances, restlessness, anxiety, and nervousness. The withdrawal phase is much shorter when patients are abusing triptans only. Seizures or hallucinations were only rarely observed, even in patients who were abusing barbiturate-containing migraine drugs.

Drug withdrawal is performed differently. Most colleagues prefer inpatient programs. Hering and Steiner abruptly withdrew the offending drugs on an outpatient basis using adequate explanation of the disorder, regular follow-up, and amitriptyline (10 mg at night) and naproxen (500 mg) for relief of headache symptoms.[63] A consensus paper by the German Migraine Society recommends outpatient withdrawal for patients who do not take barbiturates or tranquilizers with their analgesics and are highly motivated.[64] Inpatient treatment should be performed in patients who take tranquilizers, codeine, or barbiturates, who failed to withdraw the drugs as outpatients, or who have a high depression score.

Treatment recommendations for the acute phase of drug withdrawal vary considerably between studies. They include fluid replacement, analgesics, tranquilizers, neuroleptics, amitriptyline, valproate, intravenous DHE, oxygen, and electrical stimulation. Valproate has been shown to have beneficial effects in the prophylactic treatment of chronic daily headache (CDH) complicated by excessive analgesic intake.[65] A recent large open trial showed that cortisone effectively reduces withdrawal symptoms, including rebound headache.[66] A double-blind study showed a single subcutaneous dose of sumatriptan to be better than placebo in the treatment of ergotamine withdrawal headache, but the headache reappeared within 12 hours.[67] An open randomized study indicated that naproxen was better than symptomatic treatment with antiemetics and analgesics.[68] Further double-blind controlled trials are needed.

A short hospital stay is recommended if MOH has lasted more than 5 years when additional tranquilizer, barbiturate, or opioid intake exists. It is further indicated in patients who have failed outpatient withdrawal or have concomitant depression or anxiety disorder. In

| Table 11–4 | Clinical Criteria Suggesting Outpatient or Inpatient Withdrawal Therapy |
|---|---|
| Outpatient withdrawal | Patient highly motivated and self-disciplined |
| | Patient overuses triptans or other monosubstance drugs only, patient does not use drugs containing barbiturates or tranquilizers, or patient uses several different drugs |
| | Other typical signs or side effects of medication overuse are absent (ergotism, peptic ulcers, sleep disturbances) |
| | Patient does not suffer from other disorders, such as depression or anxiety |
| Inpatient withdrawal | Patient already underwent outpatient withdrawal |
| | Patient overuses drugs containing barbiturates or tranquilizers or uses several different drugs |
| | Patient suffers from other signs or side effects of medication overuse, such as ergotism, peptic ulcers, diarrhea, anemia |
| | Patient suffers from depression or anxiety |

the hospital, all pain or headache medication is stopped abruptly. Fluids should be replaced by infusion if frequent vomiting occurs. Vomiting can be treated with antiemetics, for example, metoclopramide or domperidone. The withdrawal headache can be treated with NSAIDs, for example, naproxen 500 mg twice daily. In some countries, aspirin is available in an injectable form, and 1,000 mg is given every 8 to 12 hours. If the headache has migrainous features and the patient has not abused ergots, DHE, or a triptan before, intravenous DHE 1 to 2 mg every 8 hours is given.[69–71] Prednisone, 100 mg on the first day, tapered by 20 mg for the following days, is very effective. Symptoms of opioid withdrawal can be treated with clonidine. The initial dose is 0.1 to 0.2 mg three times daily, and this is titrated up or down based on withdrawal symptoms (tachycardia, tremor, sleeping disturbances). Some patients may require anxiolytic medication; this should be given for no longer than a week. Patients need support by the treating physicians and nurses, as well as encouragement from family and friends. Behavioral techniques, such as relaxation therapy and stress management, should be initiated as soon as the withdrawal symptoms fade.

Outpatient treatment is advised for patients who take monosubstances or analgesic mixtures not containing barbiturates or codeine. Patients whose original headache is migraine (and who are scheduled for withdrawal therapy as an outpatient) can start prophylactic medication 4 weeks before withdrawal. β-blockers will improve withdrawal symptoms, such as restlessness, tachycardia, or tremor. Patients who have CTTH may be started on a tricylic antidepressant 4 weeks prior to detoxification (eg, amitriptyline 10 mg increasing to 25 to 75 mg at night). Ergots, triptans, and nonopioid drugs should be stopped abruptly. Opioids and barbiturates should be withdrawn more slowly depending on the dose and duration of intake. Withdrawal headache after ergots and triptans can be treated with oral or parenteral NSAIDs (eg, 500 mg naproxen three times daily for 5 to 7 days).

If a patient experiences more than three migraine attacks a month after withdrawal, medical and behavioral prophylaxis should be initiated. Clinical experience shows that many patients respond to prophylactic treatment with β-blockers, flunarizine, or valproic acid after drug withdrawal despite the fact that these drugs had been unsuccessful before. Ergotamine, triptans, and possibly analgesics counteract the action of prophylactic therapy and will not improve drug-induced headache. The same phenomenon can be observed for the action of amitriptyline and behavioral therapy in patients with tension-type headache.

## PREVENTION

The most important preventive measure is proper instruction and appropriate surveillance of patients. The migraine patients at risk often have a mixture of migraine and tension-type headaches and should be carefully instructed to use specific antimigraine drugs for migraine attacks only. This point was already stressed in 1951 by Peters and Horton concerning ergotamine abuse, that is, complications can be avoided if enough time is taken for proper instruction of the patient so that he or she can distinguish between "vasodilating" and "nondilating headache."[2]

Restricting the dose of ergotamine per attack (4 mg ergotamine), per week (no more than twice per week), and per month (no more than 20 mg ergotamine) is also helpful in avoiding dependency. In a similar way, the number of doses of triptans should be limited per attack and to 10 single doses per month.[72] Migraine drugs that contain barbiturates, caffeine, codeine, or tranquilizers, as well as mixed analgesics, should be avoided. Patients who take over-the-counter medication should be advised to avoid caffeine combinations. A headache diary is important for patients with frequent headache to detect a further increase of attack frequency or medication use as early as possible. Early migraine prophylaxis, either by medical or behavioral treatment, can be a preventive measure to avoid MOH.

## PROGNOSIS

The mean success rate of withdrawal therapy within a time window of 1 to 6 months is 72.4% (17 studies; $N$ = 1,101 patients). Success is defined as no headache or an improvement of more than 50% in terms of headache days. Three older studies (pretriptan era) had a longer observation period (between 9 and 35 months).[11,55,73] The success rates in these studies were 60%, 70%, and 73%, respectively. A 5-year follow-up study found a relapse rate of 40%.[73] Recent studies included patients with MOH following the misuse of triptans as well.[29,74,75] Two prospectively conducted studies indicated relapse rates for the first year after successful withdrawal therapy to be 38% and to be around 42% after 4 years.[29,75] This suggests that patients are at the greatest risk of suffering from a relapse within the first 12 months but, on the other hand, have a low risk of experiencing a relapse when they succeed in avoiding medication overuse for at least 12 months after withdrawal therapy. Interestingly, a subgroup analysis revealed that the risk of relapse mainly depends on two aspects: the type of primary headache and the type of drug that was overused.[75] Patients with tension-type headache as their primary headache entity had a significant higher relapse rate than patients with migraine (73% versus 22%, respectively). Moreover, patients who initially overuse analgesics (mostly combination analgesics) showed significantly higher relapse rates than patients overusing ergots or triptans (58% versus 22% versus 19%, respectively, for the first 12 months). Unexpectedly, other predictors, such as the duration of drug overuse, the duration of disorder, and the presence of prophylactic treatment, did not influence the relapse rate, neither within the first 12 months nor within 48 months.

Although some data are available regarding the prevalence of MOH and the prognosis after withdrawal therapy, the question to which extent patients with migraine are at risk of developing MOH has not been clarified completely. This question, however, was recently addressed by a prospective study on over 600 consecutive migraine patients without MOH or CDH.[76] Patients were prospectively followed up for 12 months. Fourteen percent of this cohort developed CDH within 1 year, and two-thirds, or almost 10%, of these patients fulfilled the criteria of MOH. Two main predictors could be identified: a high initial frequency of headache events and medication overuse. This confirms findings that have been reported from population-based studies suggesting that analgesic overuse predicted the persistence of CDH.[39,40] In one of the few prospective population-based studies, Zwart and colleagues showed that overuse of analgesics strongly predicted chronic pain associated with analgesic overuse 11 years later, particularly among those with chronic migraine.[41] More recently, the same group in a follow-up study could convincingly show that analgesic overuse is significantly more associated with chronic headache than with other chronic pain conditions, such as chronic neck pain or chronic low back pain.[77] These findings again highlight the need for a clear restriction of acute medication and early initiation of preventive medication in patients with headache.

Finally, it should be mentioned that many patients with CDH do not overuse their medication. In these cases, other biologic and psychological pathomechanisms, as well as other risks, may play a pivotal role.[78] It is hoped that the uncovering of those mechanisms leading to pain chronification in humans will be one of the most interesting and rewarding pieces of medical science in the near future.

## ACKNOWLEDGMENTS

This work was supported in part by the German Headache Consortium, funded by the Bundesministerium für Bildung und Forschung (BMBF) (01EM0117). This chapter is an updated version of a review: Diener HC and Limmroth V.[5]

## REFERENCES

1. Mihatsch MJ. Das Analgetikasyndrom. Stuttgart: Thieme; 1986.

2. Peters GA, Horton BT. Headache: with special reference to the excessive use of ergotamine preparations and withdrawal effects. Proc Staff Meet Mayo Clin 1951;26:153–61.

3. Horton BT, Peters GA. Clinical manifestations of excessive use of ergotamine preparations and management of withdrawal effect: report of 52 cases. Headache 1963;3:214–26.

4. Diener HC, Wilkinson M, editors. Drug-induced headache. Berlin: Springer; 1988.

5. Diener HC, Limmroth V. Medication-overuse headache: a worldwide problem. Lancet Neurol 2004;3:475–83.

6. Kaube H, May A, Diener HC, Pfaffenrath V. Sumatriptan misuse in daily chronic headache. BMJ 1994;308:1573.

7. Limmroth V, Kazarawa S, Fritsche G, Diener HC. Headache after frequent use of new 5-HT agonists, zolmitriptan and naratriptan. Lancet 1999;353:378.

8. Headache Classification Committee, International Headache Society. Classification and diagnostic criteria for headache disorders, cranial neuralgias and facial pain. Cephalalgia 1988;8 Suppl 7:1–93.

9. Olesen J, Bousser M-G, Diener H, et al, for the International Headache Society. The international classification of headache disorders. 2nd edition. Cephalalgia 2004;24 Suppl 1:1–160.

10. Rapoport A, Weeks R, Sheftell F. Analgesic rebound headache: theoretical and practical implications. In: Olesen J, Tfelt-Hansen P, Jensen K, editors. Proceedings of the Second International Headache Congress, Copenhagen. Copenhagen: International Headache Society; 1985. p. 448–9.

11. Baumgartner C, Wessely P, Bingöl C, et al. Longterm prognosis of analgesic withdrawal in patients with drug-induced headaches. Headache 1989;29:510–4.

12. Micieli G, Manzoni GC, Granella F, et al. Clinical and epidemiological observations on drug abuse in headache patients. In: Diener HC, Wilkinson M, editors. Drug-induced headache. Berlin: Springer; 1988. p. 20–8.

13. Diener HC, Bühler K, Dichgans J, et al. Analgetikainduzierter Dauerkopfschmerz. Existiert eine kritische Dosis? Arzneimitteltherapie 1988;6:156–64.

14. Mathew NT, Kurman R, Perez F. Drug induced refractory headache—clinical features and management. Headache 1990;30:634–8.

15. Catarci T, Fiacco F, Argentino C, et al. Ergotamine-induced headache can be sustained by sumatriptan daily intake. Cephalalgia 1994;14:374–5.

16. Gaist D, Hallas J, Sindrup SH, Gram LF. Is overuse of sumatriptan a problem? A population-based study. Eur J Clin Pharmacol 1996;3:161–5.

17. Gaist D, Tsiropoulus I, Sindrup SH, et al. Inappropriate use of sumatriptan: population based register and interview study. Br J Med 1998;316:1352–3.

18. Pini LA, Trenti T. Case report: does chronic use of sumatriptan induce dependence? Headache 1994;34:600–1.

19. Katsarava Z, Fritsche G, Diener HC, Limmroth V. Drug-induced headache (DIH) following the use of different triptans [abstract]. Cephalalgia 2000;20:293.

20. Olesen J, Diener H, Husstedt IW, et al, for the BIBN 4096 BS Clinical Proof of Concept Study Group. Calcitonin gene-related peptide (CGRP) receptor antagonist BIBN4096BS is effective in the treatment of migraine attacks. N Engl J Med 2004;350:1104–10.

21. Diener HC, Katsarava Z. Analgesic/abortive overuse and misuse in chronic daily headache. Curr Pain Headache Rep 2001;5:545–50.

22. Diener HC, Dahlöf CGH. Headache associated with chronic use of substances. In: Olesen J, Tfelt-Hansen P, Welch KMA, editors. The headaches. 2nd ed. Philadelphia: Lippincott, Williams & Wilkins; 1999. p. 871–8.

23. Lance F, Parkes C, Wilkinson M. Does analgesic abuse cause headache de novo? Headache 1988;38:61–2.

24. Bahra A, Walsh M, Menon S, Goadsby PJ. Does chronic daily headache arise de novo in association with regular use of analgesics? Headache 2003;43:179–90.

25. Dobson CF TY, Diksic M, Hamel E. Effects of acute or chronic administration of anti-migraine drugs sumatriptan and zolmitriptan on serotonin synthesis in the rat brain. Cephalalgia 2004;24:2–11.

26. Reuter U, Salome S, Ickenstein G, Waeber C. Effects of chronic sumatriptan and zolmitriptan treatment on 5-HT receptor expression and function in rats. Cephalalgia 2004;24:398–407.

27. Saucier C, Morris S, Albert P. Endogenous serotonin-2A and -2C receptors in Balb/c-3T3 cells revealed in serotonin-free medium: desensitization and down-regulation by serotonin. Biochem Pharmacol 1998;56:1347–57.

28. Weksler BB. Regulation of prostaglandin synthesis in human vascualr cells. Ann N Y Acad Sci 1987;509:142–8.

29. Katsarava Z, Fritsche G, Muessig M, et al. Clinical features of withdrawal headache following overuse of triptans and other headache drugs. Neurology 2001;57:1694–8.

30. Griffiths RR, Woodson PP. Reinforcing properties of caffeine: studies in humans and laboratory animals. Pharmacol Biochem Behav 1988;29:419–27.

31. Griffiths RR, Woodson PP. Caffeine physical dependence: a review of human and laboratory animal studies. Psychopharmacology 1988;94:437–51.

32. Silverman K, Evans SM, Strain EC, Griffiths RR. Withdrawal syndrome after the double-blind cessation of caffeine consumption. N Engl J Med 1992;327:1109–14.

33. van Dusseldorp M, Katan MB. Headache caused by caffeine withdrawal among moderate coffee drinkers switched from ordinary to decaffeinated coffee: a 12 week double blind trial. BMJ 1990;300:1558–9.

34. Fisher MA, Glass S. Butorphanol (Stadol): a study in problems of current drug information and control. Neurology 1997;48:1156–60.

35. Ziegler DK. Opiate and opioid use in patients with refractory headache. Cephalalgia 1994;14:5–10.

36. Seller EM, Busto UE, Kaplan HL, et al. Comparative abuse liability of codeine and naratriptan. Clin Pharmacol Ther 1998;63:121.

37. Saper JR, Jones JM. Ergotamine tartrate dependency: features and possible mechanisms. Clin Neuropharmacol 1986;9:244–56.

38. Fanciullacci M, Alessandri M, Pietrini U, et al. Long-term ergotamine abuse: effect on adrenergically induced mydriasis. Clin Pharmacol Ther 1992;51:302–7.

39. Lu SR, Fuh JL, Chen WT, et al. Chronic daily headache in Taipei, Taiwan: prevalence, follow-up and outcome predictors. Cephalalgia 2001;21:980–6.

40. Wang SJ, Fuh JL, Lu SR, et al. Chronic daily headache in Chinese elderly—prevalence, risk factors, and biannual follow-up. Neurology 2000;54:314–9.

41. Zwart J, Dyb G, Hagen K, et al. Analgesic use: a predictor of chronic pain and medication overuse headache: The Head-HUNT Study. Neurology 2003;61:160–4.

42. Castillo J, Munoz P, Guitera V, Pascual J. Epidemiology of chronic daily headache in the general population. Headache 1999;39:190–6.

43. Hershey AD. Chronic daily headaches in children. Exp Opin Pharmacother 2003;4:485–91.

44. Hering-Hanit R, Cohen A, Horev Z. Successful withdrawal from analgesic abuse in a group of youngsters with chronic daily headache. J Child Neurol 2001;16:448–9.

45. Symon DN. Twelve cases of analgesic headache. Arch Dis Child 1998;78:555–6.

46. Granella F, Farina S, Malferrari G, Manzoni GC. Drug abuse in chronic headache: a clinico-epidemiologic study. Cephalalgia 1987;7:15–9.

47. Rapoport A, Stang P, Gutterman DL, et al. Analgesic rebound headache in clinical practice: data from a physician survey. Headache 1996;36:14–9.

48. Mathew N. Early intervention with almotriptan improves sustained pain-free response in acute migraine. Headache 2003;43:1075–9.

49. Pascual J, Cabarrocas X. Within-patient early versus delayed treatment of migraine attacks with almotriptan: the sooner the better. Headache 2002;42:28–31.

50. Ryan RE, Diamond S, Giammarco RAM, et al. Efficacy of zolmitriptan at early time points for acute treatment of migraine and treatment of recurrence. CNS Drugs 2000;13:215–26.

51. Cady RK, Sheftell F, Lipton RB, et al. Effect of early intervention with sumatriptan on migraine pain: retrospective analyses of data from three clinical trials. Clin Ther 2000;22:1035–48.

52. Mihatsch MJ, Knüsli C. Phenacetin abuse and malignant tumors. Klin Wochenschr 1982;60:1339–49.

53. Mihatsch MJ, Hofer HO, Gudat F, et al. Capillary sclerosis of the urinary tract and analgesic nephropathy. Clin Nephrol 1983;20:285–301.

54. Andersson PG. Ergotism—the clinical picture. In: Diener HC, Wilkinson M, editors. Drug-induced headache. Heidelberg: Springer; 1988. p. 16–9.

55. Diener HC, Dichgans J, Scholz E, et al. Analgesic-induced chronic headache: long-term results of withdrawal therapy. J Neurol 1989;236:9–14.

56. Schwartz BS, Stewart WF, Simon D, Lipton RB. Epidemiology of tension-type headache. JAMA 1998;279:381–3.

57. Diener H, Kaube H, Limmroth V. A practical guide to the management and prevention of migraine. Drugs 1998;56:811–24.

58. Goadsby PJ. How do the currently used prophylactic agents work in migraine? Cephalalgia 1997;17:85–92.

59. Tfelt-Hansen P. Prophylactic treatment of migraine: evaluation of clinical trials and choice among drugs. Cephalalgia 1995; 15 Suppl 1:29–32.

60. Newman LC, Lipton RB, Russell M, Solomon S. Hemicrania continua: attacks may alternate sides. Headache 1992;32:237–8.

61. Newman LC, Lipton RB, Solomon S. Hemicrania continua: 7 new cases and a literature review. Headache 1993;32:267.

62. Diaz-Mitoma F, Vanast WJ, Tyrrell DL. Increased frequency of Epstein-Barr-virus excretion in patients with new daily persistent headaches. Lancet 1987;i:411–4.

63. Hering R, Steiner TJ. Abrupt outpatient withdrawal of medication in analgesic-abusing migraineurs. Lancet 1991;337:1442–3.

64. Haag G, Baar H, Grotemeyer KH, et al. Prophylaxe und Therapie des medikamenteninduzierten Dauerkopfschmerzes. Schmerz 1999;13:52–7.

65. Mathew NT, Ali S. Valproate in the treatment of persistent chronic daily headache. An open label study. Headache 1991;31:71–4.

66. Krymchantowski AV, Barbosa JS. Prednisone as initial treatment of analgesic-induced daily headache. Cephalalgia 2000;20:107–13.

67. Diener HC, Haab J, Peters C, et al. Subcutaneous sumatriptan in the treatment of headache during withdrawal from drug-induced headache. Headache 1990;31:205–9.

68. Mathew NT. Amelioration of ergotamine withdrawal with naproxen. Headache 1987;27:130–3.

69. Silberstein SD, Schulman EA, McFaden Hopkins M. Repetitive intravenous DHE in the treatment of refractory headache. Headache 1990;30:334–9.

70. Silberstein SD, Silberstein JR. Chronic daily headache: long-term prognosis following inpatient treatment with repetitive i.v. DHE. Headache 1992;32:439–45.

71. Raskin NH. Repetitive intravenous dihydroergotamine as therapy for intractable migraine. Neurology 1986;36:995–7.

72. Limmroth V, Katsarava Z, Fritsche G, et al. Features of medication overuse headache following overuse of different acute headache drugs. Neurology 2002;59:1011–4.

73. Schnider P, Aull S, Baumgartner C, et al. Long-term outcome of patients with headache and drug abuse after inpatient withdrawal: five year follow-up. Cephalalgia 1996;16:481–5.

74. Fritsche G, Eberl A, Katsarava Z, et al. Drug-induced headache: long-term follow-up of withdrawal therapy and persistence of drug misuse. Eur Neurol 2001;45:229–35.

75. Katsarava Z, Limmroth V, Finke M, Diener HC, Fritsche G. Rates and predictors for relapse in medication overuse headache: a 1-year prospective study. Neurology 2003;60:1682–3.

76. Katsarava Z, Schneeweiss S, Kurth T, et al. Incidence and predictors for chronicity of headache in patients with episodic migraine. Neurology 2004;62:788–90.

77. Zwart J, Dyb G, Hagen K, et al. Analgesic overuse among subjects with headache, neck, and low back pain. Neurology 2004;62:1540–4.

78. Scher AI, Stewart WI, Ricci JA, Lipton RB. Factors associated with the onset and remission of chronic daily headache in a population-based study. Pain 2003;106:81–9.

# Headaches of Cervical Origin: Focus on Anatomy and Physiology

Nikolai Bogduk, MD, PhD, DSc, Dip Pain Med, and Thorsten Bartsch, MD

Headaches of cervical origin have been recognized in the literature for nearly a century. For most of this period, various authors proclaimed that certain headaches had cervical causes, but they did not provide objective and compelling evidence of those causes or means by which such causes could be verified. For these reasons, the entity was not embraced by mainstream practitioners and remained controversial. Only in the last 20 years have headaches of cervical origin attracted serious attention. That period has seen studies that addressed clinical diagnosis, mechanisms, sources, and means of diagnosis and treatment. Headaches of cervical origin are among the best-understood types of headache, yet they still remain the least accepted.

## HISTORICAL BACKGROUND

Some investigators have traced the earliest reference to headaches and the neck to a series of lectures given by Hilton in 1860 to 1862, in which he proposed that pain in the forehead could arise from the greater or lesser occipital nerves and disease between the first and second cervical vertebrae.[1,2] The earliest, accessible publication by an eminent authority dates back to 1913, when Gordon Holmes asserted that headaches could arise from the neck.[3] He described headaches associated with tender nodules in the posterior neck muscles, which he attributed to fibrositis. This gave rise to the notion of "rheumatic headache," which contemporaries of Holmes also described.[4,5] Some 30 years later, this notion was resurrected[6] and extended to include headaches caused by trigger points[7,8] or weakened fibro-osseous insertions.[9,10]

This early literature, however, did not provide scientific data. The cardinal diagnostic criterion for headache of cervical origin was tenderness in the neck, and the recommended treatment was injection of local anesthetics or sclerosants into the tender sites. However, no publications defined the cause of pain or demonstrated its pathology; nor were the reliability and validity of the diagnostic criteria established. The alleged efficacy of treatment was never tested in controlled studies.

Tenderness is neither a valid nor a reliable criterion for the cause of pain. Tender points in various muscles of the neck and head occur in many forms of headache, including migraine,[11–14] and are not indicative specifically of a cervical source of pain. Nor are expert assessors able to agree on the presence or absence of a trigger point in the neck.[15]

In 1949, Hunter and Mayfield introduced a different idiom. They announced that occipital neuralgia could be caused by compression of the occipital nerve between the posterior arch of the atlas and the lamina of C2.[16] They recommended treatment by greater occipital neurectomy. This triggered a fashion for greater occipital nerve blocks and greater occipital neurectomy for the treatment of occipital headaches.[17–21]

The practice of occipital neurectomy has been challenged,[22,23] and it has since been shown[24,25] that the greater occipital nerve cannot be damaged in the manner proposed by Hunter and Mayfield. Moreover, exponents of greater occipital neurectomy were not deterred by a later report by Mayfield in which he was more reserved about his earlier enthusiasm for greater occipital neurectomy and its success rate.[26]

In 1926, a different concept was initiated by Barré. He proposed that headaches could be caused by irritation of the vertebral nerve by arthritis of the cervical spine.[27] Others endorsed this notion, adding that a variety of lesions in the neck could cause headache by this mechanism.[28–33] Most authors did not elaborate the proposed mechanism of pain beyond referring to "irritation of the vertebral nerve." Only Pawl ventured that irritation of the vertebral nerve by cervical disk lesions or other lesions produces an autonomic barrage, which results in spasm of the vertebrobasilar system, which produces pain in the head by causing ischemia of the vessel walls.[33]

This mechanism has been refuted. Electrical stimulation of the vertebral nerve does not influence vertebral blood flow.[34] Moreover, the vertebrobasilar system is remarkably resistant, even to intra-arterial injections of vasoactive agents.[34] Thus, not only is physiologic evidence lacking for the theory of vertebral nerve irritation, but the available evidence denies it. The physiologic data support clinical opinions that there is no basis for belief in Barré syndrome, which is also known as migraine cervicale.[35,36] This lack of evidence, however, has not prevented contemporary authors from promoting the concept.[37]

Another concept has been that headaches can be caused by cervical spondylosis. The mechanism of pain is purported to be spasm of the posterior neck muscles that attach to the occiput,[33,38–41] but this mechanism has not been verified electromyographically or otherwise, nor has any study shown that cervical spondylosis is significantly more common in patients with headache than in asymptomatic subjects.

An alternate view has been that headache can be pain referred from the upper cervical joints.[42–48] This remains the leading explanation for the basis of headaches of cervical origin.

## NEUROANATOMIC BASIS

The pars caudalis of the spinal nucleus of the trigeminal nerve is continuous longitudinally with the outer laminae (laminae I to V) of the dorsal horns of the upper three to four segments of the cervical spinal cord.[49–55] Collectively, this column of gray matter constitutes the trigeminocervical nucleus. This nucleus, however, is not defined by any distinctive cytoarchitecture or by any intrinsic boundaries. Rather, it is defined by its afferents. This column of gray matter receives afferents from the trigeminal nerve and from the upper three cervical spinal nerves (Figure 12–1). Within the nucleus, second-order neurons receive afferents from the trigeminal nerve and from the upper three cervical spinal nerves. This convergence provides for various patterns of referred pain.

Convergence between cervical spinal afferents from the vertebral column and cervical afferents from the occiput provides for cervical-cervical referral of pain. Thereby, pain from upper cervical spinal structures may be perceived in regions of the head innervated by cervical nerves, such as the external occiput or posterior cranial fossa. Convergence between cervical afferents and trigeminal afferents provides for cervical-trigeminal referral. Thereby, pain from upper cervical spinal structures can be perceived in the frontal region of the head, the orbit, or the parietal region.

## PERIPHERAL ANATOMY

The possible sources of cervical spinal pain that might be referred to the head are dictated by the distribution of the three upper cervical spinal nerves. Through their various branches, these nerves innervate the joints and ligaments of the median atlantoaxial,[56] atlanto-occipital,[57] and lateral atlantoaxial joints[57,58]; the C2–3 zygapophyseal joint[59]; the suboccipital and upper posterior neck muscles[59]; the upper prevertebral muscles[60]; the spinal dura mater and the dura mater of the posterior cranial fossa[56]; the vertebral artery[61–63]; the C2–3 intervertebral disk[64,65]; and the trapezius and sternocleidomastoid muscles.[63] Collectively, these structures constitute the possible sources of headache referred from the cervical spine.

## HUMAN EXPERIMENTAL EVIDENCE

Studies in human volunteers have demonstrated the patterns of referred pain that can occur from cervical structures to the head. Electrical stimulation of the dorsal rootlets of C1 produces frontal headache.[66] Noxious stimulation of the greater occipital nerve produces headache in the ipsilateral, frontal, and parietal regions.[67] Noxious stimulation of the suboccipital muscles of the neck produces pain in the forehead.[68–71] Noxious stimulation of the C2–3 intervertebral disk, but not the lower disks, produces pain in the occipital region.[72,73] Distending the C2–3 zygapophyseal joint with injections of contrast medium produces pain in the occipital region,[74] as does distending the lateral atlantoaxial joint or the atlanto-occipital joint.[75] In normal volunteers, all segments from the occiput to C4–5 are capable of producing referred pain to the occiput. Referral to the forehead and orbital regions more commonly occurs from the uppermost segments, C1 and C2.[69]

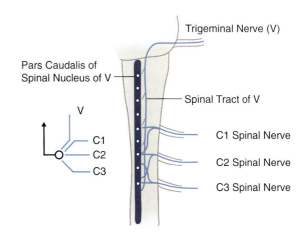

**Figure 12–1**   A schematic representation of the pattern of convergence between cervical and trigeminal afferents in the dorsal gray column of the spinal nucleus of the trigeminal nerve and the upper three cervical spinal cord segments.

Complementary studies in patients with headache have shown that headache can be relieved by anesthetizing cervical structures. Anesthetizing the C2–3 zygapophyseal joint[76-78] or the lateral atlantoaxial joint[79-82] relieves frontal and occipital headache in certain patients. Systematic studies have shown that when headache is the dominant symptom, the source is most commonly the C2–3 zygapophyseal joint and, occasionally, the joint at C3–4.[83] In patients with predominantly neck pain, but in whom headache is also a feature but not the dominant complaint, zygapophyseal joints as low as C5–6 can be the source of pain.[83]

## LABORATORY EVIDENCE

Early physiologic studies, using a cat model, demonstrated that various sites in the spinal cord at the C1–2 level respond to electrical stimulation of either the trigeminal nerve or the roots of the C1 or C2 spinal nerve.[84] These sites, however, were diverse. They extended to regions of the ventral horn and were not restricted to the dorsal horn.

More recent studies showed that neurons in the lateral cervical nucleus respond to electrical stimulation of either the superior sagittal sinus or the greater occipital nerve.[85] These studies prompted more detailed investigations of convergence between the dura mater of the skull and the greater occipital nerve.

Two complementary studies in the rat found neurons in the C2 spinal cord that received convergent input from both trigeminal and cervical afferents.[86,87] The neurons included wide dynamic-range neurons and nociceptive specific neurons located in laminae V and VI and laminae I and II of the dorsal horn at C2. The convergent input involved Aδ and C fibers. The trigeminal afferents were stimulated at the dura mater of the parietal bone but had receptive fields that extended to the cutaneous territories predominantly of the ophthalmic but also the maxillary and mandibular divisions of the trigeminal nerve. The cervical afferents were stimulated in the greater occipital nerve but had receptive fields in the cutaneous territory of this nerve and in the muscles that it innervates.

These studies demonstrated not only convergence but also functional interaction between trigeminal and cervical afferents.[86,87] Electrical or chemical stimulation of trigeminal afferents sensitized the central neurons and increased their responses to cervical stimulation. Reciprocally, electrical or chemical stimulation of cervical afferents sensitized the neurons to trigeminal input. These observations established that either trigeminal or cervical stimulation could produce central sensitization of the trigeminocervical nucleus. Furthermore, this effect was differentially sensitive to input from different types of nerves and from different peripheral tissues.

Stimulation of C fibers in cervical afferents produced greater and more enduring increases in central sensitization than did stimulation of Aδ fibers.[86] Cervical afferent input from muscle produced a greater and longer-lasting increase in neural excitability than did cutaneous input.[86] Other studies have also observed this latter phenomenon. Inflammation of ventral neck muscles by application with mustard oil leads to an enlargement of both deep and cutaneous receptive fields; in contrast, its application to skin leads only to expansion of cutaneous receptive fields.[88] This differential effect may be related to the difference in neuropeptide content between muscle and cutaneous afferents.[89]

Conversely, stimulation of trigeminal afferents from the dura mater facilitated the response to electrical stimulation of the greater occipital nerve and sensitized the response of cervical muscles to noxious mechanical stimulation.[87] These observations underscore the fact that cervical-trigeminal interactions are reciprocal. Not only can cervical nociception facilitate trigeminal sensation, but trigeminal nociception facilitates cervical perception.

Consequently, the neurophysiologic data support not only the referral of cervical pain to the head but also the generation of cervical features in patients with trigeminal sources of headache. Proponents of a cervical source of headaches, therefore, need to be alert to the possibility that signs, which they infer to indicate a cervical origin for pain, may instead be secondary phenomena of trigeminal origin. In experimental animals, stimulation of the dura mater increases electromyographic activity in suboccipital paraspinal muscles.[90] Migraine patients can complain of neck discomfort during the premonitory phase[91] or during their attacks[92] and can exhibit hypersensitivity and increased electromyographic activity in their neck muscles.[93-95]

## DIFFERENTIAL DIAGNOSIS

### Aneurysm

Because they are innervated by cervical nerves, disorders of the vertebral artery and the internal carotid artery are among the possible cervical causes of headache. However, because there are no means by which arteries can be selectively anesthetized, there are no data that directly implicate disorders of these vessels in the cause of headache. Nevertheless, there is circumstantial evidence.

Headache is the most common presenting feature of internal carotid artery dissection[96,97] and may occur together with neck pain.[97] Headache is also the cardinal presenting feature of vertebral artery dissection. In both instances, some 60 to 70% of patients present with headache, typically in the occipital region, although not exclusively so.[96,98,99]

Aneurysm of either the internal carotid artery or the vertebral artery is, therefore, an important differential diagnosis of cervical causes of headache when the headache is acute, that is, of recent onset. However, the rapid evolution of cerebrovascular symptoms and signs declares the nature of the condition. Consequently, aneurysm is not a differential diagnosis of chronic headache in the absence of cerebrovascular features.

### Diseases of the Posterior Fossa

The posterior cranial fossa is not commonly regarded as part of the neck. Consequently, diseases of the posterior fossa, notably tumors and aneurysms, might not be considered intuitively as part of the differential diagnosis of headaches of cervical origin. However, because the posterior cranial fossa is innervated by cervical nerves, it falls within the neurologic catchment area for cervical causes of headache. Diseases of the posterior cranial fossa, therefore, should not be neglected in the differential diagnosis.

### Trigger Points

Many authors have asserted or endorsed that trigger points in the neck muscles can cause headache. The muscles implicated are the trapezius, sternocleidomastoid, and splenius capitis.[7,8,100–103] The diagnosis rests on finding by palpation the characteristic features of a trigger point. These are a tender band within the muscle that, when palpated, elicits a twitch response in the muscle, reproduces the patient's pain, and causes them to react—the so-called jump sign.[104]

In the context of neck pain and headache, this explanation of the cause of pain is difficult to sustain. Examination of the literature reveals that trigger points in the neck are exempt from the conventional diagnostic criteria. In the posterior neck muscles, instead of a palpable band, the trigger point is no more than a tender mass, from which a twitch response cannot be elicited.[105] No studies have demonstrated that the diagnosis of trigger points, as a cause of headache, is either reliable or valid. Conspicuously, these tender points typically overly zygapophyseal joints.[106] Therefore, they cannot be distinguished from underlying painful and tender joints.[106]

### Cervicogenic Headache

Sjaastad and colleagues described cervicogenic headache as an ostensibly distinctive type of headache defined by its clinical features.[107] The diagnostic criteria were unilateral headache, provoked by neck movements or by pressure over points in the neck, associated with neck pain and reduced range of motion of the neck.[108] The headache is said to be characterized by nonclustering episodes, varying duration, and pain of a nonthrobbing quality emanating from the neck and spreading into the oculofrontotemporal regions of the head. The headaches may be accompanied by nausea, vomiting, dizziness, phonophobia, photophobia, blurred vision, and difficulties in swallowing.[108] Early clinical studies focused on distinguishing cervicogenic headache from cluster headache with respect to forehead sweating[109] and pupillometry[110] and looking for distinctive radiographic features, none of which were found.[111,112]

The frailty of this entity is that its definition and diagnosis rely entirely on clinical features, none of which, nor any combination thereof, are unique to headaches of cervical origin. The same features can occur in migraine and tension-type headache, and even in cluster headache and chronic paroxysmal hemicrania. The features said to indicate a cervical origin of the pain are not specific. For example, neck rotation is significantly more reduced in patients diagnosed as having cervicogenic headache than in those with migraine, but the ranges of reduction overlap substantially in all three types of headache, and the feature is not unique to cervicogenic headache.[113] Similarly, pressure-pain threshold is significantly less in patients with cervicogenic headache, but the range of values overlaps considerably with those seen in migraine and tension-type headache.[114] Forward head posture, muscle weakness, and abnormal responses to stretching of the neck muscles are more common in patients with headache said to be of cervical origin, but the distribution of abnormalities overlaps considerably with that found in asymptomatic individuals.[115,116]

For such reasons, investigators have challenged the validity of the diagnostic criteria and have been unable to distinguish cervicogenic headache from other forms of headache.[117–119] Even observers who achieve good agreement in applying the diagnostic criteria for cervicogenic headache disagree on whether the diagnosis is migraine in 10% of cases or tension-type headache in 12% of cases.[120]

The response to diagnostic blockade of cervical structures or nerves is an available diagnostic criterion by which to establish that headaches arise from the neck.[121] Although originally not included as an essential criterion for the diagnosis of cervicogenic headache,[108] it has been promoted in the revised criteria to a major criterion that is obligatory in scientific works.[122] Initial observations[123] and subsequent studies[111,124] found that many, but not all, patients diagnosed clinically as having cervicogenic headache could be temporarily relieved of their pain by blocking the greater occipital nerve, the C2 spinal nerve, or the C2–3 zygapophyseal joint. None of these studies, however, used controlled blocks to establish the validity of the response, nor was complete relief of pain required to define a positive response. Therefore, the studies have not provided conclusive evidence of a cervical source of pain for this clinical entity.

## Occipital Neuralgia

The International Association for the Study of Pain (IASP) defines occipital neuralgia as "pain, usually deep and aching, in the distribution of the second cervical dorsal root."[125] The International Headache Society (IHS) defines it as "paroxysmal jabbing pain in the distribution of the greater or lesser occipital nerves, accompanied by diminished sensation or dysesthesia in the affected area."[126] However, although the IHS stipulates sensory abnormalities in its definition, these are not listed among the diagnostic criteria.

These definitions differ in one critical respect: the IHS stipulates that the pain must be paroxysmal and jabbing, whereas the IASP describes it as deep and aching pain and only sometimes stabbing in nature. The IASP states that "nerve block may give relief," but the IHS insists that temporary relief by anesthetic block is a mandatory diagnostic criterion.

The inconsistency, conflict, and contradiction are characteristic of the literature on occipital neuralgia. There is no consensus on the definition or diagnostic criteria, and the rubric is used loosely, if not arbitrarily, to refer to any pain felt in the occipital region.

The term "neuralgia" explicitly means pain stemming from a nerve and should be reserved for such conditions. Paroxysmal lancinating pain is the hallmark of neuralgia and should be an essential diagnostic criterion for occipital neuralgia if that term is to be used. In this respect, the definition of the IASP is in error. Deep, aching pain in the occiput can arise from a variety of sources and causes, not the least of which are diseases of the posterior cranial fossa and base of the skull[45] and the upper cervical joints.[76–80] Indeed, the IHS comments that occipital neuralgia must be distinguished from occipital referral of pain from the atlantoaxial or upper zygapophyseal joints.[126]

The IASP definition would include these latter conditions even though they do not involve irritation or compression of the greater occipital nerve or even the C2 spinal nerve. Deep, aching pain in the occiput is nothing more than deep, aching pain in the occiput for which a specific cause should be found. The habit of attributing such pain to irritation of the greater occipital nerve stems from an era when neurologists and neurosurgeons were oblivious to somatic referred pain and ascribed any and every pain to irritation of a nerve.

There is no compelling evidence that occipital pain is due to irritation of the greater occipital nerve. Lancinating occipital neuralgia has been recorded as a feature of temporal arteritis,[127] in which case inflammation of the occipital artery could affect the companion nerve. However, in the majority of cases of so-called occipital neuralgia, no such pathology is evident.

The commonly held view is that occipital neuralgia is caused by entrapment of the greater occipital nerve where it pierces the trapezius. Surgical studies do not provide circumstantial evidence of this. Liberation of the nerve initially relieves headache in some 80% of cases, but the relief has a median duration of only 3 to 6 months.[128] Excision of the greater occipital nerve provides relief in some 70% of patients, but this has a median duration of only 244 days.[129]

The cardinal diagnostic criterion seems to be the response to blocks of the greater occipital nerve, but these blocks are not target specific when they involve volumes such as 5 mL[128] or 10 mL.[130,131] In such volumes, they do not selectively implicate the greater occipital nerve. No studies using more discrete blocks have implicated the greater occipital nerve as the source of pain.

## C2 Neuralgia

A distinctive form of headache can be caused by lesions affecting the C2 spinal nerve. This nerve runs behind the lateral atlantoaxial joint, resting on its capsule.[58,132] Inflammatory or other disorders of the joint may result in the nerve becoming incorporated in the fibrotic changes of chronic inflammation.[133,134] Release of the nerve relieves the symptoms. Otherwise, the C2 spinal nerve and its roots are surrounded by a sleeve of dura mater and a plexus of epiradicular veins, lesions of which can compromise the nerve. These include meningioma,[135] neurinoma,[134] and anomalous vertebral arteries,[136] but the majority of reported cases have involved venous abnormalities ranging from single to densely interwoven dilated veins surrounding the C2 spinal nerve and its roots[137] to U-shaped arterial loops or angiomas compressing the C2 dorsal root ganglion.[133,137,138]

Nerves affected by vascular abnormalities exhibit a variety of features indicative of neuropathy, such as myelin breakdown, chronic hemorrhage, axon degeneration and regeneration, and increased endoneurial and pericapsular connective tissue.[137] It is not clear, however, whether the vascular abnormality causes these neuropathic changes or is only coincident with them.

C2 neuralgia is characterized by intermittent, lancinating pain in the occipital region associated with lacrimation and ciliary injection. The pain typically occurs in association with a background of dull occipital pain and dull, referred pain in the temporal, frontal, and orbital regions. Most often, this latter pain is focused on the fronto-orbital region but encompasses all three regions when severe. However, the distinguishing feature of this condition is a cutting or tearing sensation in the occipital region, which is the hallmark of its neurogenic basis. In this regard, C2 neuralgia probably represents what previously had been called occipital neuralgia, as defined by the IHS.[126]

The frequency of attacks varies from four to five per day to two to seven per week, alternating with pain-free intervals of days, weeks, or months.[133,137] Some 75% of patients suffer the associated features of ipsilateral conjunctival and ciliary injection and lacrimation.[133,137] Blurred vision, rhinorrhea, and dizziness are less common accompaniments. Neurologic examination is normal. In particular, hypoesthesia in the territory of the trigeminal or cervical nerves is not present.

C2 neuralgia is distinguished from referred pain from the neck by its neurogenic quality, its periodicity, and its association with lacrimation and ciliary injection. The latter association has attracted the appellation of "cluster-like" headache.[135] The cardinal diagnostic feature is complete relief of pain following local anesthetic blockade of the suspected nerve root—typically the C2 spinal nerve but occasionally the C3 nerve. These blocks are performed under radiologic control and employ discrete amounts (0.6 to 0.8 mL) of a long-acting local anesthetic to block the target nerve selectively.[133]

### Neck-Tongue Syndrome

Neck-tongue syndrome is a disorder characterized by acute unilateral occipital pain precipitated by sudden movement of the head, usually rotation, and accompanied by a sensation of numbness in the ipsilateral half of the tongue.[139] The pain appears to be caused by temporary subluxation of a lateral atlantoaxial joint, whereas the numbness of the tongue arises because of impingement, or stretching, of the C2 ventral ramus against the edge of the subluxated articular process.[132] The numbness occurs because proprioceptive afferents from the tongue pass from the ansa hypoglossi into the C2 ventral ramus.[139] Neck-tongue syndrome can occur in patients with rheumatoid arthritis or with congenital joint laxity.[140] Hypomobility in the contralateral lateral atlantoaxial joint may predispose the individual to the condition.[141]

### Rheumatoid Arthritis

Headache is a common feature of patients with rheumatoid arthritis of the upper cervical spine.[141–145] By inference, these headaches represent referred pain from inflamed atlantoaxial joints. Technically, these constitute headache of cervical origin, but the distinctive circumstances in which they occur—in patients with overt rheumatoid arthritis—excludes them from the differential diagnosis of headache. Rheumatoid arthritis does not present with isolated headache. Rather, headache becomes a feature of patients with established rheumatoid arthritis when the disease extends to involve the C2 region.

### Median Atlantoaxial Arthritis

Some authors have attributed headache to osteoarthritis of the median atlantoaxial joint.[146–148] The evidence for this association, however, is barely circumstantial. Whereas some patients with radiographically evident osteoarthritis do have occipital headache, others do not. The only statistical data pertain to an association between arthritic changes in the median atlantoaxial joint and suboccipital pain.[149] No such association has been demonstrated for headache. Detecting arthritis of the median atlantoaxial joint, therefore, is not diagnostic of a cervical source of headache because radiography alone cannot distinguish symptomatic osteoarthritic changes from asymptomatic age changes. A technique for verifying that a median atlantoaxial joint is painful has not been developed.

### Congenital Anomalies

Headache has been noted in cases of atlantoaxial dislocation, separation of the odontoid, and occipitalization of the atlas.[150,151] There is no evidence, however, that these abnormalities, per se, are symptomatic. Indeed, they can be asymptomatic. Their presence and identification do not provide a diagnosis. They may predispose the individual to mechanical disorders of the neck, but they may be totally incidental findings.

### Lateral Atlantoaxial Joint Pain

Studies in normal volunteers have shown that noxious stimulation of the lateral atlantoaxial joint can produce referred pain to the head.[75] Clinical studies have shown that headache in certain patients can be relieved by anesthetizing this joint.[79–82] Therefore, there would appear to be sufficient evidence to implicate the lateral atlantoaxial joint as one possible cervical source of headache. No studies, however, have established what the pathology may be. One study attributed the pain to radiographically evident osteoarthritis,[79] but such arthritis is not always evident. A postmortem study has indicated that, in post-traumatic cases, the responsible lesions might include capsular rupture, intra-articular hemorrhage, and bruising of intra-articular meniscoids or small fractures through the superior articular process of the axis.[152]

The prevalence of lateral atlantoaxial joint pain is not known, but it may not be uncommon. One study traced the source of pain to the lateral atlantoaxial joints in 16% of patients presenting with headache, but not all patients were investigated for this condition, which suggests that 16% may be an underestimate.[82]

Diagnostic blocks are the only means of establishing the diagnosis. They involve injecting a small volume of local anesthetic into the joint under fluoroscopic guidance. Certain clinical features may be suggestive of lateral atlantoaxial joint pain, but they are not diagnostic in their own right. These include pain in the occipital or suboccipital region, together with maximal or focal tenderness in the suboccipital region, maximal or focal tenderness over the tip of the left or right transverse process of C1, restricted rotation of C1 on C2 on manual examination of that segment, and aggravation of the accustomed headache by passive rotation of the C1 vertebra to the left or right.[82]

### Third Occipital Headache

The C2–3 zygapophyseal joint is innervated by the third occipital nerve.[59] This nerve crosses the joint laterally and innervates it through articular branches from its deep surface (Figure 12–2). The joint can be anesthetized by blocking the third occipital nerve under fluoroscopic guidance (Figure 12–3). Therefore, headache stemming from the C2–3 zygapophyseal joint can be relieved by third occipital nerve blocks and, accordingly, has been named third occipital headache.

Initial studies describing third occipital headache were conducted using single diagnostic blocks with no controls.[76,77] A subsequent study used controlled diagnostic blocks and confirmed the existence of this entity.[78] Moreover, that study established the prevalence of third occipital headache. In patients with headache after whiplash, the prevalence of third occipital headache was 27%. Among patients in whom headache was the dominant complaint, the prevalence was 53% (95% confidence interval 37–68%).

There are no clinical features that are diagnostic of third occipital headache. Tenderness over the C2–3 joint is suggestive but has a positive likelihood ratio of only 2.1.[78] Controlled diagnostic blocks are the only means of establishing the diagnosis with confidence.[78]

### TREATMENT

Despite the wide and varied interest in headaches of cervical origin, few studies have provided a treatment. For rare and unusual causes, such as aneurysms, lesions of the posterior cranial fossa, and rheumatoid arthritis, standard vascular, neurosurgical, rheumatologic, or orthopedic interventions are available and appropriate. For the majority of remaining cases, a proven treatment has not been established.

### Trigger Points

The treatment of trigger points, with injections of local anesthetic, has not been subjected to any form of scientific study. Indeed, a systematic review found no evidence that needling therapies have any efficacy beyond that of placebo.[153]

### Cervicogenic Headache

Few studies have addressed the treatment of cervicogenic headache. One purported to show that radiofrequency neurotomy of the cervical zygapophyseal joints could be successful.[154] In this study, however, diagnostic blocks were expressly not performed to select a target level, and denervation was performed at all levels, from C3 to C6. Even so, only 1 of 15 patients achieved complete relief of pain. An additional 11 patients were described as having good relief of pain, but this outcome was not defined.

A recent randomized placebo-controlled study of radiofrequency neurotomy showed no benefit for patients with cervicogenic headache diagnosed on the basis of clinical features.[155] This outcome underscores the lack of validity of clinical diagnosis for this condition and highlights the importance of achieving com-

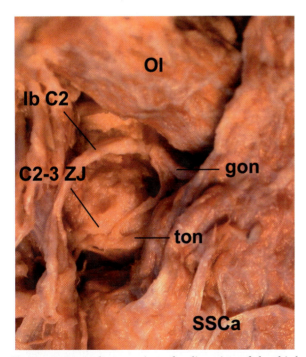

**Figure 12–2** A close-up view of a dissection of the third occipital nerve (ton) where it crosses the C2–3 zygapophyseal joint (ZJ). gon = greater occipital nerve; lb C2 = lateral branch of C2 dorsal ramus; OI = obliquus inferior; SSCa = semispinalis capitis.

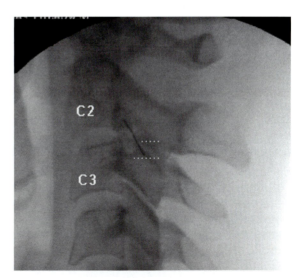

**Figure 12–3** Lateral radiograph showing a needle in place for a third occipital nerve block. The dotted lines demarcate the range of locations of this nerve.

plete relief of pain from controlled diagnostic blocks as the indication for radiofrequency neurotomy.[156]

In another study, patients were selected for surgery if they satisfied the clinical criteria for cervicogenic headache and obtained relief of headache from diagnostic blockade of the C2 spinal nerve.[157] They underwent decompression and microsurgical neurolysis of the C2 spinal nerve, with excision of the scar and ligamentous and vascular elements that compressed the nerve. Fourteen of 31 patients were rendered pain free. Details on the remaining patients are incomplete, but, ostensibly, 51% gained what was called "adequate" relief, and 11% suffered a recurrence. The authors reported finding venous compression or a scarred atlantoepistrophic ligament in the majority of their cases. However, the incomplete success rate of surgery calls into question the significance and relevance of these findings.

## Manual Therapy

Various forms of physical and manual therapy have been advocated for headaches believed to be of cervical origin. Most of the literature, however, consists of case reports or case series.[2] The few randomized controlled studies provided follow-up of only 1 or 3 weeks[158–160] and conflicting results.[2]

The largest and most recent study provided encouraging results.[161] It showed that treatment with manual therapy, specific exercises, or manual therapy plus exercises was significantly more effective at reducing headache frequency and intensity than was no specific care by a general practitioner. Manual therapy alone, however, was not more effective than exercises alone, and combining the two interventions did not achieve better outcomes. Some 76% of patients achieved > 50% reduction in headache frequency at the 7-week follow-up, and 35% achieved complete relief. At 12 months, 72% had a > 50% reduction in headache frequency, but the proportion who had complete relief was not reported. Corresponding figures for a reduction in pain intensity were not reported.

## Occipital Neuralgia

Reports about the treatment of intractable, idiopathic, occipital neuralgia are mixed. Dorsal rhizotomy at C1–3 or C1–4 has provided some patients with complete relief for 1 to 4 years, but some patients, nevertheless, suffer recurrences.[162] Partial posterior rhizotomy at C1–3 appears to achieve good relief while preserving touch sensation, but not all patients respond adequately.[163] Unfortunately, these procedures are so radical that they provide us with little insight into the mechanisms of occipital neuralgia except to warn that even complete deafferentation of the affected region does not guarantee relief of pain.

There is no evidence that C2 neuralgia responds to pharmacotherapy.[137] Surgery appears to be the only definitive means of treatment. Nerves entrapped by scarring may be liberated[134]; meningiomas may be excised.[135] With respect to venous anomalies, resection of the vascular abnormality alone does not reliably relieve the pain; resection or thermocoagulation of the nerve appears to be necessary to guarantee relief of pain.[137] This calls into question whether the vascular anomaly is really the responsible lesion, particularly in view of the fact that in 50% of cadavers, the C2 roots are surrounded by a dense venous network.[164]

A cognate study described the result of C2 ganglionectomy, not expressly for patients with C2 neuralgia but for patients with occipital pain.[165] Nineteen of 39 patients (49%) obtained > 90% relief of their pain. However, outcomes were better in certain subgroups. A successful outcome was achieved in 64% of 22 patients with a history of trauma and in 78% of 23 patients with shooting, stabbing, or burning pain. These latter patients would seem to correspond to those with C2 neuralgia described in other studies.

## Neck-Tongue Syndrome

Data on the treatment of neck-tongue syndrome are limited to case reports. Some investigators have found immobilization by a soft collar to be adequate therapy[166]; others have used spinal manipulation.[167] Some have resorted to atlantoaxial fusion[141] or resection of the C2 spinal nerves.[168] Operative findings have confirmed that the syndrome involves compression of the C2 spinal nerves by the lateral atlantoaxial joint.[168]

## Lateral Atlantoaxial Joint Pain

There are no conservative treatments for lateral atlantoaxial joint pain, nor have intra-articular injections of corticosteroids been shown to be effective. However, arthrodesis of the joint has been reported as producing complete and lasting relief of pain.[169,170]

## Third Occipital Headache

No form of pharmacologic or physical therapy has ever been tested for this type of headache, and none has been proposed to work. Nevertheless, it is not resistant to treatment. The treatment, however, requires invasive procedures.

One study reported that some patients could obtain relief from intra-articular injection of corticosteroids.[171] At 19 months following such injections, 11% of patients were free of pain. A further 50% had a reduced frequency of headaches. That study, however, was not controlled. Consequently, it is not evident if the administration of corticosteroids, or simply the act of injection into the joint, is the active component of the therapeutic effect. Nevertheless, intra-articular

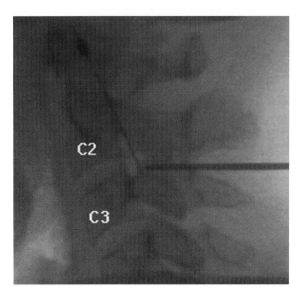

**Figure 12–4** Lateral radiograph showing an electrode in place for a third occipital radiofrequency neurotomy.

injection would seem to be a safe and expedient intervention that could benefit some patients.

It is possible to denervate the C2–3 zygapophyseal joint percutaneously by radiofrequency neurotomy of the third occipital nerve. The procedure involves placing an electrode parallel to the nerve where it crosses the joint (Figure 12–4) and using it to coagulate the nerve. The cardinal indication for the procedure is complete relief of pain following controlled diagnostic blocks of the third occipital nerve.

An early study found that radiofrequency neurotomy of the third occipital nerve did not reliably achieve relief of pain.[172] The authors warned that radiofrequency neurotomy should not be adopted until the technical deficiencies of the procedure have been overcome. That has now been achieved.

A recent study reported improvements in the technique of percutaneous radiofrequency neurotomy of the third occipital nerve,[173] which improved its success rate. The revisions included holding the electrode in place during coagulation and ensuring that multiple lesions are made to encompass all possible locations of the nerve.

Using the revised technique, complete relief of pain could be achieved in 88% of patients. The median duration of relief was 297 days, with some patients still having continuing relief at the time of review. For patients in whom headaches recurred, relief could be reinstated by repeating the neurotomy. By repeating neurotomy as required, some patients have been able to maintain relief of their headache for longer than 2 years. A randomized placebo-controlled trial showed that responses to radiofrequency neurotomy are not due to placebo effects.[174] Its success in the treatment of third occipital headache, therefore, cannot be dismissed as a placebo effect.

## DISCUSSION

It is evident from the literature that headaches of cervical origin have a sound anatomic and physiologic basis. Experimental studies in normal volunteers have shown that pain from upper cervical structures can be referred to the head. Animal studies have shown that convergence occurs between trigeminal and cervical afferents, which constitutes the physiologic substrate for referral of pain from the neck to the head.

It is in the clinical arena that the literature, and practice, has been deficient. Headaches of cervical origin are not a singular phenomenon. Any number of structures might be the source of pain. Unless that source is established, in each and every case, the diagnosis cannot be legitimately sustained.

Relying on clinical features has not proved valid, nor should it be expected to be valid. Nowhere else in the musculoskeletal system are clinical features such as pain patterns, tenderness, range of movement, or muscle spasm both reliable and valid signs of any particular diagnostic entity. Moreover, the assessment of headache is confounded by noncervical causes being capable of producing pain, muscle reactions, and impaired movements in the cervical spine. These secondary features may be mistaken as signs of a cervical cause of headache.

For a headache to be deemed to have a cervical origin, the source of the pain, or its cause, needs to be demonstrated. Yet this has rarely been the case in the history of headaches of cervical origin. Too often, authorities have relied on eminence-based medicine[175] instead of evidence. They have been content to assert that certain features constitute the criteria for a cervical cause of headache but have not provided an objective means of verifying this assertion.

In principle, conventional diagnostic criteria would be acceptable if certain patterns of pain were unique to headaches of cervical origin or if features such as tenderness, range of movement, and joint stiffness could be reliably detected and were pathognomonic of a cervical cause of pain. The evidence, to date, shows that they are not.

Diagnostic blocks are one means of pinpointing a cervical source of pain, but to be valid, they must be performed under controlled conditions.[176] However, most studies that have reported the use of diagnostic blocks have not used controlled injections, nor have they insisted that complete relief of pain be the diagnostic criterion. Under such conditions, the responses cannot be distinguished from random or placebo responses, and the data that these studies provide do not constitute evidence of a cervical source of pain.

For these reasons, the revised criteria for cervicogenic headache, as prescribed by the IHS,[177] have been strengthened. They require clinical, laboratory, and/or imaging evidence of a disorder or lesion within the cervical spine or soft tissues of the neck known to be, or generally accepted as, a valid cause of headache, or evidence that the pain can be attributed to the neck disorder or lesion based on demonstration of clinical signs that implicate a source of pain in the neck or abolition of headache following diagnostic blockade of a cervical structure or its nerve supply using placebo or other adequate controls. The accompanying notes stipulate that cervical spondylosis is not a valid cause and require that any clinical signs used to make the diagnosis must have demonstrated reliability and validity.

The only entity that has satisfied these criteria is third occipital headache. Only for this condition have controlled diagnostic blocks been found to provide complete relief of pain. Only for this condition is the prevalence known and a treatment been validated. Radiofrequency neurotomy is the only treatment, for any form of headache of cervical origin, that has been shown consistently to produce complete relief of pain.

Despite the available evidence, headaches of cervical origin remain unaccepted as a legitimate entity.[178] Several reasons may account for this:

1.  Because, and as long as, practitioners are not taught about this condition, they do entertain the diagnosis. Therefore, they do not seek the diagnosis and do not make it.
2.  The diagnosis cannot be made on conventional clinical grounds or by simple imaging tests. Therefore, practitioners cannot and do not make the diagnosis.
3.  The diagnosis cannot be made using bedside diagnostic blocks. The diagnosis requires fluoroscopically guided, controlled diagnostic blocks. Few practitioners know how to perform these blocks, and the facilities required are not always readily available. Most practitioners, therefore, will be unable to make the diagnosis. Perplexingly, however, these practitioners seem reluctant to refer their patients to others who are able to perform the blocks. Compounding this problem further, credentialing is an issue. Not everyone who claims to do these blocks necessarily performs them correctly or assesses the response to them properly. In the absence of credentialing, practitioners who might refer patients cannot tell if the service to which they refer is valid.

The same problems apply to treatment. Although radiofrequency neurotomy is the one validated treatment, it is not widely available. Moreover, only one technique has been validated. Practitioners wanting to avail their patients of this treatment need a means of determining if their provider practices the correct technique.

On review, it is apparent that a lack of acceptance of the concept of headaches of cervical origin is not due to a lack of evidence. The reasons are sociologic. What needs to be done can be done but is not. Practitioners are reluctant to embrace new attitudes and procedures that allow the condition to be diagnosed and treated. They prefer instead to ignore the entity or wish it to conform to traditional modes of practice, which, to date, it has defied.

## REFERENCES

1.  Pearce JM. Cervicogenic headache: and early description. J Neurol Neurosurg Psychiatry 1995;58:698.

2.  Haldeman S, Dagenais S. Cervicogenic headaches: a critical review. Spine J 2001;1:31–46.

3.  Holmes G. Headaches of organic origin. Practitioner 1913;1:968–84.

4.  Patrick HT. Indurative or rheumatic headache. JAMA 1913;71:82–6.

5.  Luff AP. The various forms of fibrositis and their treatment. BMJ 1913;1:756–60.

6.  Kelly M. Headaches, traumatic and rheumatic: the cervical somatic lesion. Med J Aust 1942;2:479–83.

7.  Travell J, Rinzler SH. The myofascial genesis of pain. Postgrad Med 1952;11:425–34.

8.  Travell J. Mechanical headache. Headache 1962;7:23–9.

9.  Hackett GS, Huang TC, Raftery A. Prolotherapy for headache. Headache 1962;2:20–8.

10. Kayfetz DO, Blumenthal LS, Hackett GS, et al. Whiplash injury and other ligamentous headache—its management with prolotherapy. Headache 1963;3:24–8.

11. Perelson HN. Occipital nerve tenderness: a sign of headache. South Med J 1947;40:653–6.

12. Oleson J. Some clinical features of the acute migraine attack. An analysis of 750 patients. Headache 1978;18:268–71.

13. Lous I, Olesen J. Evaluation of pericranial tenderness and oral function in patients with common migraine, muscle contraction headache and combination headache. Pain 1982;12:385–93.

14. Langemark M, Olesen J. Pericranial tenderness in tension headache. Cephalalgia 1987;7:249–55.

15. Wolfe F, Simons DG, Fricton J, et al. The fibromyalgia and myofascial pain syndromes: a preliminary study of tender point and trigger points in persons with fibromyalgia, myofascial pain and no disease. J Rheumatol 1992;19:944–51.

16. Hunter CR, Mayfield FH. Role of the upper cervical roots in the production of pain in the head. Am J Surg 1949;78:743–9.

17. Chambers WR. Posterior rhizotomy of the second and third cervical nerves for occipital pain. JAMA 1954;155:431–2.

18. Cusson D, King A. Cervical rhizotomy in the management of some cases of occipital neuralgia. Guthrie Clin Bull 1960;29:198–208.

19. Knight G. Post-traumatic occipital headache. Lancet 1963;i:6–8.

20. Murphy JP. Occipital neurectomy in the treatment of headache. Md State Med J 1969;18:62–6.

21. Hammond SR, Danta G. Occipital neuralgia. Clin Exp Neurol 1978;15:258–70.

22. Weinberger LM. Cervico-occipital pain and its surgical treatment. Am J Surg 1978;135:243–7.

23. Bogduk N. Greater occipital neuralgia. In: Long DM, editor. Current therapy in neurological surgery. 2nd ed. Philadelphia: BC Decker; 1989. p. 263–7.

24. Bogduk N. The anatomy of occipital neuralgia. Clin Exp Neurol 1980;17:167–84.

25. Bilge O. An anatomic and morphometric study of C2 nerve root ganglion and its corresponding foramen. Spine 2004;29:485–99.

26. Mayfield FH. Symposium on cervical trauma. Neurosurgical aspects. Clin Neurosurg 1955;2:83–90.

27. Barré N. Sur un syndrome sympathique cervicale posterieure et sa cause frequente: l'arthrite cervicale. Rev Neurol (Paris) 1926;33:1246–8.

28. Gayral L, Neuwirth E. Oto-neuro-opthalmologic manifestations of cervical origin. Posterior cervical sympathetic syndrome of Barre-Lieou. N Y State J Med 1954;54:1920–6.

29. Neuwirth E. Neurologic complications of osteoarthritis of the cervical spine. N Y State J Med 1954;54:2583–90.

30. Kovacs A. Subluxation and deformation of the cervical apophyseal joints. Acta Radiol 1955;43:1–16.

31. Stewart DY. Current concepts of "Barre syndrome" or the "posterior cervical sympathetic syndrome." Clin Orthop 1962;24:40–8.

32. Dutton CD, Riley LH. Cervical migraine. Not merely a pain in the neck. Am J Med 1969;47:141–8.

33. Pawl RP. Headache, cervical spondylosis, and anterior cervical fusion. Surg Ann 1977;9:391–408.

34. Bogduk N, Lambert G, Duckworth JW. The anatomy and physiology of the vertebral nerve in relation to cervical migraine. Cephalalgia 1981;1:1–14.

35. Lance JW. Mechanism and management of headache. 4th ed. London: Butterworths; 1982.

36. Bartschi-Rochaix W. Headaches of cervical origin. In: Vinken PJ, Bruyn GW, editors. Handbook of clinical neurology. Vol 5. New York: Elsevier; 1968. p. 192–203.

37. Tamura T. Cranial symptoms after cervical injury. Aetiology and treatment of the Barre-Lieou syndrome. J Bone Joint Surg Br 1989;71B:283–7.

38. Raney AA, Raney RB. Headache: a common symptom of cervical disc lesions. Arch Neurol Psychiatry 1948;59:603–21.

39. Schultz EC, Semmes RE. Head and neck pains of cervical disc origin. Laryngoscope 1950;60:338–43.

40. Peterson DI, Austin GM, Dayes LA. Headache associated with discogenic disease of the cervical spine. Bull Los Angeles Neurol Soc 1975;40:96–100.

41. Chirls M. Retrospective study of cervical spondylosis treated by anterior interbody fusion in 505 patients performed by the Cloward technique. Bull N Y Hosp Joint Dis 1978;39:74–82.

42. Dugan MC, Locke S, Gallagher JR. Occipital neuralgia in adolescents and young adults. N Engl J Med 1962;267:1166–72.

43. Brain Lord. Some unsolved problems of cervical spondylosis. BMJ 1963;1:771–7.

44. Trevor-Jones R. Osteoarthritis of the paravertebral joints of the second and third cervical vertebrae as a cause of occipital headache. S Afr Med J 1964;30:392–4.

45. Sigwald J, Jamet F. Occipital neuralgia. In: Vinken PJ, Bruyn GW, editors. Handbook of clinical neurology. Vol 5. New York: Elsevier; 1968. p. 368–74.

46. Wilkinson M. Symptomatology. In: Wilkinson M, editor. Cervical spondylosis. 2nd ed. London: Heinemann; 1971. p. 59–67.

47. Poletti CE. Proposed operation for occipital neuralgia: C-2 and C-3 root decompression. Neurosurgery 1983;12:221–4.

48. Ehni G, Benner B. Occipital neuralgia and the C1–2 arthrosis syndrome. J Neurosurg 1984;61:961–5.

49. Humphrey T. The spinal tract of the trigeminal nerve in human embryos between 7 1/2 and 8 1/2 weeks of menstrual age and its relation to early fetal behaviour. J Comp Neurol 1952;97:143–209.

50. Torvik A. Afferent connections to the sensory trigeminal nuclei, the nucleus of the solitary tract and adjacent structures. J Comp Neurol 1956;106:51–141.

51. Kerr FWL. Structural relation of the trigeminal spinal tract to upper cervical roots and the solitary nucleus in the cat. Exp Neurol 1961;4:134–48.

52. Taren JA, Kahn EA. Anatomic pathways related to pain in face and neck. J Neurosurg 1962;19:116–21.

53. Goadsby PJ, Hoskin KL. The distribution of trigemino-vascular afferents in the nonhuman primate brain *Macaca nemestrina*: a c-*fos* immunocytochemical study. J Anat 1997;190:367–75.

54. Kaube H, Keay KA, Hoskin KL, et al. Expression of c-*fos*-like immunoreactivity in the caudal medulla and upper cervical spinal cord following stimulation of the superior sagittal sinus in the cat. Brain Res 1993;629:95–102.

55. Strassman AM, Potrevbic S, Maciewicz RJ. Anatomical properties of brainstem trigeminal neurons that respond to electrical stimulation of dural blood vessels. J Comp Neurol 1994;346:349–65.

56. Kimmel DL. Innervation of the spinal dura mater and dura mater of the posterior cranial fossa. Neurology 1960;10:800–9.

57. Lazorthes G, Gaubert J. L'innervation des articulations interapophysaire vertebrales. Comptes Rendues Assoc Anatomist 1956;43:488–94.

58. Bogduk N. Local anaesthetic blocks of the second cervical ganglion: a technique with application in occipital headache. Cephalalgia 1981;1:41–50.

59. Bogduk N. The clinical anatomy of the cervical dorsal rami. Spine 1982;7:319–30.

60. Williams PL, Warwick R, Dyson M, Bannister LH, editors. Gray's anatomy. 37th ed. Edinburgh: Churchill Livingstone; 1989.

61. Hovelacque A. Anatomie des nerfs craniens et rachidiens et du systeme grand sympathique. Paris: Doin; 1927.

62. Bogduk N, Lambert G, Duckworth JW. The anatomy and physiology of the vertebral nerve in relation to cervical migraine. Cephalalgia 1981;1:1–14.

63. Kimmel DL. The cervical sympathetic rami and the vertebral plexus in the human foetus. J Comp Neurol 1959;112:141–61.

64. Bogduk N, Windsor M, Inglis A. The innervation of the cervical intervertebral discs. Spine 1989;13:2–8.

65. Mendel T, Wink CS, Zimny ML. Neural elements in human cervical intervertebral discs. Spine 1992;17:132–5.

66. Kerr FWL. A mechanism to account for frontal headache in cases of posterior fossa tumors. J Neurosurg 1962;18:605–9.

67. Piovesan EJ, Kowacs PA, Tatsui CE, et al. Referred pain after painful stimulation of the greater occipital nerve in humans: evidence of convergence of cervical afferences on trigeminal nuclei. Cephalalgia 2001;21:107–9.

68. Cyriax J. Rheumatic headache. BMJ 1938;2:1367–8.

69. Campbell DG, Parsons CM. Referred head pain and its concomitants. J Nerv Ment Dis 1944;99:544–51.

70. Feinstein B, Langton JBK, Jameson RM, Schiller F. Experiments on referred pain from deep somatic tissues. J Bone Joint Surg Am 1954;36A:981–97.

71. Wolff HG. Headache and other head pain. 2nd ed. New York: Oxford University Press; 1963. p. 582–616.

72. Schellhas KP, Smith MD, Gundry CR, Pollei SR. Cervical discogenic pain: prospective correlation of magnetic resonance imaging and discography in asymptomatic subjects and pain sufferers. Spine 1996,21:300–12.

73. Grubb SA, Kelly CK. Cervical discography: clinical implications from 12 years of experience. Spine 2000,25:1382–9.

74. Dwyer A, Aprill C, Bogduk N. Cervical zygapophysial joint pain patterns I: a study in normal volunteers. Spine 1990;15:453–7.

75. Dreyfuss P, Michaelsen M, Fletcher D. Atlanto-occipital and lateral atlanto-axial joint pain patterns. Spine 1994;19:1125–31.

76. Bogduk N, Marsland A. On the concept of third occipital headache. J Neurol Neurosurg Psychiatry 1986;49:775–80.

77. Bogduk N, Marsland A. The cervical zygapophysial joints as a source of neck pain. Spine 1988;13:610–7.

78. Lord S, Barnsley L, Wallis B, Bogduk N. Third occipital headache: a prevalence study. J Neurol Neurosurg Psychiatry 1994;57:1187–90.

79. Ehni G, Benner B. Occipital neuralgia and the C1–2 arthrosis syndrome. J Neurosurg 1984;61:961–5.

80. McCormick CC. Arthrography of the atlanto-axial (C1-C2) joints: technique and results. J Intervent Radiol 1987;2:9–13.

81. Busch E, Wilson PR. Atlanto-occipital and atlanto-axial injections in the treatment of headache and neck pain. Reg Anesth 1989;14 Suppl 2:45.

82. Aprill C, Axinn MJ, Bogduk N. Occipital headaches stemming from the lateral atlanto-axial (C1–2) joint. Cephalalgia 2002;22:15–22.

83. Lord SM, Bogduk N. The cervical synovial joints as sources of post-traumatic headache. J Musculoskel Pain 1996;4:81–94.

84. Kerr FWL. Trigeminal nerve volleys. Arch Neurol 1961;5:171–8.

85. Angus-Leppan H, Lambert GA, Michalicek J. Convergence of occipital nerve and superior sagittal sinus input

in the cervical spinal cord of the cat. Cephalalgia 1997;17:625–30.

86. Bartsch T, Goadsby PJ. Stimulation of the greater occipital nerve induces increased central excitability of dural afferent input. Brain 2002;125:1496–509.

87. Bartsch T, Goadsby PJ. Increased responses in trigeminocervical nociceptive neurons to cervical input after stimulation of the dura mater. Brain 2003;126:1801–13.

88. Yu XM, Sessle BJ, Hu JW. Differential effects of cutaneous and deep application of inflammatory irritant on mechanoreceptive field properties of trigeminal brainstem nociceptive neurons. J Neurophysiol 1993;70:1704–7.

89. O'Brien C, Woolf CJ, Fitzgerald M, et al. Differences in the chemical expression of rat primary afferent neurons which innervate skin, muscle, or joint. Neuroscience 1989;32:493–502.

90. Hu JW, Vernon H, Tatourian I. Changes in neck electromyography associated with meningeal noxious stimulation. J Manipulative Physiol Ther 1995;18:577–81.

91. Giffin NJ, Ruggiero L, Lipton RB, et al. Premonitory symptoms in migraine: an electronic diary study. Neurology 2003;60:935–40.

92. Goadsby PJ, Lipton RB, Ferrari MD. Migraine—current understanding and treatment. N Engl J Med 2002;346:257–70.

93. Bakal DA, Kaganov JA. Muscle contraction and migraine headache: psychologic comparison. Headache 1977;17:208–15.

94. Drummond PD. Scalp tenderness and sensitivity to pain in migraine and tension headache. Headache 1987;27:45–50.

95. Selby G, Lance JW. Observation on 500 cases of migraine and allied vascular headache. J Neurol Neurosurg Psychiatry 1960;23:23–32.

96. Silbert PL, Makri B, Schievink WI. Headache and neck pain in spontaneous internal carotid and vertebral artery dissections. Neurology 1995;45:1517–22.

97. Biousse V, D'Anglejan-Chatillon J, Massiou H, Bousser MG. Head pain in non-traumatic carotid artery dissection: a series of 65 patients. Cephalalgia 1994;14:33–6.

98. Sturzenegger M. Headache and neck pain: the warning symptoms of vertebral artery dissection. Headache 1994;34:187–93.

99. Mokri B, Houser W, Sandok BA, Piepgras DG. Spontaneous dissections of the vertebral arteries. Neurology 1988;38:880–5.

100. Travell J. Referred pain from skeletal muscle. The pectoralis major syndrome of breast pain and soreness and the sternomastoid syndrome of headache and dizziness. N Y State J Med 1955;55:331–40.

101. Bonica JJ. Management of myofascial pain syndromes in general practice. JAMA 1957;164:732–8.

102. Berges PU. Myofascial pain syndromes. Postgrad Med 1973;53:161–8.

103. Rubin D. Myofascial trigger point syndromes: an approach to management. Arch Phys Med Rehabil 1981;62:107–10.

104. Simons DG. Myofascial pain syndromes; where are we; where are we going? Arch Phys Med Rehabil 1988;69:207–12.

105. Travell JG, Simons DG. Myofascial pain and dysfunction. The trigger point manual. Baltimore: Williams & Wilkins; 1993. p. 305–20.

106. Bogduk N, Simons DG. Neck pain: joint pain or trigger points. In: Vaeroy H, Merskey H, editors. Progress in fibromyalgia and myofascial pain. Amsterdam: Elsevier; 1993. p. 267–73.

107. Sjaastad O, Saunte C, Hovdahl H, et al. "Cervicogenic" headache. An hypothesis. Cephalalgia 1983;3:249–56.

108. Sjaastad O, Fredriksen TA, Pfaffenrath V. Cervicogenic headache: diagnostic criteria. Headache 1990;30:725–6.

109. Fredriksen TA. Cervicogenic headache: the forehead sweating pattern. Cephalalgia 1988;8:203–9.

110. Fredriksen TA, Wysocka-Bakowska MM, Bogucki A, Antonaci F. Cervicogenic headache. Pupillometric findings. Cephalalgia 1988;8:93–103.

111. Pfaffenrath V, Dandekar R, Pollmann W. Cervicogenic headache—the clinical picture, radiologic findings and hypotheses on its pathophysiology. Headache 1987;27:495–9.

112. Fredriksen TA, Fougner R, Tangerund A, Sjaastad O. Cervicogenic headache. Radiological investigations concerning head/neck. Cephalalgia 1989;9:139–46.

113. Zwart JA. Neck mobility in different headache disorders. Headache 1997;37:6–11.

114. Bovim G. Cervicogenic headache, migraine, and tension-type headache. Pressure-pain threshold measurements. Pain 1992;51:169–73.

115. Watson DH, Trott PH. Cervical headache: an investigation of natural head posture and upper cervical flexor muscle performance. Cephalalgia 1993;13:272–84.

116. Jull G, Barret C, Magee R, Ho P. Further clinical clarification of the muscle dysfunction in cervical headache. Cephalalgia 1999;19:179–85.

117. Leone M, D'Amico D, Moschiano F, et al. Possible identification of cervicogenic headache among patients with migraine: an analysis of 374 headaches. Headache 1995;35:461–4.

118. Leone M, D'Amico D, Grazzi L, et al. Cervicogenic headache: a critical review of the current diagnostic criteria. Pain 1998;78:1–5.

119. Antonaci F, Ghirmai S, Bono G, et al. Cervicogenic headache: an evaluation of the original diagnostic criteria. Cephalalgia 2001;21:573–83.

120. van Suijlekom JA, de Vet HCW, van den Berg SGM, Weber WEJ. Interobserver reliability of diagnostic criteria for cervicogenic headache. Cephalalgia 1999;19:817–23.

121. Bogduk N. Headache and the cervical spine. Cephalalgia 1984;4:167–70.

122. Sjaastad O, Fredriksen TA, Pfaffenrath V. Cervicogenic headache: diagnostic criteria. Headache 1998;38:442–5.

123. Sjaastad O, Fredriksen TA, Stolt-Nielsen A. Cervicogenic headache, C2 rhizopathy, and occipital neuralgia: a connection? Cephalalgia 1986;6:189–95.

124. Bovim G, Berg R, Dale LG. Cervicogenic headache: anaesthetic blockades of cervical nerves (C2-C5) and facet joint (C2/C3). Pain 1992;49:315–20.

125. Merskey H, Bogduk N, editors. Classification of pain. Descriptions of chronic pain syndromes and definitions of pain terms. 2nd ed. Seattle (WA): International Association for the Study of Pain; 1994.

126. Headache Classification Committee, International Headache Society. Classification and diagnostic criteria for headache disorders, cranial neuralgias and facial pain. Cephalalgia 1988;8 Suppl 7:1–96.

127. Jundt JW, Mock D. Temporal arteritis with normal erythrocyte sediment rates presenting as occipital neuralgia. Arthritis Rheum 1991;34:217–9.

128. Bovim G, Fredriksen TA, Stolt-Nielsen A, Sjaastad O. Neurolysis of the greater occipital nerve in cervicogenic headache. A follow up study. Headache 1992;32:175–9.

129. Anthony M. Headache and the greater occipital nerve. Clin Neurol Neurosurg 1992;94:297–301.

130. Saadah HA, Taylor FB. Sustained headache syndrome associated with tender occipital nerve zones. Headache 1987;27:201–5.

131. Gawel MJ, Rothbart PJ. Occipital nerve block in the management of headache and cervical pain. Cephalalgia 1992;12:9–13.

132. Bogduk N. An anatomical basis for neck tongue syndrome. J Neurol Neurosurg Psychiatry 1981;44:202–8.

133. Jansen J, Markakis E, Rama B, Hildebrandt J. Hemicranial attacks or permanent hemicrania—a sequel of upper cervical root compression. Cephalalgia 1989;9:123–30.

134. Poletti CE, Sweet WH. Entrapment of the C2 root and ganglion by the atlanto-epistrophic ligament: clinical syndrome and surgical anatomy. Neurosurgery 1990;27:288–91.

135. Kuritzky, A. Cluster headache-like pain caused by an upper cervical meningioma. Cephalalgia 1984;4:185–6.

136. Sharma RR, Parekh HC, Prabhu S, et al. Compression of the C-2 root by a rare anomalous ectatic vertebral artery. J Neurosurg 1993;78:669–72.

137. Jansen J, Bardosi A, Hildebrandt J, Lucke A. Cervicogenic, hemicranial attacks associated with vascular irritation or compression of the cervical nerve root C2. Clinical manifestations and morphological findings. Pain 1989;39:203–12.

138. Hildebrandt J, Jansen J. Vascular compression of the C2 and C3 roots—yet another cause of chronic intermittent hemicrania? Cephalalgia 1984;4:167–70.

139. Lance JW, Anthony M. Neck tongue syndrome on sudden turning of the head. J Neurol Neurosurg Psychiatry 1980;43:97–101.

140. Bland JH, Davis PH, London MG, et al. Rheumatoid arthritis of the cervical spine. Arch Intern Med 1963;112:892–8.

141. Bertoft ES, Westerberg CE. Further observations on the neck-tongue syndrome. Cephalalgia 1985;5 Suppl 3:312–3.

142. Cabot A, Becker A. The cervical spine in rheumatoid arthritis. Clin Orthop 1978;131:130–40.

143. Robinson HS. Rheumatoid arthritis: atlanto-axial subluxation and its clinical presentation. Can Med Assoc J 1966;94:470–7.

144. Sharp J, Purser DW. Spontaneous atlanto-axial dislocation in ankylosing spondylitis and rheumatoid arthritis. Ann Rheum Dis 1961;20:47–77.

145. Stevens JS, Cartlidge NEF, Saunders M, et al. Atlanto-axial subluxation and cervical myelopathy in rheumatoid arthritis. QJM 1971;159:391–408.

146. Fournier AM, Rathelot P. L'arthrose atlo-odontoidienne. Presse Med 1960;68:163–5.

147. Harata S, Tohno S, Kawagishi T. Osteoarthritis of the atlanto-axial joint. Int Orthop 1981;5:277–82.

148. Zapletal J, Hekster REM, Straver JS, Wilmink JT. Atlanto-odontoid osteoarthritis. Appearance prevalence at computed tomography. Spine 1995;20:49–53.

149. Zapletal J, Hekster REM, Straver JS, et al. Relationship between atlanto-odontoid osteoarthritis and idiopathic suboccipital neck pain. Neuroradiology 1996;38:62–5.

150. McRae DL. The significance of abnormalities of the cervical spine. AJR Am J Roentgenol 1960;84:3–25.

151. McRae DL. Bony abnormalities of the cranio-spinal junction. Clin Neurosurg 1968;16:356–75.

152. Schonstrom N, Twomey L, Taylor J. The lateral atlanto-axial joints and their synovial folds: an in vitro study of soft tissue injuries and fractures. J Trauma 1993;35:886–92.

153. Cummings TM, White AR. Needling therapies in the management of myofascial trigger point pain: a systematic review. Arch Phys Med Rehabil 2001;82:986–92.

154. van Suijlekom HA, van Kleef M, Barendse GAM, et al. Radiofrequency cervical zygapophyseal joint neurotomy for cervicogenic headaches: a prospective study of 15 patients. Funct Neurol 1998;13:297–303.

155. Stovner LJ, Kolstad F, Helde G. Radiofrequency denervation of facet joints C2-C6 in cervicogenic headache: a randomised, double-blind, sham-controlled study. Cephalalgia 2004;24:821–30.

156. Bogduk N. Editorial cervicogenic headache. Cephalalgia 2004;24:819–20.

157. Pikus HJ, Phillips JM. Characteristics of patients successfully treated for cervicogenic headache by surgical decompression of the second cervical root. Headache 1995;35:621–9.

158. Nillson N. A randomized controlled trial of the effect of spinal manipulation in the treatment of cervicogenic headache. J Manipulative Physiol Ther 1995;18:435–40.

159. Nillson N, Christensen HW, Hartvigsen J. The effect of spinal manipulation in the treatment of cervicogenic headache. J Manipulative Physiol Ther 1997;2:326–30.

160. Vernon HT. Spinal manipulation and headaches of cervical origin. J Manipulative Physiol Ther 1989;12:455–68.

161. Jull G, Trott P, Potter H, et al. A randomized controlled trial of exercise and manipulative therapy for cervicogenic headache. Spine 2002;27:1835–43.

162. Horowitz MB, Yonas H. Occipital neuralgia treated by intradural dorsal nerve root sectioning. Cephalalgia 1993;13:354–60.

163. Dubuisson D. Treatment of occipital neuralgia by partial posterior rhizotomy at C1–3. J Neurosurg 1995;82:581–6.

164. Bovim G, Bonamico L, Fredriksen TA, et al. Topographic variations in the peripheral course of the greater occipital nerve. Spine 1991;16:475–8.

165. Lozano A, Vanderlinden G, Bachoo R, Rothbart P. Microsurgical C-2 ganglionectomy for chronic intractable occipital pain. J Neurosurg 1998;89:359–65.

166. Fortin C J, Biller J. Neck tongue syndrome. Headache 1985;25:255–8.

167. Cassidy JD, Diakow PRP, de Korompay VL, et al. Treatment of neck-tongue syndrome by spinal manipulation: a report of three cases. Pain Clin 1986;1:41–6.

168. Elisevich K, Stratford J, Bray G, Finlayson M. Neck tongue syndrome: operative management. J Neurol Neurosurg Psychiatry 1984;47:407–9.

169. Joseph B, Kumar B. Gallie's fusion for atlantoaxial arthrosis with occipital neuralgia. Spine 1994;19:454–5.

170. Ghanayem AJ, Leventhal M, Bohlman HH. Osteoarthrosis of the atlanto-axial joints—long-term follow-up after treatment with arthrodesis. J Bone Joint Surg Am 1996;78A:1300–7.

171. Slipman CW, Lipetz JS, Plastara CT, et al. Therapeutic zygapophyseal joint injections for headache emanating from the C2–3 joint. Am J Phys Med Rehabil 2001;80:182–8.

172. Lord SM, Barnsley L, Bogduk N. Percutaneous radiofrequency neurotomy in the treatment of cervical zygapophysial joint pain: a caution. Neurosurgery 1995;36:732–9.

173. Govind J, King W, Bailey B, Bogduk N. Radiofrequency neurotomy for the treatment of third occipital headache. J Neurol Neurosurg Psychiatry 2003;74:88–93.

174. Lord SM, Barnsley L, Wallis BJ, et al. Percutaneous radio-frequency neurotomy for chronic cervical zygapophysial-joint pain. N Engl J Med 1996;335:1721–6.

175. Isaacs D, Fitzgerald D. Seven alternatives to evidence based medicine. BMJ 1999;319:1618.

176. Bogduk N. Diagnostic nerve blocks in chronic pain. Best Pract Res Clin Anaesthesiol 2002;16:565–8.

177. International Headache Society. The international classification of headache disorders, 2nd edition. Cephalalgia 2004;24 Suppl 1:115–6.

178. Gobel H, Edmeads JG. Disorders of the skull and cervical spine. In: Olesen J, Tfelt-Hansen P, Welch KMA, editors. The headaches. 2nd ed. Philadelphia: Lippincott Williams & Wilkins; 2000. p. 891–8.

# CHAPTER 13

# Headache due to Cervical Disease: Clinical Implications

Julio Pascual, MD, PhD

## THE NECK AND HEADACHE

As reviewed in Chapter 12, "Headaches of Cervical Origin," abnormalities of various neck structures, mainly the synovial joints, intervertebral disks, ligaments, muscles, nerve roots, and the vertebral artery, have all been implicated as a source of headache. Headaches, especially those with a posterior location, are often connected with disorders of the cervical spine. However, the question as to whether disease or dysfunction of the structures of the neck can give rise to true headache has been discussed for over a century.[1] In its operational 1988 diagnostic criteria, the International Headache Society (IHS) defined "headache associated with disorder of the neck" as "a pain localized to [the] neck and occipital region radiating to [the] forehead, orbital region, temples, vertex or ear, precipitated or aggravated by special neck movements or sustained neck posture."[2] In addition, at least one of the following three criteria must be fulfilled: (1) resistance or limitation of passive neck movements; (2) changes in neck muscle contour, texture, tone, or response of the neck musculature to active and passive stretching and contraction; (3) abnormal tenderness of neck muscles. Also mandatory was a "pathological finding in a radiological examination of: a) movement abnormalities in flexion/extension; b) abnormal posture; or c) a clear symptomatic cause (fractures, arthritis, etc)." Spondylosis or osteochondrosis was not sufficient for classification. Hence, a chronic headache of cervical origin persisting for more than 1 month or a headache without radiologic pathology of the cervical spine could not be defined according the 1988 IHS criteria.

The new IHS classification now accepts three varieties of "headache attributed to disorder of the neck": (1) cervicogenic headache, (2) headache attributed to retropharyngeal tendonitis, and (3) headache attributed to cranial dystonia.[3] The IHS diagnostic criteria of the main variety, cervicogenic headache, appear in Table 13–1. The diagnosis of these headache varieties becomes definite only when pain resolves after effective treatment or spontaneous remission. If the cervical disorder is effectively treated or remits spontaneously but headache does not resolve or markedly improves after 3 months, the headache has other mechanisms. Additionally, the entity "chronic post-craniocervical disorder headache" is now described in the appendix of the new IHS classification. Headaches meeting these criteria clinically exist but have been poorly studied, and the appendix entry is intended to stimulate further research into such headaches and their mechanisms. The true debate on the concept of "cervicogenic headache" was provoked by Sjaastad and colleagues, when they proposed that the neck is the origin of a somewhat uniform pain profile frequently experienced by headache patients.[4] In this chapter, headaches with a potential origin in the neck are reviewed. The well-demonstrated cervical causes of headache are commented on first, and then the most controversial cervical entities possibly leading to headache, including Sjaastad and colleagues' cervicogenic headache, are discussed.

## WELL-DEMONSTRATED CERVICAL CAUSES OF HEADACHE

The accepted cervical causes of headache are listed in Table 13–2.

## DEVELOPMENTAL ANOMALIES OF THE CRANIOVERTEBRAL JUNCTION

The developmental anomalies of the craniovertebral junction and upper cervical spine frequently cause headaches.[5] More than three decades ago, headache was reported as the presenting complaint in a quarter of patients with anomalies such as basilar invagination,

**Table 13–1** International Headache Society Criteria for Cervicogenic Headache

| | |
|---|---|
| A. | Pain referred from a source in the neck and perceived in one or more regions of the head and/or face, fulfilling criteria C and D |
| B. | Clinical, laboratory, and/or imaging evidence of a disorder or lesion within the cervical spine or soft tissues of the neck known to be, or generally accepted as, a valid cause of headache |
| C. | Evidence that the pain can be attributed to the neck disorder or lesion based on at least 1 of the following: |
| | 1. Demonstration of clinical signs that implicate a source of pain in the neck |
| | 2. Abolition of headache following diagnostic blockade of a cervical structure or its nerve supply using placebo or other adequate controls |
| D. | Pain resolves within 3 mo after successful treatment of the causative disorder or lesion |

Tumors, fractures, infections, and rheumatoid arthritis of the upper cervical spine have not been validated formally as causes of headache but are nevertheless accepted as valid causes when demonstrated to be so in individual cases. Cervical spondylosis and osteochondritis are not accepted as valid causes fulfilling criterion B. When myofascial tender spots are the cause, the headache should be coded as "tension-type headache."

Clinical signs acceptable for criterion C1 must have demonstrated reliability and validity. The future task is the identification of such reliable and valid operational tests. Clinical features, such as neck pain, focal neck tenderness, a history of neck trauma, mechanical exacerbation of pain, unilaterality, coexisting shoulder pain, reduced range of motion in the neck, nuchal onset, nausea, vomiting, and photophobia, are not unique to cervicogenic headache. These may be features of cervicogenic headache, but they do not define the relationship between the disorder and the source of the headache.

Abolition of headache means complete relief of headache, indicated by a score of zero on a visual analog scale (VAS). Nevertheless, acceptable as fulfilling criterion C2 is a > 90% reduction in pain to a level of < 5 on a 100-point VAS.

congenital atlantoaxial dislocation, or separate odontoid process.[6] With the advent of magnetic resonance imaging (MRI), we now know that most of these patients also have soft-tissue anomalies, such as Chiari malformation type I.[7] These neural abnormalities are key contributors to headache because isolated bony anomalies unassociated with neural malformations (ie, Klippel-Feil syndrome) are not associated with head pain. These patients experience headaches that are typically provoked (not aggravated) by activities—coughing, sneezing, laughing, crying, heavy lifting, straining at stool, or bending over—that incorporate a Valsalva's maneuver. "Cough" headaches are sudden in onset, reach a peak intensity rapidly, and then either disappear or fade to a dull ache, which may remain for several hours. The pain is moderate to severe in intensity, usually with a sharp or stabbing quality, bilateral, and not associated with nausea or vomiting. The major locus of pain is the occipital-suboccipital regions, but vertex or frontal radiation is commonly seen. These patients are usually pain free between attacks (Figure 13–1).[7] There can be a genetic basis for anomalies of the craniocervical junction in some families.[8]

The acute onset of headache with the Valsalva's maneuver is most likely explained by increased intracranial venous pressure.[9,10] The Valsalva's maneuver increases intrathoracic and intra-abdominal pressure, which is transmitted to epidural veins, producing a pressure wave that moves cerebrospinal fluid rostrally. The headache may be caused by the temporary impaction of the cerebellar tonsils with traction on the pain-sensitive dura. This sudden obstruction of the free flow of cerebrospinal fluid in the subarachnoid space was recently confirmed in Chiari malformation type I patients with cough headache versus controls before surgery. Cough headache disappeared after surgery when intrathecal pressure became normalized.[11]

Cough headache secondary to anomalies of the craniovertebral junction are differentiated from "benign" cough headache (ie, unassociated with intracranial pathology) already on clinical grounds. Benign cough headache is almost exclusive to elderly men, is not associated with posterior fossa or upper cervical symptoms or signs, and responds to indomethacin. Reconstructive suboccipital craniectomy, but not indomethacin, relieves pain in cough headache owing to Chiari malformation type I.[12]

## ACQUIRED LESIONS OF THE CRANIOVERTEBRAL JUNCTION

These acquired disorders also produce occipital headaches, which are also triggered and worsened by neck movements or straining.[13,14] They include primary tumors (schwannoma, meningioma, ependymoma), multiple myeloma, metastatic tumors, Paget's disease of

**Table 13–2** Cervical Causes of Headache*

I. Well-demonstrated causes:

    A. Developmental anomalies of the craniocervical junction and upper cervical spine with or without neural anomalies (mainly Chiari malformation type I)

    B. Acquired lesions:

        1. Tumors of craniovertebral junction and upper cervical spine

        2. Paget's disease of the skull with secondary basilar invagination

        3. Osteomyelitis of the upper cervical vertebrae

        4. Rheumatoid arthritis of the upper cervical spine

        5. Ankylosing spondylitis of the upper cervical spine

        6. Traumatic subluxation of the upper cervical vertebrae

        7. Retropharyngeal tendonitis

        8. Craniocervical dystonias

II. Controversial causes:

        1. Cervical disk disease

        2. Spondylosis

        3. "Whiplash" injuries

III. Unaccepted causes:

        1. Posterior cervical syndrome of Barré

        2. Migraine cervical syndrome of Bartschi-Rochaix

Adapted from Gobel H and Edmeads JG.[13]

*Sjaastad's cervicogenic headache and Bogduk's third occipital headache are not specific headache entities but rather syndromes or reaction patterns said to result from a variety of lesions.

the skull with secondary basilar invagination, and osteomyelitis of the upper cervical column. All of these conditions may produce headache by erosion of the pain-sensitive structures or traction of the upper cervical nerve roots. Rheumatoid arthritis and ankylosing spondylitis of the upper cervical spine are capable of inducing headache through a variety of mechanisms, including inflammation of the synovial atlantoaxial and atlanto-occipital joints and stretching of the upper cervical ligaments and nerve roots caused by atlantoaxial subluxation secondary to attenuation of the transverse ligament of the odontoid process. Blows to the head or even forceful sneezing may produce rotatory subluxation of the atlas, which, through irritation of the synovial joints, can cause daily occipital headache. When examining these patients with rheumatoid arthritis who also experience headache, care should be taken when asking them to flex the neck because fatalities have resulted from compression of the medulla by the odontoid, which, no longer bound to the atlas by

the transverse ligament, fails to move away from the brainstem on anteflexion of the cervical spine.[15–17]

## RETROPHARYNGEAL TENDONITIS

This is a very uncommon condition of unknown etiology characterized by the acute onset of occipital and upper cervical pain aggravated by neck movements and accompanied by pain on swallowing and tenderness in the upper neck, mild to moderate fever, and usually an elevated erythrocyte sedimentation rate.[18] Current IHS diagnostic criteria for this exceptional entity are listed in Table 13–3.

## HEADACHE ATTRIBUTED TO CRANIAL DYSTONIA

Focal dystonias of the head and neck can be accompanied by headache. According to the current IHS classification, pharyngeal dystonia, spasmodic torticollis, mandibular dystonia, lingual dystonia, and a combination of cranial

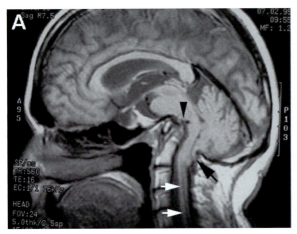

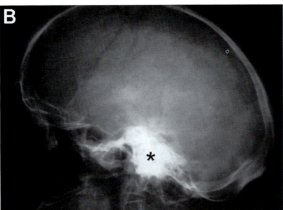

**Figure 13–1**  *A*, Magnetic resonance image of a 38-year-old woman who meets International Headache Society (IHS) criteria for cervicogenic headache disclosing severe basilar invagination (*arrowhead*), tonsilar descent (*black arrow*), and syringomyelia (*white arrows*). *B*, Skull radiographs of her mother also showing severe basilar invagination (the *asterisk* points out the top of the odontoid process). She had been admitted to our hospital 35 years earlier owing to cervical pain and headache aggravated by coughing and died from obstructive hydrocephalus. These cases illustrate two typical examples of cervicogenic headache according to the current IHS classification and show that most patients with developmental anomalies of the craniovertebral junction also have neural malformations, for which there can be a genetic basis.

and cervical dystonias (segmental craniocervical dystonia) can by accompanied by pain somewhere in the head. Pain from craniocervical dystonia is either due to continuous muscle contraction or may occur as a result of secondary irritation of neural structures, for example, where the occipital nerve emerges.[3]

The operational IHS criteria for this entity appear in Table 13–4. With the current criteria, abnormal dystonic movements are not strictly necessary for the diagnosis of headache attributed to dystonia but only a defective posture of the head and neck. In our experience, more than 80% of patients suffering from these craniocervical dystonias complain of local pain, and almost two-thirds meet the criteria for either tension-type headache or migraine.[19] In fact, migraine itself

seems more common than that expected in such patients. All of this has stimulated a debate with two, not necessarily opposed, views regarding the relationship of this headache to primary headaches. One possibility might be that some patients with apparent primary headaches would actually have headache owing to defective neck postures. Alternatively, this defective muscle postural hyperactivity, seen in some patients with primary headaches, would only be a secondary phenomenon, with no direct pathophysiologic role. Further research, using the new diagnostic criteria, is needed to clarify this debate.

There is no specific curative therapy for craniocervical dystonia. Physiotherapy, local injections of an anesthetic plus corticosteroids and oral analgesics, nonsteroidal anti-inflammatory drugs (NSAIDs), and muscle relaxants have been employed as symptomatic therapy with, at most, some relief. Local injections of botulinum toxin have brought a dramatic improvement in this condition, with a success rate in more than two-thirds of segmental dystonic patients. Specific effects on pain are particularly successful, being achieved in nearly all patients and to a higher degree and earlier than the benefit in the movement disorder.[20] Interestingly, primary headaches in dystonic patients also seem to improve with botulinum toxin injections,[19] which, again, might suggest a role of dystonia in the pathophysiology of primary headaches in these patients.

## CONTROVERSIAL CERVICAL CAUSES OF HEADACHE

### Cervical Disk Disease and Spondylosis

A relationship between these two conditions and headache remains unproven.[6,13,14,21] In those over 40 years of age, disk space narrowing and posterior osteophytes are increasingly common, from C3–4 to C7–T1 and especially at C5–6. Because they involve the lower cervical disks and vertebrae, a pathophysiologic referral of the pain to the head would be difficult to explain. Hypothetically, the restriction of movement in these lower cervical regions would lead to excessive work in the C2–4 joints, and this could refer pain to the head.

Clinically, these patients may complain of attacks, lasting days or even weeks, of dull aching pain in the neck and occiput on one or both sides, which may radiate to the vertex or the frontoparietal area. Headache is common on waking and diminishes spontaneously within hours. Unilaterality is not an essential feature, but some may complain of more obvious hemicranial radicular pains precipitated by coughing or sneezing.

### Whiplash Injuries

Cervical trauma as an origin of chronic headaches is not discussed here in detail for two reasons: whiplash

**Table 13–3** International Headache Society Criteria for Headache Attributed to Retropharyngeal Tendonitis

Diagnostic criteria:

A.  Unilateral or bilateral nonpulsating pain in the back of the neck, radiating to the back of the head or to the whole head and fulfilling criteria C and D

B.  Swollen prevertebral soft tissues in adults measuring > 7 mm at the level between C1 and C4 (a special radiographic technique may be required)

C.  Pain is aggravated severely by bending the head backward

D.  Pain is alleviated within 2 wk of treatment with NSAIDs in their recommended doses

*Comments:* Body temperature and erythrocyte sedimentation rate are usually elevated. Although retroflexion of the neck most consistently aggravates pain, this also usually happens with rotation and swallowing. The transverse processes of the upper three vertebrae are usually tender to palpation.

In several cases, amorphous calcified material has been aspirated from the swollen prevertebral tissues. Thin calcification in prevertebral tissues is best seen on computed tomography.

Upper carotid dissection should be ruled out.

NSAID = nonsteroidal anti-inflammatory drug.

**Table 13–4** International Headache Society Criteria for Headache Attributed to Craniocervical Dystonia

Diagnostic criteria:

A.  Sensation of cramp, tension, or pain in the neck, radiating to the back of the head or to the whole head and fulfilling criteria C and D

B.  Abnormal movements or defective posture of neck or head due to muscular hyperactivity

C.  Evidence that pain is attributed to muscular hyperactivity based on at least 1 of the following:

  1.  Demonstration of clinical signs that implicate a source of pain in the hyperactive muscle (eg, pain is precipitated or exacerbated by muscle contraction, movements, sustained posture, or external pressure)

  2.  Simultaneous onset of pain and muscular hyperactivity

D.  Pain resolves within 3 mo after successful treatment of the causative disorder

*Comment:* Focal dystonias of the head and neck accompanied by pain are pharyngeal dystonia, spasmodic torticollis, mandibular dystonia, lingual dystonia, and a combination of the cranial and cervical dystonias (segmental craniocervical dystonia). Pain is caused by local contractions and secondary changes.

is not a recognized cause of chronic headache,[6,13,14,21,22] and there is a chapter on headache and cranial trauma in this book (see Chapter 16, "Headaches Associated with Head Trauma (Postconcussive Headache)"). It is a clinical reality that many people with an extension-flexion injury of the neck do complain of occipitofrontal dull or shooting pain. This pain subsides within 3 to 6 weeks in most patients. In these cases, a mechanical sprain involving traction and tearing of long neck muscles and interspinous ligaments is a more than reasonable explanation for this transient headache. The specific unexplained problem remains with those with "chronic whiplash syndrome" when headache and stiffness of the neck continue after 6 months, together with other physical and emotional complaints. These headaches are primarily posterior, although they may radiate anteriorly, predominantly unilateral, aggravated by neck movement, and associated with palpable spasm or nodule formation in the cervical muscles. Some investigators think that chronic whiplash syndrome is a psychological illness reinforced by legal and social sanction because evidence indicates that the reported incidence of "whiplash" can be reduced by minor legislative changes. Others believe that shearing injuries of the long axons in the pain brainstem and upper cervical cord nuclei would disrupt regulatory mechanisms, bringing headache on. Such a mechanism would account for the typical migraine following some neck sprains and showing benefit to preventive antimigraine medications, despite ongoing litigation. Finally, occult severe injuries are very infrequent. In this minority subgroup, MRI discloses lesions of the annulus, vertebrae and plates, anterior longitudinal ligaments, and zygapophyseal joints, with focal hemorrhages in the prevertebral space, muscles, and facet joint capsules.[23]

Patients with acute whiplash usually respond to ice for 24 hours followed by heat applications, analgesics and NSAIDs, and muscle relaxants. Not without controversy, cervical collars, active physiotherapy, and tractions should probably be avoided in the acute phase. Treatment of chronic whiplash syndrome usually gives little relief, often lasting but a few days.[13,14,21,24] Many patients are not cured by legal settlement. Physical therapy, local depot corticosteroids, botulinum toxin, acupuncture, and transcutaneous nerve stimulators are often recommended to reduce pain.[24,25] Such claims are based more on optimism and a desire to do something than on any objective and independent appraisal of results.

## SYNDROMES NOT GENERALLY ACCEPTED

### Third Occipital Headache

Bogduk and Marsland's third occipital headache is an entity of uncertain status.[26] This nerve, the superficial medial branch of the C3 dorsal ramus, supplies the C3 dermatome, part of the semispinalis capitis muscle, and the C2–3 zygapophyseal joint. Bogduk and Marsland, in a group of patients with occipital headaches radiating frontally and at least one feature that could suggest a cervical origin for the pain (eg, history of neck injury, triggering of pain by neck movement), blocked this nerve and recorded pain relief in two-thirds of patients.[26] They interpreted their results as suggesting that disease of the C2–3 zygapophyseal joints may produce headache by irritating or compressing the third occipital nerve. The small number of patients and the absence of radiologic evidence of local anomalies, however, are disturbing. Alternatively, the nerve blocks could relieve headache in a nonspecific fashion by cutting impulses to the central trigeminal system.[6,13,14,21]

### Barré's Syndrome and Cervical Migraine Syndrome

In Barré's posterior cervical sympathetic syndrome, symptoms of headache, neck discomfort, dizziness, visual blurring, psychological disturbances, and impaired hearing are believed to be caused by osteophytes irritating the sympathetic nerve plexus that invests the vertebral arteries.[27] In the cervical migraine syndrome of Bartschi-Rochaix, similar symptoms are believed to be due to actual compression of the vertebral artery by osteophytes or trauma.[28] Trauma is considered a frequent precipitant of these syndromes. Physical findings in both syndromes are suboccipital tenderness, palpable spasm of neck muscles, limitation of neck movement, and reproduction or intensification of these symptoms by neck movements. Sensory changes in the territory of C2 dermatome have occasionally been described. The similarities of these syndromes to the whiplash syndrome are striking. Impeding the acceptance of these syndromes is the failure to demonstrate that stimulation of the posterior sympathetic syndrome can, indeed, induce these symptoms.

### Sjaastad's Cervicogenic Headache

#### Description

The term "cervicogenic headache" was first introduced to the medical literature by Sjaastad and colleagues in 1983.[4] In 1990, Sjaastad's group published very specific and detailed diagnostic criteria for cervicogenic headache. This was followed by the publication of less stringent diagnostic criteria by the International Association for the Study of Pain in 1994 and by the Quebec Headache Study of Pain.[29,30] In 1998, Sjaastad and colleagues revised their diagnostic criteria for cervicogenic headache based on more extensive clinical research. These revised criteria are listed in Table 13–5.

Currently, there is a debate about the validity of the concept of cervicogenic headache as proposed by Sjaastad and colleagues.[13,14,24,31–33] The Sjaastad school, however, carefully stipulates that cervicogenic headache is not a "disease" or entity sui generis but a reaction pattern.[4,31,34,35] Thus, in a sense, the concept of cervicogenic headache simply reiterates what has been reviewed in this chapter: that some headaches may result from neck dysfunction or disease and that these headaches may show clinical characteristics suggesting a neck origin. None of this is actually controversial. Sjaastad and colleagues have drawn criticism, however, because of their position that cervicogenic headache may be extremely common and their consideration of neural blockade as a major diagnostic criterion.

#### Differential Diagnosis

Following Sjaastad and colleagues' experience, cervicogenic headache is, in principle, a strict unilateral headache, but it may also be bilateral ("unilaterality on the two sides"). Otherwise, this headache will be confused with tension-type headache or migraine without aura. The duration of the solitary attack—or an exacerbation—varies from a few hours to a few weeks. In the initial phase, the headache is usually episodic; later, it frequently becomes chronic-fluctuating. Symptoms and signs referable to the neck are essential, such as a reduced range of motion in the neck or mechanical precipitation of attacks. "Migrainous" symptoms, such as nausea and photophobia, are, when present, generally not marked. A positive response to appropriate anesthetic blockades is essential. No specific radiologic abnormalities have been identified according to Sjaastad's group, in contradiction to the inclusion of radio-

**Table 13–5**  Sjaastad and Colleagues' Diagnostic Criteria for Cervicogenic Headache

Major (mandatory) criteria

    I. Symptoms and signs of neck involvement:

        a. Precipitation of head pain, similar to the usually occurring one

        b. Restriction of the range of motion in the neck

        c. Ipsilateral neck, shoulder, or arm pain of a rather vague, nonradicular nature or, occasionally, arm pain of a radicular nature

    II. Confirmatory evidence by diagnostic anesthetic blockades

    III. Unilaterality of the head pain, without side shift

Head pain characteristics

    IV. a. Moderate-severe, nonthrobbing, and nonlancinating pain, usually starting in the neck

        b. Episodes of varying duration

        c. Fluctuating, continuous pain

Other characteristics of some importance

    V. a. Only marginal effect or lack of effect of indomethacin

        b. Only marginal effect or lack of effect of ergotamine and sumatriptan

        c. Female sex

        d. Not infrequent occurrence of head or indirect neck trauma by history, usually of more than only medium severity

Other features of lesser importance

    VI. Various attack-related phenomena, only occasionally present and/or moderately expressed when present:

        a. Nausea

        b. Phonophobia and photophobia

        c. Dizziness

        d. Ipsilateral "blurred vision"

        e. Difficulties swallowing

        f. Ipsilateral edema, mostly in the periocular area

logic abnormalities as an obligatory criterion by the current IHS classification.[36]

The scarcity of autonomic symptoms and signs distinguishes this headache from cluster headache, as do other features, such as the temporal pattern, severity, and female preponderance. Hemicrania continua and cervicogenic headache have many traits in common as far as clinical manifestations and developmental patterns are concerned. Both disorders frequently begin with a remitting headache, which may eventually develop into a chronic type and predominate in females. However, precipitation mechanisms are not an integral part of hemicrania continua, and the response to indomethacin is a decisive factor in the differential diagnosis. Sjaastad's group states that the dif-

ferential diagnosis versus migraine is also possible, taking into account that migraine attacks are accompanied to a higher extent by photophobia, phonophobia, pulsating pain, and aggravation on minor physical activity. Migraine pain most frequently starts in the anterior parts of the head, not infrequently shifts side, and is not abated by local anesthetic blockades of cervical nerves.[35] It does not appear that any specific clinical finding or test can be used to define patients with cervicogenic headache versus migraine without aura or even tension-type headache. I agree with the proposal that cervicogenic headache versus tension-type headache and migraine without aura should be considered only when a pattern of unilateral pain without side shift exists, with the initial pain located at the posterior area, and failure to be classified by diagnostic criteria for other headaches.

### Epidemiology

As a result of the heterogeneity of diagnostic criteria, the variation in the perceived prevalence of cervicogenic headache ranges from 0% of patients with migraine headache to 80% of patients with headache. In headache centers, prevalence estimates range from 0.4 to 80%.[24] In the general population, prevalence rates varied from 0.4 to 2.5%, whereas studies looking at all patients with a complaint of headache reported estimates of 15 to 20%.[37] Analysis of patient descriptive data from these studies reveals that patients with cervicogenic headache conform to a fairly homogeneous population, with a mean age of 43 years, a clear female predominance (4:1), and a mean duration of symptoms of around 7 years.[38,39]

### Treatment

Haldeman and Dagenais recently reviewed in depth all of the medical literature in this particular aspect.[24] Their conclusion was that treatment recommended to patients with a clinical picture compatible with Sjaastad and colleagues' cervicogenic headache is usually not supported by science or research but is more dependent on the specialty and experience of the treating physician. For example, there are no controlled studies to support the use of any surgical procedure (eg, radiofrequency neurotomy or decompression procedures) for the management of cervicogenic headache, the current justification for surgery being based on the anecdotal experience of the surgeon.[40] There is only one randomized controlled trial on the use of transcutaneous electrical nerve stimulation suggesting slight temporary symptom relief.[41]

The prevalence of cervicogenic headache within chiropractic patients is high (up to one-quarter), indicating the frequency with which these headaches are treated by manipulation. Even though the shortcomings of most studies on cervical manipulation are similar to those after surgery, some more rigorous studies have shown that spinal manipulation was, in the short term, more effective than massage in reducing the frequency and severity of headaches and the amount of analgesic use. Several authors, examining randomized controlled trials on manipulation, have concluded that there is moderate evidence for the efficacy of cervical manipulation and neck exercise (low-intensity endurance training) in the management of cervicogenic headache.[24,42,43]

Therapeutic injections are another common treatment approach. There are a number of small case series on the injection of the occipital nerves in which short-term improvement was noted in 50 to 90% of patients.[24] Again, these studies suffer from the same shortcomings as those on surgery and manipulation. One randomized study compared bupivacaine and betamethasone and found that intra-articular injection of betamethasone in the zygapophyseal joints is not an effective therapy for chronic cervical pain after a whiplash injury.[44] Injections of depot methylprednisolone, however, produced complete pain relief in 169 of 180 patients with cervicogenic headache who had not suffered from whiplash or head injury.[45] Recently, a randomized controlled trial comparing botulinum toxin with saline injection into the cervical paraspinal muscles found a significant decrease in pain and increased cervical spine range of motion in the botulinum toxin group.[46,47] There are no studies on the use in cervicogenic headache of other, very popular treatments, such as massage, biofeedback, exercise and nutrition.

## ACKNOWLEDGMENTS

This article was supported by the "Centro de Investigación de Enfermedades Neurológicas," Nodo HUMV/UC, ISCIII, Spain. I am grateful to Professor José Berciano for helpful suggestions on the manuscript.

## REFERENCES

1. Lance JW. Mechanism and management of headache. 4th ed. London: Butterworth Scientific; 1982.

2. Headache Classification Committee, International Headache Society. Classification and diagnostic criteria for headache disorders, cranial neuralgias and facial pain. Cephalalgia 1998;8 Suppl 7:1–96.

3. Headache Classification Subcommittee, International Headache Society. The international classification of headache disorders. 2nd edition. Cephalalgia 2004;24 Suppl 1:1–160.

4. Sjaastad O, Saunte C, Hovdal H, et al. Cervicogenic headache: a hypothesis. Cephalalgia 1983;3:249–56.

5. MacRae DL. Bony abnormalities at the craniospinal junction. Clin Neurosurg 1969;16:356–75.

6. Edmeads J. The cervical spine and headache. Neurology 1988;38:1874–8.

7. Pascual J, Oterino A, Berciano J. Headache in type I Chiari malformation. Neurology 1992;42:1519–21.

8. Speer MC, George TM, Enterline DS, et al. A genetic basis for Chiari I malformation with and without syringomyelia. Neurosurg Focus 2000;8:1–4.

9. Williams B. Cerebrospinal fluid changes in response to coughing. Brain 1976;99:331–46.

10. Williams B. Cough headache due to craniocerebrospinal pressure dissociation. Arch Neurol 1980;37:226–30.

11. Sansur CA, Heiss JD, DeVroom LH, et al. Pathophysiology of headache associated with cough in patients with Chiari malformation. J Neurosurg 2003;98:453–8.

12. Pascual J, Iglesias F, Oterino A, et al. Cough, exertional, and sexual headaches. An analysis of 72 benign and symptomatic cases. Neurology 1996;46:1520–4.

13. Gobel H, Edmeads JG. Disorders of the skull and cervical spine. In: Olesen J, Tfelt-Hansen P, Welch KMA, editors. The headaches. 2nd ed. Philadelphia: Lippincott Williams & Wilkins, 2000. p. 891–8.

14. Edmeads JG. Disorders of the neck. In: Silberstein SD, Lipton RB, Dalessio DJ, editors. Wolff's headache. New York: Oxford University Press; 2001. p. 447–58.

15. Sharp J, Puser DW. Spontaneous atlanto-axial dislocation in ankylosing spondylitis and rheumatoid arthritis. Ann Rheum Dis 1961;20:47–77.

16. Bland JH. Rheumatoid arthritis of the cervical spine. Bull Rheum Dis 1967;18:471–5.

17. Conlon PW, Isdale IC, Rose BS. Rheumatoid arthritis of the cervical spine: an analysis of 333 cases. Ann Rheum Dis 1966;25:120–6.

18. Fahlgren R. Retropharyngeal tendonitis. Cephalalgia 1986;6:169–74.

19. Pascual J. Influence of botulinum toxin treatment on previous primary headaches in patients with cranio-cervical dystonia. Cephalalgia 2003;23:706.

20. Jankovic J, Orman J. Botulinum toxin for cranial-cervical dystonia: a double-blind, placebo-controlled study. Neurology 1987;37:616–23.

21. Bogduk N. Headache and the neck. In: Goadsby PJ, Silberstein SD, editors. Headache. Boston: Butterworth-Heinemann; 1997. p. 369–82.

22. Berger M, Gerstenbrand F. Cervicogenic headache. In: Vinken PJ, Bruyn GW, Klawans HL, Rose FC, editors. Handbook of clinical neurology. Vol 4(48). Headache. Amsterdam: Elsevier Science Publishers; 1986. p. 405–12.

23. Radanov BP, Sturzenegger M, Di Stefano G. Long-term outcome after whiplash injury. A 2-year follow-up considering features of injury mechanism and somatic, radiologic, and psychosocial findings. Medicine 1995;74:281–97.

24. Haldeman S, Dagenais S. Cervicogenic headaches: a critical review. Spine J 2001;1:31–46.

25. Freund BJ, Schwartz M. Treatment of chronic cervical-associated headache with botulinum toxin A: a pilot study. Headache 2000;40:231–6.

26. Bogduk N, Marsland A. On the concept of third occipital headache. J Neurol Neurosurg Psychiatry 1986;49:775–80.

27. Barré JA. Sur un syndrome sympathique cervical postérieur et sa cayse fréquente, l'arthrite cervicale. Rev Neurol (Paris) 1926;33:1246–8.

28. Bartschi-Rochaix W. Headache of cervical origin. In: Vinken PJ, Bruyn GW, Klawans HL, Rose FC, editors. Handbook of clinical neurology. Vol 5. Headache. Amsterdam: North-Holland; 1968. p. 192–203.

29. Merskey H, Bogduk N, editors. Classification of chronic pain. Descriptions of chronic pain syndromes and definitions of pain terms. Cervicogenic headache. 2nd ed. Seattle (WA): IASP; 1994.

30. Meloche J, Bergeron Y, Bellavance A, et al. Painful intervertebral dysfunction: Robert Maigne's original contribution to headache of cervical origin. The Quebec Headache Study Group. Headache 1993;33:328–34.

31. Sjaastad O. Cervicogenic headache: the controversial headache. Clin Neurol Neurosurg 1992;94 Suppl:147–9.

32. Pearce JM. Cervicogenic headache: a personal view. Cephalalgia 1995;15:463–9.

33. Pollmann W, Keidel M, Pfaffenrath V. Headache and the cervical spine. A critical review. Cephalalgia 1997;17:817–21.

34. Sjaastad O, Fredriksen TA, Pfaffenrath V. Cervicogenic headache: diagnostic criteria. Headache 1990;30:725–6.

35. Sjaastad O, Fredriksen TA, Pfaffenrath V, on behalf of the Cervicogenic Headache International Study Group. Cervicogenic headache: diagnostic criteria. The Cervicogenic Headache International Study Group. Headache 1998;38:442–5.

36. Sjaastad O, Bovim G. Cervicogenic headache: the differentiation from common migraine. An overview. Funct Neurol 1991;6:93–100.

37. Nilsson N. The prevalence of cervicogenic headache in a random sample of 20–59 year olds. Spine 1995;20:1884–8.

38. Sjaastad O, Fredriksen TA. Cervicogenic headache: criteria, classification and epidemiology. Clin Exp Rheumatol 2000;18 Suppl 19:3–6.

39. Antonaci F, Fredriksen TA, Sjaastad O. Cervicogenic headache: clinical presentation, diagnostic criteria, and differential diagnosis. Curr Pain Headache Rep 2001;5:387–92.

40. Jansen J. Surgical treatment of non-responsive cervicogenic headache. Clin Exp Rheumatol 2000;18 Suppl 19:67–70.

41. Farina S, Granella F, Malferrari G, Manzoni GC. Headache and cervical spine disorders: classification and treatment with transcutaneous eletrical nerve stimulation. Headache 1986;26:431–3.

42. Hurwitz EL, Aker PD, Adams AH, et al. Manipulation and mobilization of the cervical spine. A systematic review of the literature. Spine 1996;21:1746–60.

43. Bronfort G, Nilsson N, Haas M, et al. Non-invasive physical treatments for chronic/recurrent headache. Cochrane Database Syst Rev 2004;3:CD001878.

44. Barnsley L, Lord SM, Wallis BJ, Bogduk N. Lack of effect of intraarticular corticosteroids for chronic pain in the cervical zygapophyseal joints. N Engl J Med 1994;330:1047–50.

45. Anthony M. Cervicogenic headache: prevalence and response to local steroid therapy. Clin Exp Rheumatol 2000;18 Suppl 19:59–64.

46. Hobson DE, Gladish DF. Botulinum toxin injection for cervicogenic headache. Headache 1997;37:253–5.

47. Borodic GE, Acquadro M, Johnson EA. Botulinum toxin therapy for pain and inflammatory disorders: mechanisms and therapeutic effects. Exp Opin Invest Drugs 2001;10:1531–44.

# CHAPTER 14

# Low–Cerebrospinal Fluid Volume Headaches

Bahram Mokri, MD

The first report on pachymeningeal enhancement in intracranial hypotension appeared only over a decade ago.[1] In this short interval, magnetic resonance imaging (MRI) has revolutionized the diagnosis of spontaneous intracranial hypotension (SIH) and cerebrospinal fluid (CSF) leaks. Far more patients are now diagnosed, and the clinicians may have wondered as to where these patients were only one or two decades ago.[2] The fact is that the diagnosis was missed in many of these patients. Although many spontaneously improved, many did not and carried on with significantly compromised quality of life, seeking help from a variety of physicians and pain management facilities. Some had even undergone suboccipital craniectomy and upper cervical decompressive laminectomies for "Chiari malformation," without much benefit. It is now known that the large majority of cases of SIH, if not all, result from spontaneous CSF leaks. The previous theories of increased CSF absorption or decreased CSF production have never been substantiated. Furthermore, SIH can no longer be simply equated with post–lumbar puncture headaches.[3] A much broader clinical and imaging spectrum of this disorder is now recognized. Although the triad of orthostatic headaches, low-CSF pressures, and diffuse pachymeningeal enhancement on MRI is the reassuring classic hallmark of this disorder, the variability is surely considerable. This includes patients who do not display meningeal enhancement, those who may not have headaches, and patients who may consistently reveal CSF opening pressures that are within normal limits. The core pathogenetic factor and the independent variable are a loss of CSF volume, whereas CSF pressures, clinical manifestations, and MRI abnormalities are variables dependent on the loss of CSF volume.

The term "spontaneous intracranial hypotension" no longer appears to be broad enough to embrace all of these variations. Therefore, terms such as "CSF hypovolemia" or "CSF volume depletion," as well as "spontaneous CSF leaks," have appeared in the literature and have been used interchangeably. In this chapter, an attempt is made to outline clinical features, diagnostic approaches, treatment, and the expectations from these treatments in patients with spontaneous CSF leaks and CSF volume depletion. Furthermore, the considerable variability that exists in clinical, imaging, and CSF findings in this disorder is demonstrated. This variability is particularly noticeable in the features of the headaches that are associated with spontaneous CSF leaks and, therefore, low-CSF volume.

## SELECTED HISTORIC LANDMARKS OF CSF HYPOTENSION AND LOW-CSF VOLUME

In 1891, Quincke introduced lumbar puncture. In 1898, Bier suffered post–lumbar puncture headaches and was the first to report them.[4] In 1938, Schaltenbrand emphasized the term "aliquorrhea," with clinical descriptions that we now recognize as the clinical picture of intracranial hypotension.[5] The patients had very low, unobtainable, or even negative CSF opening pressures. This had been described earlier in the French literature under the terms "hypotension of spinal fluid" and "ventricular collapse." Schaltenbrand, who should be credited for drawing attention to spontaneous occurrence to this entity, tended to think that decreased CSF production was the cause.[6] Of course, the technology of the time would not have allowed him or his contemporaries to study patients properly for CSF leak.

From 1950 to 1990, the details of clinical manifestations of intracranial hypotension and CSF leak were described in several publications.[7] The introduction of radioisotope cysternography provided more information on CSF dynamics and its leaks. Myelography and computed tomography (CT) myelography using water-soluble contrast emerged as a useful and reliable diagnostic test to demonstrate CSF leaks.

In the 1990s, MRI features of intracranial hypotension and CSF leaks were recognized.[8–10] Detection of more cases and broadening of the clinical and imaging spectrum of the disease followed and continue.[11,12]

## ETIOLOGY

The etiologies of CSF volume loss are listed in Table 14–1. Total body water loss (a true hypovolemic state) or holes or rents in the sites of dural puncture or traumatic dural tears, whether post–epidural catheterization or postsurgical, that may cause leakage of CSF, all can lead to a decrease in CSF volume. The most challenging, however, is the spontaneous group, which needs to be addressed in more depth. Often the exact cause of spontaneous CSF leaks remains unclear. Two factors should be considered: trivial trauma and weakness of the dural sac. A previous trivial trauma, such as coughing, lifting, pushing, trivial falls, etc., is reported by a minority of patients. Evidence for weakness of the dural sac is increasingly recognized. Dural sac abnormalities and ectasia, meningeal diverticula, and CSF leaks have been noted in Marfan syndrome,[13,14] a disorder known to be related to abnormality of elastin and fibrillin. Stigmata of connective tissue disorder, particularly disorders of fibrillin or elastin, have been observed in a notable minority of the patients with spontaneous CSF leaks.[15,16] Single or multiple meningeal diverticula are frequently noted in patients with spontaneous CSF leaks, as well as in certain heritable disorders of connective tissue. It is likely that a combination of a weakened thecal sac and a trivial trauma might lead to occurrence of "spontaneous" CSF leaks in some patients. Uncommonly, a dural tear from a spondylotic spur[17,18] or disk herniation[19] may cause CSF leaks.

## CLINICAL MANIFESTATIONS

### Headaches

The most common clinical manifestation is headache. This is often orthostatic (present when the patient is upright and relieved by recumbency), may or may not be throbbing (usually is not), and is typically, but not always, bilateral. It may be frontal, fronto-occipital, or occipital. Sometimes it may be holocephalic or begin as a focal or unilateral headache and evolve into a holocephalic headache if the patient continues to be up and about or in an upright position. The headaches are often aggravated by Valsalva-type maneuvers. At this juncture, it should be emphasized that orthostatic headaches and intracranial hypotension or CSF leaks ought not be considered synonymous: not all orthostatic headaches are due to CSF leaks or intracranial hypotension, and not all headaches in CSF leaks are orthostatic. They may have a variety of different features:

- Orthostatic headaches may be accompanied by posterior neck or intrascapular pain.
- Cervical or intrascapular pain may precede the orthostatic headaches by days or weeks.
- In some patients with chronicity (after months or more), orthostatic headaches may be transferred into chronic lingering headaches.
- Lingering nonorthostatic headaches may precede typical orthostatic headaches by days or weeks.
- Headache may have an acute thunderclap-like onset mimicking a subarachnoid hemorrhage[20] before the orthostatic features become manifest.
- Rarely, a paradoxical postural headache may occur. These headaches are present in recumbency and are relieved in the upright position.
- A second-half-of-the-day headache can sometimes be seen in patients with CSF leaks, presumably in those with slow flow or intermittent leaks. These headaches with clear or not so clear orthostatic features are absent in the morning and usually begin by late morning or early afternoon and increase in severity if the patient continues to be up and about.
- Although headaches of CSF leaks are often aggravated by Valsalva-type maneuvers, sometimes exertional headaches in isolation might be the only type of headache noted in patients with CSF leaks.[21]
- In intermittent CSF leaks, headaches with whatever features they might have may appear and

| Table 14-1   Etiology of Cerebrospinal Fluid Volume Loss |
|---|
| True hypovolemic state (reduced total body water) |
| CSF shunt over drainage |
| CSF leaks |
|    Traumatic |
|       Definite trauma (eg, MVAs, sports injuries) |
|       Lumbar punctures |
|       Epidural catheterization |
|       Spinal or cranial surgeries |
|    Spontaneous |
|       Unknown cause (often) |
|       Weakness of the dural sac |
|          Meningeal diverticula |
|          Abnormalities of connective tissue matrix |

CSF = cerebrospinal fluid.

disappear for variable periods of time.

- Sometimes patients with documented CSF leaks or overdraining CSF shunts and with the typical MRI abnormalities of CSF volume depletion may have no headaches.[22]

## Other Clinical Manifestations

Although headache is the most common clinical manifestation, it is often associated with a variety of other manifestations, which are listed in Table 14–2.[23–37] Sometimes one or more of these may be the dominant clinical picture, and, on rare occasions, they may be the only clinical manifestation and occasionally without the presence of any headaches. In recent years, reports on unusual manifestations of spontaneous CSF leaks have appeared in the literature, and, undoubtedly, more cases will be reported in the future. Subdural hematomas may occur in CSF leaks but much less frequently than subdural collections of CSF. These hematomas are frequently asymptomatic, but, uncommonly, they may be large and symptomatic, causing compression of the underlying brain and shift of the midline.

**Table 14–2**  Clinical Manifestations of Cerebrospinal Fluid Hypovolemia

| |
|---|
| Headache |
| Pain or stiff feeling of neck (sometimes orthostatic) |
| Interscapular pain, less commonly low back pain |
| Nausea with or without emesis (often orthostatic) |
| Horizontal diplopia due to unilateral or bilateral sixth CN palsy[23] |
| Diplopia due to third CN and, rarely, fourth CN palsy or a combination of these or with sixth CN palsy[24–27] |
| Change in hearing (echoed, distant, muffled) |
| Visual blurring |
| Photophobia |
| Upper limb numbness, paresthesias, aches |
| Facial numbness or weakness* |
| Encephalopathy,[28] stupor,[29] coma[30]* |
| Frontotemporal dementia[31]* |
| Parkinsonism, ataxia, bulbar manifestations[32]* |
| Galactorrhea[33]* |
| Meniere's disease–like syndrome[34]* |
| Gait unsteadiness[35]* |
| Upper limb radiculopathy[36]* |
| Trouble with bowel and bladder control[37]* |

CN = cranial nerve.

*Only a single or a few case reports.

## DIAGNOSIS

In CSF leaks, CSF findings show considerable variability, not only in the opening pressures but also in the cell counts[9] and protein concentration[38] (Table 14–3).

### Computed Tomography

Head CT in CSF leaks is often normal and therefore of very limited diagnostic value. Only infrequently may it show subdural fluid collections or increased tentorial contrast enhancement.

### Radioisotope Cisternography

Indium 111 is the radioisotope of choice. It is introduced intrathecally via a lumbar puncture, and its dynamics are followed by sequential scanning at various intervals, up to 24 or even 48 hours. Normally, by 24 hours but often earlier, abundant radioactivity can be detected over the cerebral convexities. Additionally, no activity outside the dura (so-called parathecal activity) is noted, unless, through technical difficulties, some of the radioisotope is injected extrathecally. In CSF leaks. the following may be noted:

- The radioactivity typically does not extend much beyond the basal cisterns; therefore, at 24 or even 48 hours, there is an absence or a paucity of activity over the cerebral convexities.[39–41] This is the most common cisternographic abnormality in CSF leaks.

- The presence of parathecal activity pointing to the level or the approximate site of the leak (Figure 14–1). Although this is a more desirable finding, unfortunately, it is far less commonly noted than a paucity of activity over cerebral convexities.

Of note is that meningeal diverticula, if large enough, may appear as foci of parathecal activity, and sometimes one may not be able to reliably distinguish them from actual sites of CSF leak. CT myelography frequently enables the differentiation, and even if a diverticulum is noted, the test is helpful in determining whether the CSF leak is from the identified diverticulum.

The early appearance of radioactivity in the kidneys and urinary bladder (in less than 4 hours versus 6 to 24 hours) is another fairly common finding. This indicates that intrathecally introduced radioisotope has extravasated and entered the venous system quickly, with subsequent early renal clearance and early appearance in the urinary bladder. This finding should not be misinterpreted as a manifestation of increased CSF absorption[39,40] because the radioisotope hardly reaches the cerebral convexities to be reabsorbed. Inadvertent extradural injections of radioisotope may cause the same finding of early appearance of radioisotope in the kidneys and urinary bladder, often even more quickly than most CSF leaks.

**Table 14–3**   Cerebrospinal Fluid Findings in Low-CSF Volume Headaches

| | |
|---|---|
| Opening pressure | Often low (sometimes atmospheric and unmeasurable, occasionally even negative) <br> Sometimes consistently within limits of normal |
| Color | Often clear <br> Sometimes xanthochromic, occasionally clear in some of the taps and xanthochromic in others in the same patient |
| Protein concentration | Normal or elevated; may be normal in some of the taps and elevated in others in the same patient protein <br> Concentrations of up to 100 mg/dL are not uncommon <br> Protein concentrations as high as 1,000 mg/dL have been recorded[38] |
| Glucose concentration | Never low |
| Leukocyte count | Normal or elevated; a primarily lymphocytic pleocytosis of up to 50 cells/mm² is common, but higher counts are not rare, and pleocytosis as high as 200 cells/mm² has been reported[9] |
| Erythrocyte count | Normal or elevated; difficult and traumatic taps are not uncommon owing to difficulty obtaining fluid in some patients; engorgement of epidural venous plexus is also a factor in obtaining blood-tinged lumbar punctures |
| Cytology and microbiology | Always normal and negative |

CSF = cerebrospinal fluid.

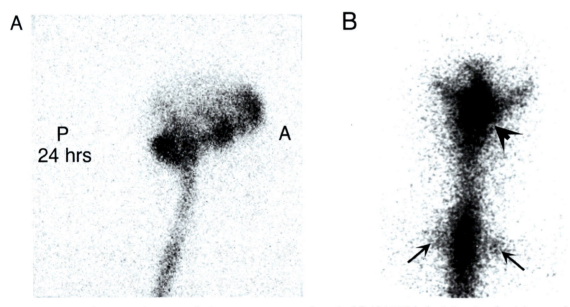

**Figure 14–1**   Indium-111 cisternography in a spontaneous cerebrospinal fluid (CSF) leak. *A*, Paucity of activity over the cerebral convexities at 24 hours. *B*, Arrowhead shows activity in the basal cistern but not beyond. Arrows demonstrate parathecal activity from extrathecal egress of CSF.

## Magnetic Resonance Imaging

Head and spine MRI abnormalities that may occur in CSF leaks and CSF hypovolemia are listed in Table 14–4.

### Head MRI Abnormalities

Diffuse pachymeningeal enhancement (Figure 14–2) without leptomeningeal involvement is the most common head MRI abnormality. The enhancement is typically linear, uninterrupted, nonnodular, bilateral, and both supratentorial and infratentorial. It is often thick and obvious but sometimes quite thin and subtle.[8,9] Descent or "sagging" or "sinking" of the brain is recognized by descent of the cerebellar tonsils (at or below the foramen magnum, sometimes mimicking Chiari malformation type I) (Figure 14–3),[42] a decrease in the size of prepontine and perichiasmatic cisterns, inferior displacement and flattening of the optic chiasm, and crowding of the posterior fossa. Subdural fluid collections may be bilateral or unilateral (Figure 14–4). They are typically noted over the cerebral convexities and are often (but not always) thin and without compression or effacement of the underlying sulci. The subdural fluid collections in this disorder are usually hygromas and if located may reveal variable signal intensity depending on the protein concentration of the fluid. They are, however, sometimes subdural hematomas, but, fortunately uncommonly, the subdural hematomas become large enough to compress and shift the brain or become symptomatic. If they do, quick attention may become necessary. Decreased ventricular size, although sometimes obvious, is often subtle and noted only in retrospect when post- and prerecovery MRIs are compared. Pituitary enlargement may mimic pituitary adenoma or hyperplasia (Figure 14–5).[43] Engorgement of cerebral venous sinuses[44] (Figure 14–6) may be obvious or more subtle, sometimes appreciated only when pre- and postrecovery MRIs are compared.

### Spine MRI Abnormalities

On spine MRI, extra-arachnoid fluid collections[45–47] may be seen. These typically extend to several levels

and, therefore, very uncommonly, may enable us to determine the exact site of the leak. Extravasation and extension of fluid into the paraspinal soft tissues sometimes may be seen. These often occur across fewer levels and sometimes may point to the actual or approximate site of the leak, a very desirable but unfortunately very uncommon finding. Meningeal diverticula may be single or multiple, may vary in size, and may or may not be the actual site of the leak. Spinal pachymeningeal enhancement[48] may be seen, usually, although not exclusively, at the cervical spinal levels. Engorgement of the epidural venous plexus can be seen at any level but more prominently at the mid- and low thoracic and lumbar levels.[47] Although spine MRI can often show the extra-arachnoid or extradural fluid, only occasionally may it reveal the actual site of the CSF leak.[49]

### Myelography and CT Myelography

Using water-soluble contrast myelography but particularly CT myelography can reveal extra-arachnoid fluid that has leaked (often extending across several spinal

---

**Table 14–4**  Magnetic Resonance Imaging Abnormalities in Cerebrospinal Fluid Leaks

Head MRI

  Diffuse pachymeningeal enhancement

  Descent ("sagging" or "sinking") of the brain

    Descent of cerebellar tonsils (may mimic Chiari malformation type I)

    Obliteration of prepontine or perichiasmatic cisterns

    Crowding of the posterior fossa

  Flattening of the optic chiasm

  Enlargement of the pituitary (may mimic pituitary tumor or hyperplasia)

Subdural fluid collections (typically hygromas, infrequently hematomas)

  Engorged cerebral venous sinuses

  Decrease in size of the ventricles ("ventricular collapse")

  Increase in anteroposterior diameter of the brainstem

Spine MRI

  Extra-arachnoid fluid collections (often extending across several levels)

  Extradural extravasation of fluid (extending to paraspinal soft tissues)

  Meningeal diverticula (single or multiple)

  Identification of level (ie, cervical, thoracic, lumbar) of the leak (not uncommonly)

  Identification of the actual site of the leak (very uncommonly)

  Spinal pachymeningeal enhancement

  Engorgement of spinal epidural venous plexus

MRI = magnetic resonance imaging.

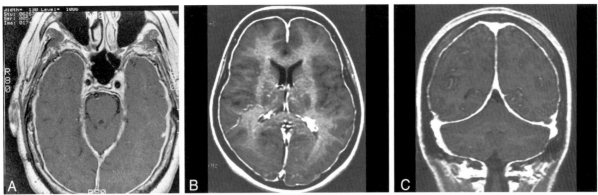

**Figure 14–2**    Gadolinium-enhanced T$_1$-weighted magnetic resonance images in spontaneous cerebrospinal fluid leak. The enhancement is diffuse, uninterrupted, and nonnodular (*A* to *C*); involves both supratentorial and infratentorial meninges (*C*); and is limited to pachymeninges without leptomeningeal involvement (note absence of leptomeningeal enhancement around the brainstem in *A* and absence of any enhancement of leptomeninges in sylvian fissures in *B*).

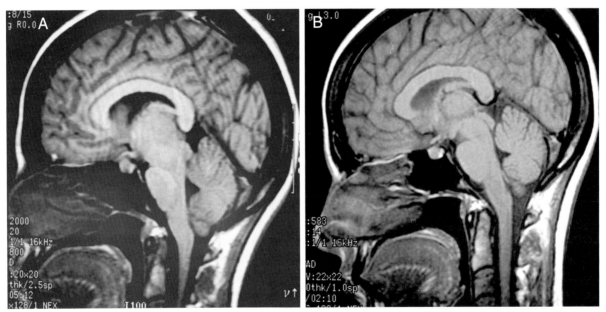

**Figure 14–3**    Unenhanced sagittal magnetic resonance images in a patient with cerebrospinal fluid leak. *A*, Descent of the cerebellar tonsils. *B*, After recovery, this abnormality is reversed.

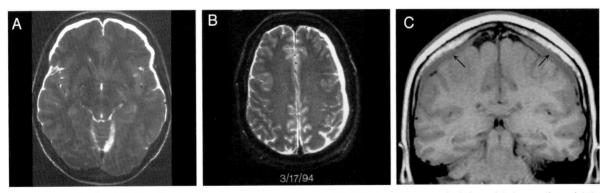

**Figure 14–4**    Subdural fluid collections in spontaneous cerebrospinal fluid leaks. These may be bilateral (*A*) or unilateral (*B*). *C*, Signal intensity may vary depending on the protein concentration or presence of blood products in the subdurally accumulated fluid (*arrows*).

levels), meningeal diverticula, and extradural egress of contrast into the paraspinal tissues. CT myelography is more reliable than other studies for locating the actual site of the leak (Figure 14–7). Because some of the leaks

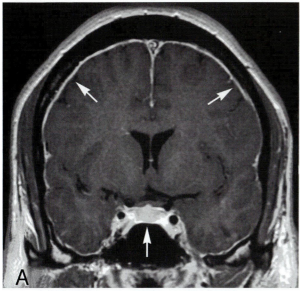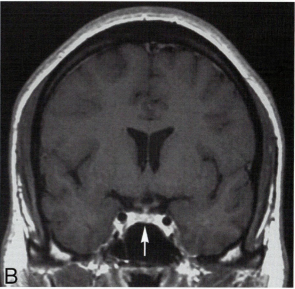

**Figure 14–5** Coronal view T₁-weighted gadolinium-enhanced magnetic resonance image (MRI) at the level of the sella and pituitary gland in a patient with spontaneous cerebrospinal fluid (CSF) leak during the symptomatic phase (*A*) and after clinical recovery (*B*). *A* demonstrates several of the MRI abnormalities seen in CSF leaks, including diffuse pachymeningeal enhancement (*upper arrows*) and enlargement of the pituitary gland (*lower arrow*). Also note flattened optic chiasm above the pituitary and partial obliteration of perichiasmatic cisterns. All of these abnormalities have reversed after cessation of the leak and with clinical recovery (*B*). Additionally, note that in *A*, the lateral ventricles are slightly smaller than in *B*, a manifestation of ventricular collapse in CSF leaks. This may be subtle (as it was in this case), but sometimes it may be quite obvious. Reproduced from Mokri B[61] with the permission of the Mayo Foundation.

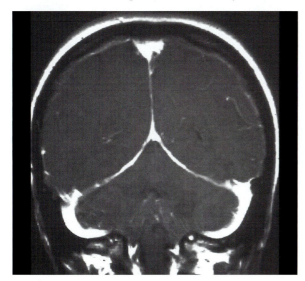

**Figure 14–6** T₁-weighted gadolinium-enhanced magnetic resonance image in a patient with spontaneous cerebrospinal fluid leak. Note engorgement of venous sinuses. Also note the thin pachymeningeal enhancement over the cerebral convexities.

can be rapid (fast flow) or slow (slow flow), each may present special diagnostic challenges.

### Fast- and Slow-Flow CSF Leaks

#### Fast-Flow CSF Leaks

CT myelography is typically done by performing a myelogram with water-soluble contrast, followed by CT scanning. Slices are obtained at each spinal level or at a selected length of the spine (if the myelogram or a previous cisternogram has revealed clues to a more limited length of the spine to be investigated). When the flow of the leak is rapid, by the time the CT is done, so much of the CSF (and therefore of the contrast) has leaked that it spreads across several spinal levels; therefore, it becomes virtually impossible to locate the exact site of the leak. One way to try to overcome this obstacle would be to bypass the myelographic part of the study and proceed with CT scanning right after the intrathecal injection of contrast. Furthermore, a high-speed multidetector spiral CT, which allows obtaining many cuts in a short period of time, is very helpful for this purpose. This technique is referred to as "dynamic CT myelography."[50]

#### Slow-Flow CSF Leaks

Slow-flow leaks create a different type of challenge. When the postmyelogram CT is carried out as the result of the slow flow of the leak, still not enough contrast has leaked to allow detection. Obtaining a delayed CT, perhaps 3 to 4 hours or so after the first one, may enable the detection of the site of the leak. Magnetic resonance myelography (spine MRI after intrathecal injection of gadolinium)[51] may prove to be a useful technique for detection of the site of the slow-flow CSF leaks.

## MECHANISM OF MRI ABNORMALITIES AND CLINICAL MANIFESTATIONS

Loss of CSF volume in compliance with the Monro-Kellie doctrine[52] requires volume compensation. This is

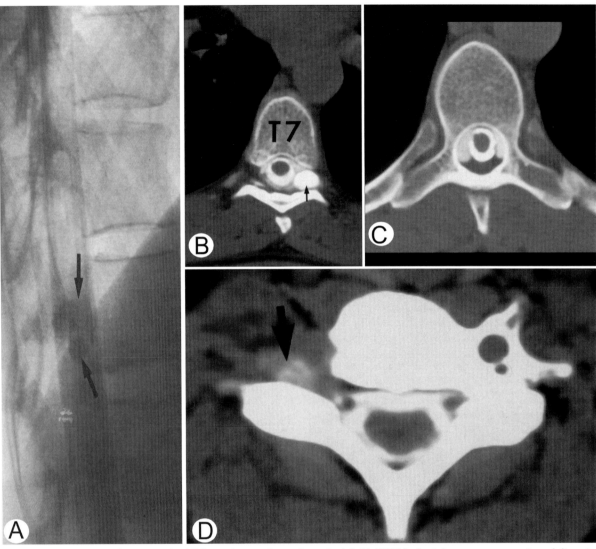

**Figure 14–7**   Computed tomography (CT)-myelogram in cerebrospinal fluid (CSF) leak. *A* demonstrates meningeal diverticulum noted in the initial myelogram (*arrows*). *B*, *C*, and *D* are CT-myelograms. In *B*, a meningeal diverticulum is seen (*arrow*). In *C*, note the extra-arachnoid fluid giving the "dog-ear" appearance in the axial view. In *D*, extradural egress of contrast (and therefore CSF) is noted extending toward the paraspinal soft tissues (*arrow*). Of note is that in the patient who had a fairly large meningeal diverticulum (*B*), the actual site of the leak was found to be at a different level away from the diverticulum (*D*). Reproduced from Mokri B[61] with the permission of the Mayo Foundation.

accommodated by collection of subdural fluids, an increase in intracranial venous blood volume (venous hypervolemia), and relative collapse of the spinal dural sac, resulting in engorgement of the epidural venous plexus. Intracranial venous hypervolemia is reflected by meningeal venous engorgement and therefore pachymeningeal gadolinium enhancement (leptomeninges have blood-brain barriers and therefore do not enhance, whereas pachymeninges lack blood-brain barriers and therefore enhance). Other MRI features that result from intracranial venous hyperemia include dilatation of cerebral venous sinuses and engorgement and enlargement of the pituitary. Histologic examination of the enhanced meninges shows findings confirming that the meningeal enhancement is a secondary phenomenon in reaction to CSF volume and pressure changes.[53]

Another consequence of CSF volume depletion is sinking of the brain and ventricular collapse. The latter results in a decrease in the size of the ventricles, and the former leads to descent of the cerebellar tonsils, crowding of the posterior fossa, and obliteration of some of the basal cisterns, in particular the prepontine and perichiasmatic cisterns, in addition to flattening of the optic chiasm. The major clinical consequence of sagging of the brain is traction on pain-sensitive suspending structures of the brain that leads to orthostatic headaches.[9,10] Similarly, traction on cranial nerves leads to various cranial nerve palsies (third, fourth, fifth, sixth, seventh, and eighth nerves).[23–27] The cochleovestibular manifestations may be related to traction on the eighth cranial nerve or, more plausibly, due to a decrease in the pressure of perilymphatic fluid.[34] Galactorrhea and increased prolactin have been attributed to distortion of the pituitary stalk,[33] frontotemporal dementia to pressure on frontotemporal regions,[31] and obtundation, stupor, and coma to pressure on diencephalic structures.[28–30] Radicular upper limb symptoms are attributed to traction of cervical nerve roots or dilatation of the epidural venous plexus.[36] Gait disorder and incontinence have been attributed to spinal cord venous congestion.[35]

## TREATMENT

When there is a true hypovolemic state, the lost body water should be replaced. Overdraining CSF shunts may require shunt valve replacement or modification. Postsurgical CSF leaks may call for surgical correction. Here I concentrate on management of spontaneous CSF leaks, for which a variety of treatment modalities have been tried (Table 14–5). The effectiveness of caffeine, and more so theophylline, is only marginal and not predictable. The effectiveness of corticosteroids is unproven and mostly anecdotal. Some patients, however, may report temporary improvement. A durable response to a course of steroid therapy would be exceptional. Traditionally, bed rest has been advocated. Given that the majority of patients have significant orthostatic symptoms, they tend to stay mostly recumbent anyway. The effectiveness of hydration or overhydration, yet another traditionally advocated measure, is undetermined, particularly when the patient is not dehydrated. Epidural saline infusion[53] has produced various results. The experience has not been extensive. It could be tried with limited expectations in some of the patients who failed repeated epidural blood patches (EBPs) and when surgery is not an option. Similarly, experience with epidural infusions of colloids such as dextran[54] and intrathecal infusions of fluid[55] is limited. With intrathecal infusions, it is not hard to predict that as long as the infusion continues, patients with CSF hypovolemia may note improvement. However, a lasting improvement after cessation of infusion, although possible, would seem less likely than otherwise. One would be concerned about infections in prolonged epidural and intrathecal infusions.

EBP has emerged as the treatment of choice for those patients who have failed the initial trial of conservative management.[56] EBP has essentially two separate effects. The first is the immediate effect simply related to volume replacement by compression of the dura. The second is the latent effect related to a sealing of the dural defect. The time interval between these two effects varies considerably. Sometimes these two effects may fuse temporally. Many patients with spontaneous CSF leaks may need more than one EBP, and some have

required several EPBs. The efficacy of each EBP is about 30%.[57] A previous failure would not guarantee future failures, and a previous success would not guarantee the success of a future EBP should it become necessary. The efficacy of EBP in post–lumbar puncture headaches is far more impressive in that the first EBP brings relief in about 90% of the patients and a second EBP brings relief in almost all of the remaining cases.[58] Even in inadvertent dural tears related to epidural catheterization, the efficacy of response to EBP is superior to spontaneous CSF leaks. Why does such a discrepancy exist? There are several reasons:

1. In spontaneous CSF leaks, many of the dural defects are in the anterior aspect of the dura or in the nerve root sleeves as opposed to the leaks that occur after lumbar puncture or epidural catheterization, where leak sites are typically in the posterior aspect of the dura.

2. EBPs in post–lumbar puncture headaches are practically always targeted at the exact site of the leak and not distant from it. The site of the leak in spontaneous CSF leaks is mostly at levels above the lumbar spine, where most of the EBPs are given. Therefore, the odds are that many of these will be nontargeted and distant from the site of the leak.

3. In spontaneous CSF leaks, the defect is often not a simple hole or rent but may be a congenitally attenuated zone or patch of dura with or without associated diverticula and with an unsupported arachnoid that has finally given away and is oozing CSF from one or more sites.

**Table 14–5** Treatment of Spontaneous CSF Leaks and CSF Hypovolemia

| |
|---|
| Bed rest |
| Caffeine |
| Theophylline |
| Corticosteroids |
| Abdominal binder |
| Epidural blood patch |
| Continuous epidural saline infusion |
| Epidural infusion of dextran |
| Epidural injection of fibrin glue |
| Intrathecal infusion of fluid |
| Surgical repairs of the leak |
| CSF shunting |

CSF = cerebrospinal fluid.

Some of the patients with spontaneous CSF leaks fail EBPs altogether. Reports on epidural injections of fibrin glue are encouraging,[59] but more experience and more studies are needed.

Surgery in well-selected cases is effective and can be tried when conservative and less invasive approaches (such as EBP) have failed. However, it should be recognized that the findings at surgery may not be entirely straightforward.[60] Sometimes the surgeon may encounter CSF that has leaked but may not be able to locate the exact site of the leak and therefore may proceed to pack the area with blood-soaked Gelfoam or muscle and hope for the best. Sometimes the surgeon may be faced with dural defects with borders that are markedly attenuated and may not yield to suturing. Furthermore, patients may leak from more than one site at different levels. Thorough preoperative studies to identify the actual site of the leak are essential before the actual surgery is undertaken.

## CSF Hypertension after Treatment of CSF Hypotension

Sometimes after treatment of spontaneous CSF leaks or CSF hypovolemia, whether by EBP or by surgery, patients may develop a symptomatic syndrome of intracranial hypertension.[61] This is likely transient (weeks, months) and self-limiting. The results of treatment with acetazolamide have been encouraging.

## Broadening of the Clinical and Imaging Spectrum of CSF Volume Loss

In spontaneous CSF leaks and CSF hypovolemia, unusual presentations have been reported, and, undoubtedly, more will be reported in the future. Overall, however, the disorder represents as one of the following four major categories:

1. *Classic form.* The three elements of headache (typically orthostatic), low CSF pressure, and pachymeningeal gadolinium enhancement are all present.
2. *Normal pressure form.* The typical clinical and imaging findings are present, but the CSF opening pressures are consistently within normal limits.[62]
3. *Normal meninges.* The typical clinical manifestations are present and CSF opening pressures are low, but no meningeal abnormalities are noted on head MRIs.[63]
4. *Acephalgic form.* The typical MRI abnormalities are present and the CSF pressures are low; however, headache is absent.[22]

The above variations point to low CSF volume (CSF hypovolemia) as the independent variable, whereas the clinical manifestations, CSF pressures, and imaging findings are variables depending on the loss of CSF volume. The term "CSF hypovolemia" or "CSF volume depletion" is proposed for this syndrome because the term "intracranial hypotension" no longer appears to be broad enough to embrace all of the variations that have emerged.[18]

## Conclusions

MRI has truly revolutionized the diagnosis, management, and follow-up of patients with spontaneous CSF leaks and CSF hypovolemia. It is now known that SIH nearly always results from spontaneous CSF leaks. Past theories of increased CSF absorption or decreased CSF production have never been substantiated. Low CSF volume, rather than low CSF pressure, is the pathogenetic core of the disorder as the independent variable. A CSF pressure that may be normal for one person may not be normal for another. The overwhelming majority of CSF leaks take place at the level of the spine. Spontaneous CSF leaks at the skull base are quite uncommon. Stigmata of disorders of connective tissue matrix are noted in a sizable minority of the patients. Considerable variability exists in the clinical manifestations, CSF findings, and imaging abnormalities. The terms "CSF hypovolemia," "CSF volume depletion," and "spontaneous CSF leaks" are gradually replacing the term "spontaneous intracranial hypotension," which no longer appears to be adequate to embrace all of the variations that have emerged. The anatomy of spontaneous CSF leaks can be complex. One should not expect to necessarily find a simple hole or rent. EBP is the treatment of choice in patients who have failed an initial trial of conservative measures. However, the results of the EBP in spontaneous CSF leaks are not as dramatic as in post–lumbar puncture headaches. Surgery can be considered in selected cases that have failed trial of less invasive measures. It is essential, however, to locate the sites of the leak before surgery is attempted. Occasionally, after treatment of CSF leaks and intracranial hypotension, whether by EBP or by surgery, symptomatic intracranial hypertension may develop, which is likely self-limiting and transient.

## References

1. Mokri B, Krueger BR, Miller GM, et al. Meningeal gadolinium enhancement in low pressure headaches [abstract]. Ann Neurol 1991;30:294–5.

2. Dillon WP, Fishman RA. Some lessons learned about the diagnosis and treatment of spontaneous intracranial hypotension [editorial[. AJNR Am J Neuroradiol 1998;19:1001–2.

3. Mokri B, Posner JB. Spontaneous intracranial hypotension. The broadening of clinical spectrum of CSF leaks [editorial]. Neurology 2000;55:1771–2.

4. Raskin NH. Lumbar puncture headache: a review. Headache 1990;30:197–200.

5. Schaltenbrand G. Neure Anschauungen zur pathophyiologic der Liquorzirkulation. Zentrabl Neurochir 1938;3:290–300.

6. Schaltenbrand VG. Normal and pathological physiology of the cerebrospinal fluid circulation. Lancet 1953;i:805–8.

7. Marcelis J, Silberstein SD. Spontaneous low cerebrospinal fluid pressure headache. Headache 1990;30:192–6.

8. Pannullo SC, Reich JB, Krol G, et al. MRI changes in intracranial hypotension. Neurology 1993;43:919–26.

9. Mokri B, Piepgras DG, Miller GM. Syndrome of orthostatic headaches and diffuse pachymeningeal gadolinium enhancement. Mayo Clin Proc 1997;72:400–13.

10. Fishman RA, Dillon WP. Dural enhancement and cerebral displacement secondary to intracranial hypotension. Neurology 1993;43:609–11.

11. Mokri B. Spontaneous cerebrospinal fluid leaks: from intracranial hypertension to cerebrospinal fluid hypovolemia—evolution of a concept. Mayo Clin Proc 1999;74:1113–23.

12. Chung SJ, Kim JS, Lee MC. Syndrome of cerebral spinal fluid hypovolemia: clinical and imaging features and outcome. Neurology 2000;55:1321–7.

13. Davenport RJ, Chataway SJ, Warlow CP. Spontaneous intracranial hypotension from a CSF leak in a patient with Marfan's syndrome. J Neurol Neurosurg Psychiatry 1995;59:516–9.

14. Fattori R, Nienaber CA, Descovich B. Importance of dural ectasia in phenotypic assessment of Marfan's syndrome. Lancet 1999;354:910–3.

15. Mokri B, Maher CO, Sencakova D. Spontaneous CSF leaks: underlying disorder of connective tissue. Neurology 2002;58:814–6.

16. Schriver I, Schievink WI, Godfrey M, et al. Spontaneous spinal cerebrospinal fluid leaks and minor skeletal features of Marfan's syndrome: a microfibrillonathy. J Neurosurg 2002;96:483–9.

17. Vishteh AG, Schievink, Baskin JJ, et al. Cervical bony spur presenting with spontaneous intracranial hypotension. Case report. J Neurosurg 1998;89:483–4.

18. Eros EJ, Dodick DW, Nelson KD. Orthostatic headache syndrome with CSF leak secondary to bony pathology of the cervical spine. Cephalalgia 2002;22:439–43.

19. Winter SCA, Martens NF, Amslow P, et al. Spontaneous intracranial hypotensions due to thoracic disc herniation. J Neurosurg 96:343–5.

20. Schievnik WI, Wijdicks EFM, Meyer FB, Sonntag VKH. Spontaneous intracranial hypotension mimicking aneurysmal subarachnoid hemorrhage. Neurosurgery 2001;28:513–7.

21. Mokri B. Spontaneous CSF leaks mimicking benign exertional headaches. Cephalalgia 2002;22:780–3.

22. Mokri B, Atkinson JLD, Piepgras DG. Absent headaches despite CSF volume depletion (intracranial hypotension). Neurology 2000;55:573–5.

23. Horton JC, Fishman RA. Neurovisual findings in the syndrome of spontaneous intracranial hypotension from dural cerebrospinal fluid leak. Ophthalmology 1994;101:244–51.

24. Brady-McCreery K, Spiedel S, Hussein MAW, Coats DK. Spontaneous intracranial hypotension with unique strabismus due to third and fourth cranial neuropathies. Binocul Vis Strabismus Q 2002;17:43–8.

25. Follens I, Evans PA, Tassignon MJ. Combined fourth and sixth cranial nerve palsy after lumbar puncture: a rare complication. Bull Soc Belge Ophtalmol 2001;281:29–33.

26. Warner GT. Spontaneous intracranial hypotension causing a partial third cranial nerve palsy: a novel observation. Cephalalgia 2002;22:822–3.

27. Ferrante E, Savino A, Briuschia A, et al. Transient oculomotor cranial nerve palsy in spontaneous intracranial hypotension. J Neurosurg Sci 1998;42:177–9.

28. Beck CE, Rizk NW, Kiger LT, et al. Intracranial hypotension presenting with severe encephalopathy. Case report. J Neurosurg 1998;89:470–3.

29. Pleasure SJ, Abosch A, Friedman J, et al. Spontaneous intracranial hypotension resulting in stupor caused by diencephalis compression. Neurology 1998;50:1854–7.

30. Evans RW, Mokri B. Spontaneous intracranial hypotension resulting in coma. Headache 2002;24:159–60.

31. Hong M, Shah GV, Adams KM, et al. Spontaneous intracranial hypotension causing reversible frontotemporal dementia. Neurology 2002;58:1285–7.

32. Pakiam AS, Lee C, Lang AE. Intracranial hypotension with parkinsonism, ataxia, and bulbar weakness. Arch Neurol 1999;56:869–72.

33. Yamamoto M, Suehiro T, Nakata H, et al. Primary low cerebrospinal fluid pressure syndrome associated with galactorrhea. Intern Med 1993;32:228–31.

34. Portier F, de Minteguiaga C, Racy E, et al. Spontaneous intracranial hypotension: a rare cause of labyrinthine hydrops. Ann Otol Rhinol Laryngol 2002;111:817–20.

35. Nowak DA, Radiek SO, Zinner J, et al. Broadening of the clinical spectrum: unusual presentation of spontaneous cerebrospinal fluid hypovolemia. Case report. J Neurosurg 2003;98:903–7.

36. Albayram S, Wasserman BA, Yousem DM, Wityk R. Intracranial hypotension as a cause of radiculopathy from cervical epidural venous engorgement. Case report. AJNR Am J Neuroradiol 2002;23:618–21.

37. Schievink WI, Meyer FB, Atkinson JLD, Mokri B. Spontaneous spinal cerebrospinal fluid leaks and intracranial hypotension. J Neurosurg 1999;84:598–605.

38. Mokri B, Parisi JE, Scheithauer BW, et al. Meningeal biopsy in intracranial hypotension: meningeal enhancement on MRI. Neurology 1995;45;1801–4.

39. Molins A, Alvarez J, Sumalla J, et al. Cisternographic pattern of spontaneous liquoral hypotension. Cephalalgia 1990;10:5–65.

40. Weber WE, Heidendahl GA, de Krom MC. Primary intracranial hypotension and abnormal radionuclide cisternography: report of a case and review of the literature. Clin Neurol Neurosurg 1991;93:55–60.

41. Bai J, Yokoyama K, Kinuya S, et al. Radionuclide cisternography in intracranial hypotension syndrome. Ann Nucl Med 2002;16:75–8.

42. Atkinson JDL, Weinshenker BF, Miller GM, et al. Acquired Chiari I malformation secondary to spontaneous spinal cerebrospinal fluid leakage and chronic intracranial hypotension syndrome in seven cases. J Neurosurg 1998;88:237–42.

43. Mokri B, Atkinson JLD. False pituitary tumor in CSF leaks. Neurology 2000;55:573–5.

44. Bakshi R, Mechtler LL, Kamran S, et al. MRI findings in lumbar puncture headache syndrome: abnormal dural-meningeal and dural venous sinus enhancement. Clin Imaging 1999;23:73–6.

45. Rabin BM, Roychowdhury S, Meyer JR, et al. Spontaneous intracranial hypotension: spinal MRI findings. AJNR Am J Neuroradiol 1998;19:1034–9.

46. Chiapparini L, Farina L, D'Incerti L, et al. Spinal radiological findings in nine patients with spontaneous intracranial hypotension. Neuroradiology 2002;44:143–50.

47. Mokri B. Headaches caused by decreased intracranial pressure: diagnosis and management. Curr Opin Neurol 2003;16:319–26.

48. Moayeri NN, Henson JW, Schaefer PW, et al. Spinal dural enhancement on magnetic resonance imaging associated with spontaneous intracranial hypotension. J Neurosurg 1998;88:912–8.

49. Mokri B. Low CSF pressure syndromes. Neurol Clin N Am 2004;22:55–74.

50. Leutmer PH, Mokri B. Dynamic CT myelography: a technique for localizing high-flow spinal cerebrospinal fluid leaks. AJNR Am J Neuroradiol 2003;24:1711–4.

51. Tali ET, Ercan N, Krumina G, et al. Intrathecal gadolinium (gadopentetate dimeglumine). Enhanced magnetic resonance myelography and cisternography. Results of a multicenter study. Invest Radiol 2002;37:152–9.

52. Mokri B. The Monro-Kellie hypothesis. Applications in CSF volume depletion. Neurology 2001;56:1746–8.

53. Gibson BE, Wedel DJ, Faust RJ, et al. Continuous epidural saline infusion for the treatment of low CSF pressure headache. Anesthesiology 1988;48:789–91.

54. Aldrete JA. Persistent post-dural-puncture headache treated with epidural infusion of dextran. Headache 1994;265–7.

55. Binder DK, Dillon WP, Fishman RA, et al. Intrathecal saline infusion in the treatment of obtundation associated with spontaneous intracranial hypotension, technical case report. Neurosurgery 2002;51:830–7.

56. Duffy PJ, Crosby ET. The epidural blood patch. Resolving the controversies. Can J Anaesth 1999;46:878–86.

57. Sencakova D, Mokri B, McClelland RL. The efficacy of epidural blood patch in spontaneous CSF leaks. Neurology 2001;57:1921–3.

58. Vilming ST, Titus F. Low cerebrospinal fluid pressure. In: Olefson J, Tpelt-Hanson P, Welch KMA, editors. The headache. New York: Raven Press; 1993. p. 687–95.

59. Cru JBP, Gerritse BM, Van Dongen RTM, Schoonderwaldt HC. Epidural fibrin glue injection stops persistent post-dural puncture headache. Anesthesiology 1999;91:576–7.

60. Schievink WI, Morreale VM, Atkinson JLD, et al. Surgical treatment of spontaneous spinal cerebrospinal fluid leaks. J Neurosurg 1998;88:243–6.

61. Mokri B. Intracranial hypertension after treatment of spontaneous cerebrospinal fluid leaks. Mayo Clin Proc 2002;77:1241–6.

62. Mokri B, Hunter SF, Atkinson JLD, Piepgras DG. Orthostatic headaches caused by CSF leak but with normal CSF pressures. Neurology 1998;51:786–90.

63. Mokri B, Atkinson JLD, Dodick DW, et al. Absent pachymeningeal gadolinium enhancement on cranial MRI despite symptomatic CSF leak. Neurology 1999;53:402–4.

# CHAPTER 15

# Raised Cerebrospinal Fluid Pressure Headache

Maria E. Santiago, MD, and James J. Corbett, MD

Of the chronic headaches that practitioners encounter in their clinical practice, more than 90% are primary headaches (see Chapter 2, "Epidemiology of Chronic Daily Headache" and Chapter 3, "Diagnostic Evaluation of Chronic Daily Headache"). A small minority of headaches are secondary to organic disease affecting the structures of the head.

Because the brain is not sensitive to pain, headache from raised intracranial pressure (ICP) is most often produced by traction on or displacement of pain-sensitive elements, including the venous sinuses, meningeal coverings, blood vessels, and intracranial portions of the trigeminal, glossopharyngeal, vagus, and upper cervical nerves.

Changes in the cerebrospinal fluid (CSF) pressure, irritation of the meninges, and disease in the blood vessels will likely cause headache. CSF is primarily formed in the choroid plexus at an estimated rate of 0.37 mL/min or 450 to 500 mL/d. The total CSF volume is renewed every 6 to 8 hours and is absorbed at the level of the arachnoid granulations in the lateral lacunae of the venous sinuses and, to a lesser extent, into pacchionian granulations at the nerve root level. This process involves flow down a pressure gradient into the venous sinus and some metabolic activity of the endothelial cell of the arachnoid villi. Venous pressure plays a very important role in CSF absorption. Changes in venous pressure affect the normal pressure gradient and the orderly disposition of CSF from the intracranial space.

The average CSF pressure, when measured in the lateral decubitus position, ranges between 70 and 200 mm of water, with an average of 150 mm $H_2O$ according to Fishman[1]; however, Corbett and Mehta recorded CSF pressures between 200 and 250 mm of water in normal controls, increasing the upper level of normal for normal patients.[2]

Because the adult skull has rigid walls, any increase in intracranial volume will cause increased ICP. Increased CSF production or decreased CSF absorption, increased venous pressure, obstruction to normal CSF circulation, a mass lesion, cerebral edema, or increased bulk or pressure within the dural structures will result in elevated ICP.

Increased ICP is not always associated with headache. There is no clear correlation between the degree of pressure elevation and the intensity of headache.

According to CSF pressure recording studies, the *rate of change* of CSF pressure may be the more critical element. Thus, brief episodes of increased ICP or plateau waves superimposed on a baseline of chronically elevated ICP are frequently associated with headache. This phenomenon may be related to traction on dural structures or distortion of the brainstem during transient episodes of asymmetric compartment pressures.[3,4]

There are many conditions reported in the literature associated with intracranial hypertension. Some of these associations are listed in Table 15–1.

## HEADACHE IN BRAIN TUMOR

Headaches are a feature of the course of illness in between 60 and 70% of patients with intracranial tumors. Infratentorial tumors that are more common in children, with the exception of cerebellopontine angle tumors, frequently have headache as the initial symptom. This is well reported by the pediatric brain tumor literature owing to the greater incidence of posterior fossa tumor in children. Supratentorial tumors are more common in adults and are frequently associated with focal neurologic deficits or seizures. Occasionally, brain tumors of considerable size exist with no symptoms at all.[5]

Frequently, the headaches of increased ICP are associated with nausea, vomiting, or nuchal rigidity. The pain is usually characterized as deep, aching, dull, generalized, and nonthrobbing. It is usually intermittent

**Table 15–1** Intracranial Hypertension Syndromes

Venous hypertension

> Cerebral venous thrombosis
> Superior vena cava syndromes
> Cor pulmonale
> Posterior fossa dural AVMs

Metabolic disorders

> Obesity
> Renal failure
> Diabetes
> Iron deficiency anemia
> Pernicious anemia
> Hypercapnia
> Galactosemia
> Maple syrup urine disease

Endocrinopathies

> Acromegaly
> Pituitary ademonas
> Cushing's disease
> Addison's disease
> Pregnancy, menstrual irregularities, and oral
>   contraceptives
> Hyper- and hypothyroidism
> Hypoparathyroidism and
>   pseudohypoparathyroidism

Head injury

Nutritional disorders

> Hypervitaminosis A
> Vitamin A deficiency

Parainfectious and immunologic conditions

> Guillain-Barré syndrome
> Poliomyelitis
> HIV
> Lyme disease
> Coxsackievirus infections
> Behçet's disease
> Systemic lupus erythematosus

Drugs and toxins

> Anabolic steroids: danazol, stanozolol, testosterone
> Herbicides and pesticides
> Tetracycline and related antibiotics
> Nalidixic acid
> Lithium
> Amiodarone
> Cimetidine
> Growth hormone
> Oxytocin
> Various retinoids

AVM = arteriovenous malformation; HIV = human immunodeficiency virus.

and may not be severe, with a variable response to common over-the-counter analgesic medications. As a rule, both the site and the intensity of the headache vary; therefore, headache has no specific localizing value.

Brain tumor headache is commonly bilateral, but it can occur on one side of the head. When headache is ipsilateral to the tumor and is causing papilledema, headache is of great value, localizing the tumor. In patients with tumor and unilateral headache, 80% had supratentorial tumors and 63% had infratentorial tumors with lateralization of the tumor to the side of the headache.[5–7] Occasionally, brain tumors may present with a migraine-like, recurrent, paroxysmal headache in association with photophobia, phonophobia, nausea, vomiting, and a visual aura.[8] In addition, the headaches are often worse with exertion or Valsalva's maneuvers, such as coughing, sneezing, or straining at stool.

Headaches may occur in the presence of brain tumors even if there is no evidence of increased ICP. There again, traction or compression of pain-sensitive structures such as dural sinuses, circle of Willis blood vessels, or cranial nerves V, VII, IX, and X may cause the headaches. The trigeminal nerve innervates the structures of the anterior and middle cranial fossa, and the pain deriving from disturbances of those structures refers to the bilateral forehead or the ipsilateral forehead or eye.

The glossopharyngeal and vagus nerves supply the undersurface of the tentorium and the transverse, straight, and sigmoid sinuses. The pain that arises from traction on these elements is localized to the occiput and ipsilateral ear. The remaining structures of the posterior fossa are supplied by the upper cervical nerves, and when stimulated, the pain is referred to the occipital and posterior cervical regions.[9]

Postural headache is a common feature of ventricular colloid cysts or other tumors of the third ventricle that may move and obstruct the CSF flow intermittently with postural changes. Although an uncommon disorder, accounting for only up to 2% of all intracranial tumors, the headache of colloid cysts of the third ventricle is classically described as paroxysmal, lasting only a few minutes at a time, both precipitated and relieved by changes in position. The pain is bifrontal or bioccipital and commonly associated with episodic vomiting, impaired consciousness, changes in mentation, encephalopathy, papilledema, gait disturbances, and drop attacks.[10]

Neoplastic meningitis results from the widespread involvement of the leptomeninges by tumor cells. It occurs in approximately 5% of all patients with cancer. Clinical series estimate that meningeal carcinomatosis occurs in 4 to 15% of patients with solid tumors, particularly breast, lung, and gastrointestinal cancers and melanoma; 7 to 15% of patients with lymphomas; 5 to 15% of patients with leukemias; and 1 to 2% of cases of primary brain tumors, especially after intracranial surgery has been performed.

Neoplastic meningitis affects all levels of the central nervous system, the cerebral hemispheres, cranial nerves, and spinal cord and roots, explaining the quite varied clinical presentation. However, headache was recorded in up to one-third of patients, closely followed by mental status change and ataxia as accompanying symptoms. The headache was often diffuse and associated with nausea, vomiting, and focal neurologic dysfunction such as weakness or paresthesias, bilateral hearing loss, and bilateral visual loss.[11]

The single most useful laboratory test in diagnosing neoplastic meningitis is a CSF examination, obtained by lumbar or cervical puncture. CSF cytology positive for malignant cells is the standard method of diagnosis of carcinomatous meningitis. In a study of 90 patients with carcinomatous meningitis, the initial CSF examination was cytology positive in 55% but increased to 80% following a second CSF examination.[12]

Neuroradiographic studies include contrast-enhanced computed tomography (CT) and magnetic resonance imaging (MRI) of the brain and spine. CT is abnormal in 25 to 56% of cases; however, gadolinium-enhanced MRI appears to have greater (1.5- to 2.0-fold) sensitivity and specificity detecting lesions when compared with CT and is the preferred imaging modality.[13]

## HEADACHE IN HYDROCEPHALUS

Hydrocephalus results from obstruction of CSF egress from the ventricular system, decreased absorption from the arachnoid villi, or rarely, excess production of CSF as seen in choroid plexus papillomas in children. Whatever the cause, the excess CSF elevates ICP and enlarges the cerebral ventricles and aqueduct of Sylvius, resulting in the clinical manifestations of hydrocephalus. The clinical presentation varies depending on the age at onset.

If hydrocephalus occurs in infancy, before the closure of the cranial sutures, it commonly results in enlargement of the skull, with associated vomiting, lethargy, and irritability in the case of acute hydrocephalus. If the onset is more insidious, the child may have macrocephaly as a sole manifestation. Assessment of headache in infants and young children is problematic and is generally seen as fussiness, trouble sleeping, and vomiting.

Ventricular obstruction after closure of the sutures leads to increased ICP. Symptoms and signs of increased ICP include headache, vomiting and diplopia, papilledema, and transient visual obscurations.

The headache may be present on awakening. It may be worse with Valsalva's maneuvers, such as coughing, sneezing, or lifting. Pain may be localized to the occipital region with neck stiffness. The headache may also be episodic and have migraine-like features with or without aura.[14]

If the hydrocephalus develops rapidly, owing to a posterior fossa tumor, for example, it can cause a rapidly progressing headache followed by vomiting, impaired consciousness, and neurologic deterioration. Slowly developing hydrocephalus may result in greatly dilated ventricles with little or no headache.

The differential diagnosis of hydrocephalus includes congenital malformations such as aqueductal stenosis, Dandy-Walker syndrome, and Chiari malformations; infectious causes, including tuberculosis, congenital syphilis, toxoplasmosis, and cytomegalovirus; neoplasms; and vascular events, such as subarachnoid hemorrhage.[15]

In communicating hydrocephalus, there is free circulation of CSF between the ventricular system and the spinal and cranial subarachnoid space. Ventricular dilation occurs because there is obstruction within the subarachnoid space over the cerebral hemispheres or around the incisura of the tentorium or impaired CSF absorption at the level of the arachnoid granulations, which is usually seen with subarachnoid hemorrhage and meningitis.

Noncommunicating or obstructive hydrocephalus results from blockage to CSF circulation within the ventricular system, which is commonly associated with congenital defects, such as aqueductal stenosis, intraventricular hemorrhage, or vascular malformations, such as vein of Galen malformation.

Oversecretion of CSF from choroid plexus papillomas produces hydrocephalus in children, typically presenting before the age of 3 years, with enlargement of head circumference. The lateral ventricles in children and the fourth ventricle in adults are the most common sites for this tumor.

During the neonatal period and early childhood period, irritability is the most common symptom of hydrocephalus. The child feeds poorly and may be lethargic. In older children, headache may be present. Vomiting, frequently in the morning, and unilateral or bilateral sixth nerve palsy result from increased pressure.

Papilledema is rarely seen in infancy because the cranial sutures spread in response to increased ICP; however, papilledema is common in older children. Chronic hydrocephalus is associated with optic nerve atrophy, which is seen as a pale optic disk with attenuated arterioles.

In the adult, symptoms of chronic hydrocephalus may also include intellectual impairment, gait difficulty, and urinary incontinence. This triad is usually attributed to normal-pressure hydrocephalus, in which enlarged ventricles are seen on CT or MRI, but lumbar puncture generally reveals a normal CSF pressure. However, patients who have undergone long-term CSF pressure monitoring with this syndrome have intermittently elevated pressures with B waves and plateau waves, especially during the night.[16]

Ventricular size in the neonate can be followed by B-mode ultrasonography at bedside or a CT scan. In the older child and adult, CT and MRI can make the diagnosis of hydrocephalus, revealing the nature and location of the obstruction.

Imaging findings in obstructive hydrocephalus vary with the site and duration of the blockage. The ventricular system enlarges proximal to the obstruction. With elevated intraventricular pressure, CSF passes through across the ependyma into the adjacent white matter. Proton density–weighted MRIs demonstrate periventricular high–signal intensity "finger-like" projections that extend outward from the ventricles.[17,18]

Treatment of hydrocephalus involves shunting CSF from the ventricles to drain fluid into another body cavity. In very young children, a ventriculoatrial shunt is often placed in the right heart. Other common shunting procedures include ventriculoperitoneal and lumboperitoneal (LP) shunts. The complications of shunt operations are subdural hematomas, shunt infections and meningitis, catheter occlusion, and, in the case of LP shunts, acquired Chiari I malformations and cervical syringomyelia.

Shunt malfunction is a complex problem faced by many patients of all ages. Most patients would present with signs and symptoms of increased ICP; however, some patients develop intermittent or chronic headaches as the only manifestation of shunt dysfunction. The headache tends to be bilateral and severe and lasts for days or weeks, presenting in a constant or episodic fashion. It may be accompanied by vomiting or behavioral changes.[19]

Neuro-ophthalmologic complications commonly reported in association with shunt failure include ocular motility abnormalities, nystagmus, and papilledema with secondary visual loss, strabismus, and amblyopia in young children. The acute development of dorsal midbrain syndrome or pretectal pseudobobbing with V-pattern convergence nystagmus should alert the clinician about shunt failure even if there is still no evidence of ventricular enlargement on neuroimaging.[20]

## HEADACHE IN IDIOPATHIC INTRACRANIAL HYPERTENSION

Idiopathic intracranial hypertension (IIH) is a disorder of increased ICP characterized by headache, papilledema, no localizing signs, and normal CSF. Less commonly, IIH may present in the absence of papilledema.[21] IIH affects primarily obese females. The incidence of IIH is 1 in 100,000 general population but increases to 19 in 100,000 obese women of childbearing age. The age at onset ranges from 14 to 60 years, with a mean age of 31 years. There is a predilection for women over men from 8:1 to 4.3:1.[22] IIH may also occur in children, with an equal incidence in boys and girls. There is no racial predilection.

The pathophysiology of IIH is still unclear. Some investigators proposed that increased venous pressure might be the key factor in the development of IIH because it is the unifying mechanism for all of the pseudotumor syndromes; others suggest that increased resistance to absorption of CSF through arachnoid granulations or vitamin A toxicity could be responsible.[23,24]

Headache is the most common symptom of IIH, seen in 94% of patients[25] and 100% of those reported by Weisberg.[26] The headache is usually daily, of variable intensity and gradual onset, although many patients identified this headache as new, different, and their most severe.[27]

The headache can be holocranial or one-sided and is frequently reported as worse with Valsalva's maneuvers, such as coughing or straining. IIH may be associated with nausea but less frequently with vomiting.

Many patients with a history of migraines described this headache as a different one, transformed into a chronic daily headache, unresponsive to recumbence, rest, or over-the-counter medication (Figure 15–1).

In a review of 82 patients with IIH, 68% of patients had a definable headache disorder, including episodic tension-type headache in 30% and migraine without aura in 20%. Patients with IIH frequently have other types of headaches as well, not necessarily related to increased ICP.[28,29]

Associated features include pain on eye movement and radicular pain into the neck and shoulders. The postulated mechanism for this is the stretching of the dural sac of the nerve root sleeves by the increased ICP. Pain and tingling in the legs are also reported (Figure 15–2).[30]

The second most common symptom reported by Guiseffi and colleagues is transient visual obscurations, which are seen in 62% of patients.[25] These obscurations are very short, lasting a few seconds, and consist of transient episodes of dimming or loss of vision, presumably owing to transient ischemia of the swollen optic nerve. These episodes may occur several times a day, unilaterally or bilaterally, and are usually provoked by postural changes.

Intracranial noise or tinnitus was reported in 60% of patients. The noise is described as a pulsatile bruit-like sound or sometimes as a whooshing or buzzing sound.

In 1990, Sismanis and colleagues reported a higher frequency of tinnitus (87%) in 31 patients with IIH.[31]

The tinnitus is believed to result from increased CSF pressure causing compression of venous structures near the ear, such as the transverse and sigmoid sinuses. This results in blood flow turbulence.

Another association is horizontal diplopia. Giuseffi and colleagues reported sixth nerve palsy in 38% cases as a false localizing sign.[25]

Papilledema is an almost constant finding in patients with IIH, although cases without papilledema have been reported (Figure 15–3).[32] This finding seems to be related to individual anatomic variations in the adequacy of the subarachnoid space of the optic nerve sheath (Figure 15–4).

Long-standing papilledema may present as a pale, gliotic, and flat optic nerve head. Optic atrophy was

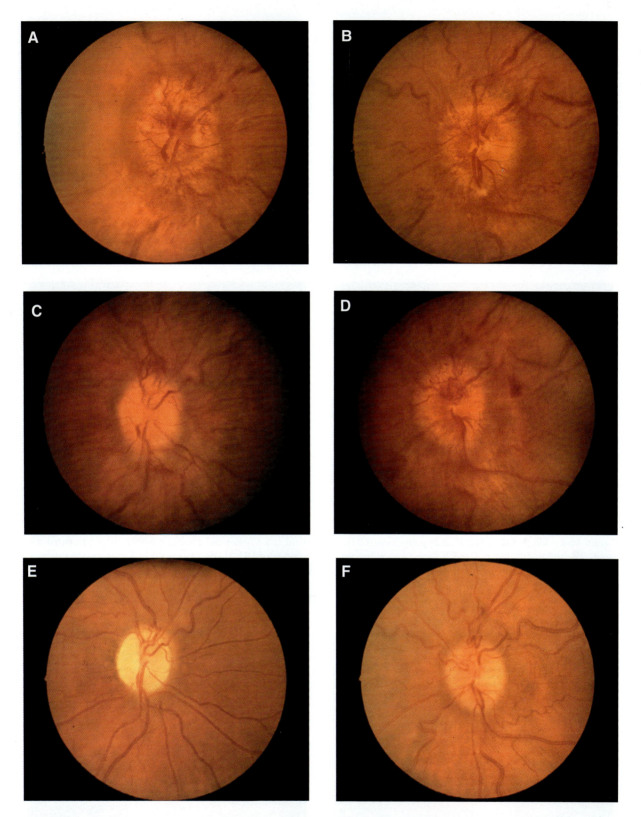

**Figure 15–1**   Papilledema owing to idiopathic intracranial hypertension. A 34-year-old obese female presented with a history of headache and transient visual obscurations in her right eye for the past 4 months. Bilateral disk elevation and an absent cup are noted at the time of diagnosis. Venous dilation and tortuosity are present, as well as obscuration of the retinal vessels as they enter the globe. There are nerve fiber layer infarcts and occasional splinter hemorrhages in *A* and *B*. In *C* and *D*, there is improvement of the papilledema 2 months after treatment with acetazolamide and weight loss. In *E* and *F*, there is complete resolution of papilledema at the 6-month follow-up.

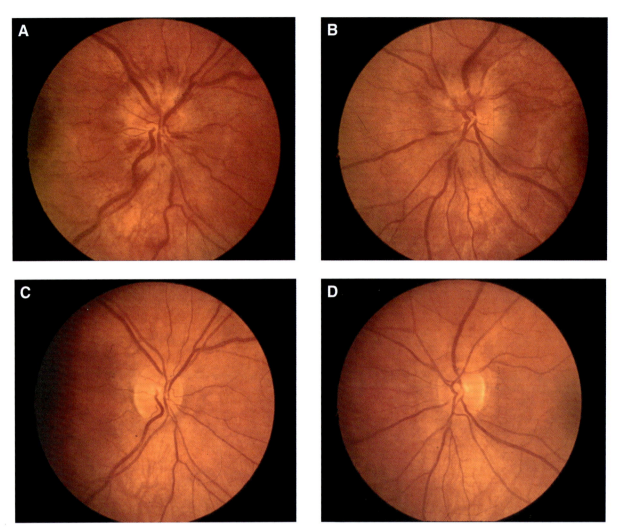

**Figure 15-2**   Idiopathic intracranial hypertension (IIH). The patient is a 27-year-old pregnant woman who presented with headaches and papilledema. *A* and *B* were taken at the time of diagnosis of IIH. *C* and *D* were taken 6 months after delivery. The optic nerves look normal, with complete resolution of papilledema.

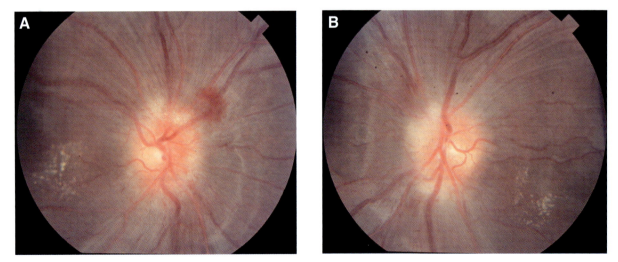

**Figure 15–3**   Papilledema caused by raised intracranial pressure. There is increased diameter of the optic nerve head, with obscuration and elevation of all borders. Obscuration of blood vessels and hemorrhages are also present at the disk.

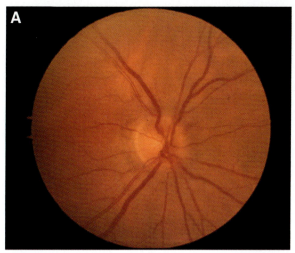
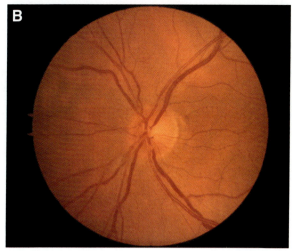

**Figure 15–4** Very early papilledema is seen in this case of idiopathic intracranial hypertension. There is the presence of C-shape blurring of the nasal, superior, and inferior borders of the disk in *A* and *B*. This patient's automated visual field-testing revealed enlarged blind spots. Her visual acuity was 20/20 in both eyes, and her neurologic examination was also normal. Magnetic resonance imaging and magnetic resonance venography of the brain were normal, and a lumbar puncture revealed an opening pressure of 340 mm of water with normal cerebrospinal fluid studies.

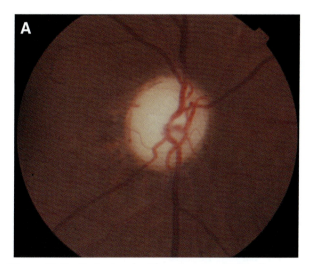
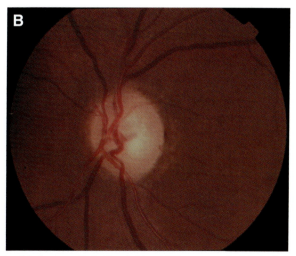

**Figure 15–5** Optic atrophy. There is asymmetric pallor more noticeable temporally in the right eye (A) compared with the left eye (B). The disk margins are sharp.

reported in 7% of patients in Wall and George's series (Figure 15–5).[27]

Visual field abnormalities range from slight blind spot enlargement to severe generalized constriction of the visual fields (Figure 15–6).

Visual acuity remains normal until very late in the course of the disease. In general, the visual loss seen in IIH is a gradual progression into blindness with chronic papilledema; however, some patients may have acute loss of vision. The risk of legal blindness is between 4 and 10%. Systemic hypertension and increased intraocular pressure increase the risk. The combination of the three is deadly to the disk.[33]

Diagnosis of IIH is made based on normal neuroimaging of the brain, including magnetic resonance venography (MRV), documented increased ICP ($> 250$ mm $H_2O$), and a normal CSF examination. The diagnostic criteria of IIH are listed in Table 15–2.

Brain MRI added the benefit over CT of being able to visualize the venous sinuses with a two-dimensional time-of-flight MRV to exclude venous sinus thrombosis. Other MRI findings include enlargement of the subarachnoid space around the anterior optic nerve, flattening of the posterior sclera, an empty sella turcica in 70% of patients, and tortuosity of the optic nerve in 40% of cases (Figure 15–7).

A recent study of 29 patients with IIH using gadolinium-enhanced three-dimensional MRV with an autotriggered elliptic centric-ordered sequence demonstrated variable degrees of cerebral venous stenosis in 90% of cases compared with normal controls. This technique is superior to the time-of-flight method.[34]

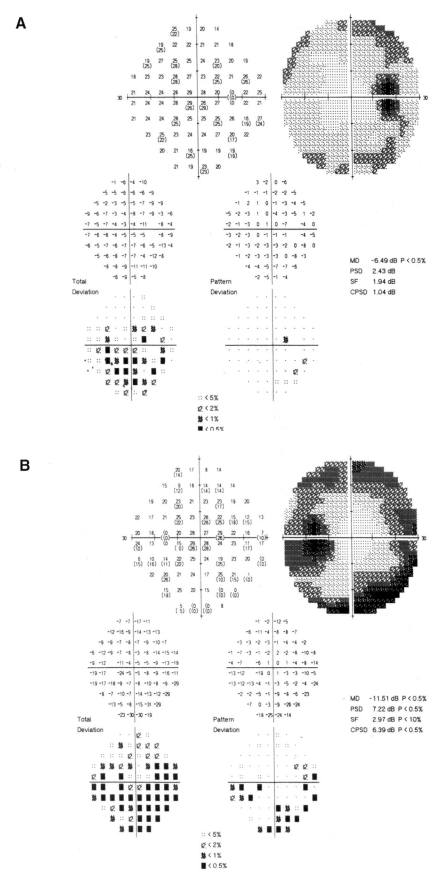

**Figure 15–6**  Visual field abnormalities in idiopathic intracranial hypertension range from blind spot enlargement (A) to severe generalized constriction of peripheral vision (B), as seen in these examples of an automated visual field test.

**Table 15–2** Diagnostic Criteria of Idiopathic Intracranial Hypertension

Increased ICP > 250 mm $H_2O$ measured by lumbar puncture or subarachnoid pressure monitoring

Symptoms and signs of increased ICP with no localizing signs

Normal neuroimaging, including magnetic resonance imaging and magnetic resonance venography

Normal cerebrospinal fluid composition

ICP = intracranial pressure.

A documented elevated CSF opening pressure is essential for a diagnosis of IIH. An opening pressure > 250 mm $H_2O$ in adults is abnormal. The opening pressure must be measured with the patient relaxed, in the lateral decubitus position, with legs extended and the neck in a neutral position at the level of the spine. CSF pressures between 200 and 250 mm are nondiagnostic, and a second lumbar puncture should be performed at another time. Long-term ICP monitoring with a transducer may be necessary if the pressures remain in the indeterminate range or in patients without papilledema.[2,35]

The CSF must have a normal chemical and cytologic composition. The presence of elevated protein, pleocytosis, or hypoglycorrhachia; other conditions, such as sarcoidosis; infections; or neoplasms should be considered (Table 15–3).

Treatment of IIH is divided into medical and surgical therapy. Weight loss is an effective treatment. According to the studies, even a relatively small weight reduction has shown improvement of vision.[36,37]

The initial medical therapy is administration of diuretics, which reduce CSF production. Acetazolamide, in particular, a potent carbonic anhydrase inhibitor, reduces the production of CSF by 50 to 60%. The effective dose of acetazolamide varies from 1 to 4 g/d in two to four divided doses.

Other diuretics, such as furosemide, used alone or in combination with acetazolamide, have been helpful. Doses range from 40 to 160 mg daily.

In patients with impending or severe visual loss despite maximum medical therapy, surgical intervention is indicated. The most commonly used procedures include optic nerve sheath fenestration and ventriculoperitoneal or LP shunts.

Optic nerve sheath fenestration produces a fistula into the orbital tissues with pressure relief to the optic nerve, decreasing papilledema, even in the opposite eye, 50% of the time. Another benefit from this procedure is headache reduction, which is reported in about half of patients.[38–40]

Shunting procedures are also effective in decreasing ICP and preventing further visual loss; however, these procedures are not without complications. Shunt revisions (many times multiple revisions), especially with LP shunts, are needed over time in over 50% of patients.

## HEADACHE IN CEREBRAL VENOUS THROMBOSIS

Cerebral venous thrombosis (CVT) is an uncommon condition being more commonly recognized. CVT is characterized by headache, papilledema, seizures, focal neurologic deficits, coma, and, potentially, death. CVT may affect all age groups but is reported more frequently in young women.[41] Thrombosis of the dural sinuses causes increased venous pressure, which alters the pressure gradient necessary for CSF absorption through the pacchionian granulations, resulting in increased ICP. This process probably begins when a thrombus partially occludes a dural sinus, and then the thrombus progresses, extending into the bridging veins proximal to the obstruction. Once the tributary cortical veins are involved, cortical hemorrhagic venous infarctions occur.[42]

The characteristic results of cerebral venous occlusion are congestion, cerebral swelling, and hemorrhagic infarcts, which are frequently accompanied by frank cerebral and subarachnoid hemorrhage. When occlusion of the superior sagittal sinus and its tributary veins results in hemorrhagic infarcts, the parietal and occipital lobes tend to be the most severely affected. The immediate parasagittal area and the mesial aspect of the cerebral hemispheres are frequently spared, indicating functioning anastomoses with the galenic system.

Thrombosis of the galenic system or internal cerebral venous system results in hemorrhagic infarcts in the thalamus, basal ganglia, corpus callosum, and medial aspects of the occipital lobes.

CVT may cause focal brain lesions or an isolated intracranial hypertension syndrome without focal signs. This seems related to the pattern of dural sinus involvement; the presence of isolated intracranial hypertension is more frequent in patients with more extended thrombosis of the dural sinuses.[43] The most commonly involved is the superior sagittal sinus, followed by the transverse, sigmoid, and cavernous sinuses (Figure 15–8).

The internal cerebral vein thrombosis is rare and clinically devastating because it affects drainage from deep gray matter nuclei, upper midbrain, and adjacent structures. Thrombosis of the galenic system causes a misleading clinical presentation characterized by a depressed level of consciousness without signs of either focal neurologic dysfunction or raised ICP.

Causes of thrombosis include local disease processes, such as sinusitis, mastoiditis, or trauma. Common systemic disorders, such as dehydration, puerperium, pregnancy, malignancy, lupus, sarcoidosis, and inflammatory bowel disease, can cause dural sinus thrombosis. Hypercoagulable states may cause occlu-

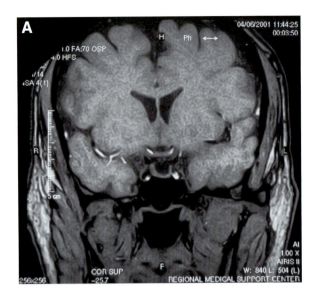

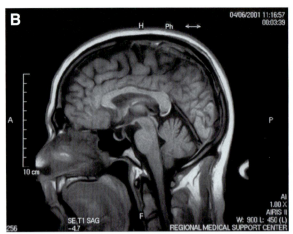

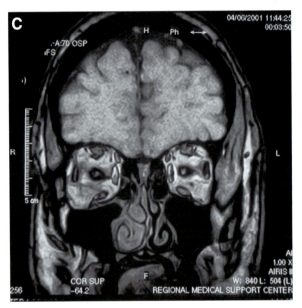

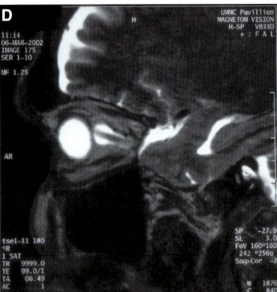

**Figure 15–7** Magnetic resonance imaging (MRI) findings in idiopathic intracranial hypertension. An empty sella turcica is commonly seen in patients with IIH. *A* and *B* demonstrate this finding. The MRI of the brain of this patient is otherwise unremarkable. *C* is a coronal section of MRI of the brain that shows optic nerve sheath dilation. *D* and *E* are T$_2$-weighted MRI sections of the brain that demonstrate flattening of the posterior sclera and enlargement of the subarachnoid space around the optic nerves.

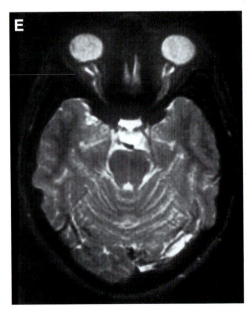

**Table 15–3   Conditions That May Mimic Idiopathic Intracranial Hypertension**

| |
| --- |
| Chronic meningitis |
| Meningeal carcinomatosis |
| Gliomatosis cerebri |
| Arteriovenous malformations |
| Cerebral venous thrombosis |
| Spinal cord tumors |
| Obstructive sleep apnea |
| Sarcoidosis |

sion, as seen in antithrombin III deficiency, anticardiolipin antibodies, protein C and protein S deficiency, mutant Leiden factor V with protein C resistance, and oral contraceptive use.

Mass lesions compressing the venous sinuses, such as meningiomas or metastases from prostate or breast tumors, as well as cerebral vascular malformations, also cause CVT (Table 15–4).

CVT has a wide spectrum of clinical presentations, but headache was the most common complaint (80%) in a series of 150 patients. Headache occurred either in isolation or associated with papilledema (50%); seizures (42%); focal neurologic deficits, such as aphasia; sensory or motor abnormalities (38%); mental sta-

tus changes, including confusion or coma (30%); and multiple cranial nerve palsies (11%).[44]

The headache of CVT has no specific characteristics; it is often diffuse but can be localized to any region of the head and neck. Its severity varies from a slight discomfort to excruciating pain. Headache can be constant or intermittent, associated with nausea or even vomiting, resembling migraine attacks. The duration of

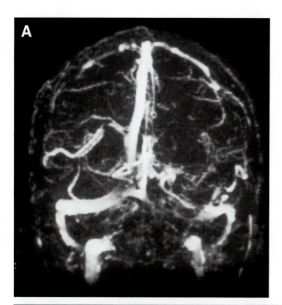

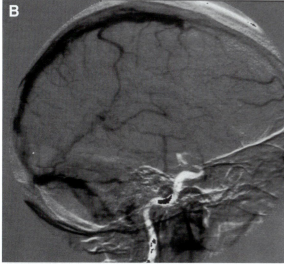

**Figure 15–8** Cerebral venous thrombosis. *A,* Coronal view of a magnetic resonance venogram of the brain in this patient with acute onset of severe headaches and seizures shows an absent lateral sinus on the left side. *B,* Cerebral angiogram of a patient with superior sagittal sinus (SSS) occlusion. Note the intraluminal filling defect in the anterior segment of the SSS.

**Table 15–4**  Cerebral Venous Thrombosis: Associated Conditions

| |
|---|
| Infections |
|        Facial/orbital/paranasal sinuses/middle ear |
| Pregnancy and puerperium |
| Dehydration |
| Congestive heart failure |
| Diabetes mellitus |
| Chronic lung disease |
| Nephrotic syndrome |
| Homocystinuria |
| Inflammatory conditions |
|        Systemic lupus erythematosus |
|        Wegener's granulomatosis |
|        Behçet's disease |
|        Polyarteritis nodosa |
|        Inflammatory bowel disease |
|        Sarcoidosis |
| Hematologic conditions |
|        Iron deficiency anemia |
|        Sickle cell disease and trait |
|        Polycythemia vera |
|        Essential thrombocythemia |
|        Paroxysmal nocturnal hemoglobinuria |
| Coagulation abnormalities |
|        Antiphospholipid syndrome |
|        Protein C and protein S deficiency |
|        Activated protein C resistance |
|        Factor V Leiden mutation |
|        Antithrombin III deficiency |
| Idiopathic |

the pain is variable. Typically, the mode of onset is sub-acute, progressing over 2 days to 1 month.

Bousser and Russell reported four distinctive presentations for CVT[41]:

1. Headache with isolated intracranial hypertension
2. Headache with focal signs
3. Subacute encephalopathy
4. Cavernous sinus thrombosis

The first group had worsening headaches over days to weeks, papilledema, and no focal neurologic signs. This variety resembles IIH or pseudotumor cerebri (Figure 15–9).

The second group of patients presented with headaches and focal neurologic deficits. This association accounts for the majority of published cases. Acute presentations mimic arterial strokes; subacute or chronic CVT may resemble abscesses or tumors.

The third group is a subacute encephalopathy, in which there is a diffuse headache in combination with a depressed level of consciousness seen frequently with deep venous thrombosis. The differential diagnosis includes encephalitis, cerebral vasculitis, and toxic-metabolic encephalopathies.

Cavernous sinus venous thrombosis is a clinically distinct entity with chemosis, proptosis, ophthalmoplegia, and visual loss. Ipsilateral facial pain and loss of V1 sensation are common.

The clinical and radiologic diagnosis of dural sinus thrombosis is sometimes difficult because of its variable, nonspecific presentation. Fortunately, with the widespread use of neuroimaging techniques such as CT and MRI, the diagnosis is made earlier, and the proper and prompt treatment has improved the prognosis.

The diagnosis of dural sinus thrombosis is not always straightforward because the thrombus and flow can produce overlapping intensities on conventional MRIs. Two-dimensional time-of-flight MRV, contrast-enhanced CT, projection venography, and digital subtraction angiography are common techniques in the diagnosis of CVT. Even today, despite its invasiveness, digital subtraction angiography is considered the standard of reference in the diagnosis of CVT, in which a thrombosed sinus appears as an empty channel devoid of contrast and surrounded by dilated collateral draining veins.

CT scans may show a hyperdense thrombus in the thrombosed sinus or vein (cord sign), or in a postcontrast study, the enhancing dura around a thrombosed superior sagittal sinus can be seen as an "empty delta sign" (Figure 15–10).

With two-dimensional time-of-flight MRV, sinus thrombosis is suspected indirectly by the absence of normal flow in a sinus.

Hypoplastic or aplastic sinuses are common variations and are difficult to distinguish from thrombosis; therefore, correlation with $T_1$- and $T_2$-weighted MRIs are essential to confirm a diagnosis of CVT. Another

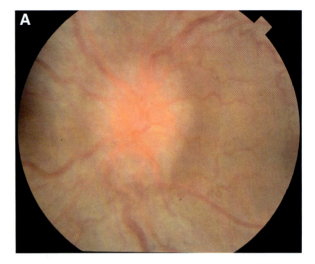

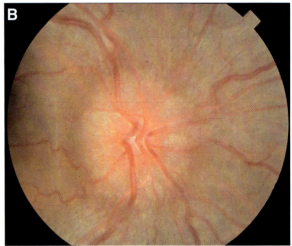

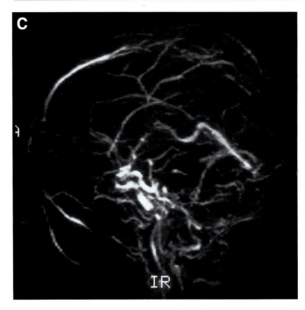

**Figure 15–9** Cerebral venous thrombosis. A 29-year-old postpartum woman with several weeks of moderately severe intermittent headache, nausea, and vomiting. *A* and *B,* Her neurologic examination was unremarkable except for the presence of papilledema. *C,* Magnetic resonance venography of her brain showed superior sagittal sinus occlusion.

common artifact relates to signal loss when there is flow in the same plane or turbulent flow.[45,46]

A new technique, gadolinium-enhanced three-dimensional MRV with an autotriggered elliptic centric-ordered sequence, is used in some institutions and provides improved visibility of venous structures (99%) compared with the time-of-flight MRV technique. One of the advantages of MRV with an autotriggered elliptic centric-ordered sequence is flow insensitivity and higher resolution to detect contrast material in the vessel lumen, allowing the visualization of small vessels.[47]

Anticoagulation with full-dose intravenous heparin remains the first-line treatment for CVT, followed by oral anticoagulation with warfarin.

Management of patients with CVT also includes seizure control and reduction of ICP. In cases of clinical worsening despite adequate anticoagulation, local thrombolysis has been reported to be useful.[48,49]

## HEADACHE IN HYPERTENSION

Numerous studies have tried to establish whether there is a relationship between headache and hypertension over the years. There is still no clear association between blood pressure and headache.

In 1952, Schottstaedt and Sokolow studied 104 patients with malignant hypertension.[50] Visual symptoms and hypertensive retinal changes, including swollen disks, exudates, and different degrees of vascular changes, are present in 90% of cases (Figure 15–11).

Headaches occurred in 85% of patients predominantly in the occipital and frontal areas, frequently throbbing but also reported as dull pain, severe in intensity, and commonly present in the morning. Nonetheless, neither the headache features nor the timing were considered absolutely typical of malignant hypertension. Seizures occurred in 18 patients, and the majority of them were uremic and had elevated ICP when a lumbar puncture was performed.

These findings corroborated earlier studies done by Wolff in 1948 in which he postulated that the headache associated with hypertension was not related in frequency or severity to blood pressure levels but resulted from dilation and distention of the branches of the external carotid artery.[9]

Some authors reported that headaches were common but unrelated to blood pressure levels in large series of target population studies.[51,52] Others concluded in a survey of 11,710 hypertensive patients that headache was, in fact, related to the blood pressure level, which could be reduced by antihypertensive treatment.[53]

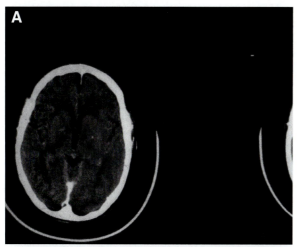
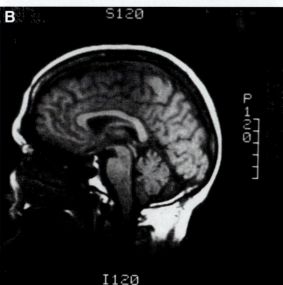

**Figure 15–10** Cerebral venous thrombosis. *A*, Axial view of computed tomographic scans of the brain shows the classic "empty delta" sign of superior sagittal sinus (SSS) thrombosis with enhancing dura around the dural sinus filled with a clot. *B*, Sagittal T1-weighted brain magnetic resonance image of the same patient shows an SSS thrombus isointense with cortex.

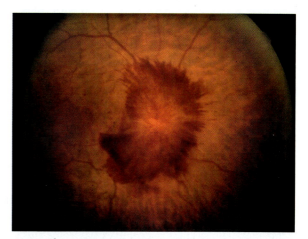

**Figure 15–11** Optic disk swelling and nerve fiber layer hemorrhages in a patient with malignant hypertension. Nerve fiber layer hemorrhages are also called "splinter hemorrhages." They are linear and follow the nerve fiber layer with a flame shape located around the disk and obscuring the blood vessels. There is also a preretinal or subhyaloid hemorrhage with a clear horizontal level. Courtesy of Marcela Hickey.

In 1978, Chester and colleagues compared clinical features and pathologic findings in patients with hypertensive encephalopathy with normal hypertensive patients.[54] The clinicopathologic study of 20 patients with hypertensive encephalopathy showed a history of severe headache and altered consciousness in the majority and both visual disturbances and seizures. Hypertensive retinopathy was present in all patients with malignant hypertension. Optic disk edema was present in 15 patients and did not always correlate with the severity of the headache or the CSF pressure.

In 1977, Hayreh showed that the optic disk swelling in severely hypertensive rhesus monkeys was, in fact, due to ischemia to the optic disk and not to increased ICP.[55] The pathologic findings included diffuse microvascular changes, including fibrinoid necrosis and thrombosis of arterioles affecting all organs, including the brain, eyes, and kidneys. They concluded that clinical manifestations of hypertensive encephalopathy correlated well with the ophthalmologic changes, and cerebral edema was not observed, even in the autopsied brains of patients with increased ICP and optic disk swelling.

Many of the changes seen in the central nervous system of patients with hypertensive encephalopathy or eclampsia are attributable to loss of autoregulation of cerebral perfusion, as seen in malignant hypertension. Autoregulation maintains a constant blood flow during wide variations of blood pressure by varying the degree of vasoconstriction. Autoregulation fails when hypertension is severe, and brain edema may develop. With a decreased vasoreactive response in the posterior circulation, severe hypertensive changes are translated into transudates, hemorrhages, and edema, causing raised ICP from vasogenic edema. In addition to seizures, eclamptic patients may have strokes, psychosis, blindness, aphasia, and coma as neurologic complications.[56]

Brain imaging studies frequently show a pattern of posterior leukoencephalopathy involving the parieto-occipital watershed areas. Common findings included an increased $T_2$-weighted magnetic resonance signal in the gray-white matter junction and deep white matter. Also, the brainstem and cerebellum had foci of increased signal. Petechial cortical hemorrhages and edema were also reported. Most of these changes resolved at follow-up scans.[57]

## HEADACHE AT HIGH ALTITUDE

Acute mountain sickness is a complex syndrome affecting people rapidly ascending to altitudes higher than 2,500 or 3,000 m. It is commonly recognized among unacclimatized mountain climbers and skiers. The symptoms typically develop 6 to 10 hours after the ascent.

Clinical features include headache, gastrointestinal symptoms, fatigue, tachycardia, and tachypnea. In severe cases, acute mountain sickness may progress to acute encephalopathy, manifested by ataxia and a depressed level of consciousness, called high-altitude cerebral edema and high-altitude pulmonary edema.

Other findings of high-altitude cerebral edema may include papilledema, retinal hemorrhages, and sixth cranial nerve palsy; however, global encephalopathy is commonly seen. Seizures are rare.[58]

In a prospective study of 60 patients performed by Silber and colleagues in 2003, 83% of individuals reported at least one episode of headache that would qualify as altitude related according to the International Headache Society criteria.[59,60] The headache characteristics included onset within 24 hours of ascending to altitude above 2,500 m, lasting less than a day and usually bilateral generalized, with a dull pressure-like quality of pain.

Headache was frequently present in the early morning and aggravated by movement, coughing, sneezing, or stooping, suggesting the presence of intracranial hypertension.

High-altitude headache responded well to treatment with several medications, including acetazolamide, acetaminophen, aspirin, codeine and codeine combinations, and other anti-inflammatory drugs, including ibuprofen.[59,61]

According to Hacket and colleagues, patients with high-altitude cerebral edema showed increased $T_2$ signal in MRI of the brain, particularly in the corpus callosum and centrum semiovale.[62] The gray matter remained normal. All patients had complete resolution of the imaging abnormalities, suggesting a reversible pattern of vasogenic edema as a possible mechanism for this condition.

## REFERENCES

1. Fishman RA Cerebrospinal fluid in diseases of the nervous system. Philadelphia: WB Saunders; 1992.

2. Corbett JJ, Mehta MP. Cerebrospinal fluid pressure in normal obese subjects and patients with pseudotumor cerebri. Neurology 1983;33:1386–8.

3. Solomon S, Wisoff H, Thorpy M. Symptoms of vascular headache triggered by intracranial hypertension. Headache 1983;23:307–12.

4. Lundberg N. Continuous recording and control of ventricular fluid pressure in neurosurgical practice. Rapid variations in the ventricular fluid pressure. Acta Psychiatr Neurol 1960;36 Suppl 149:81–177.

5. Kunkle EC, Ray BS, Wolff HG. Studies on headache: the mechanisms and significance of the headache associated with brain tumor. Bull N Y Acad Med 1942;18:400–22.

6. Suwanwela N, Phanthumchinda K, et al. Headache in brain tumor: a cross-sectional study. Headache 1994;34:435–8.

7. Jaeckle KA. Clinical presentations and therapy of nervous system tumors. In: Bradley WG, Daroff RB, Fenichel GM, et al, editors. Neurology in clinical practice. Boston: Butterworth-Heinemann; 1991. p. 1008–30.

8. Schlake HP, Grotemeyer KH, Husstedt IW, et al. "Symptomatic migraine": intracranial lesions mimicking migrainous headache—a report of three cases. Headache 1991;31:661–5.

9. Wolff HG. Headache and other head pain. New York: Oxford University Press; 1948.

10. Nitta M, Symon L. Colloid cysts of the third ventricle. A review of 36 cases. Acta Neurochir 1985;76:99–104.

11. Chamberlain MC. Neoplastic meningitis: a guide to diagnosis and treatment. Curr Opin Neurol 2000;13:641–8.

12. Wasserstrom W, Glass J, Posner J. Diagnosis and treatment of leptomeningeal metastases from solid tumors experience with 90 patients. Cancer 1982;49:759–72.

13. Chamberlain M, Sandy A, Press G. Leptomeningeal metastasis: a comparison of gadolinium-enhanced MR and contrast-enhanced CT of the brain. Neurology 1990;40:435–8.

14. James HE, Nowak TP. Clinical course and diagnosis of migraine headaches in hydrocephalic children. Pediatr Neurosurg 1991;17:310–6.

15. Welch K. The etiology and classification of hydrocephalus in childhood. Z Kinderchir 1980;31:331–5.

16. Abbott R, Epstein FJ, Wisoff JH. Chronic headache associated with a functioning shunt: usefulness of pressure monitoring. Neurosurgery 1991;28:72–7.

17. Kitagaki H, Mori E, Ishii K, et al. CSF spaces in idiopathic normal pressure hydrocephalus: morphology and volumetry. AJNR Am J Neuroradiol 1998;19:1277–84.

18. Suh DY, Gaskill-Shipley M, Nemann MW, et al. Corpus callosal changes associated with hydrocephalus: a report of two cases. Neurosurgery 1997;41:488–94.

19. Baskin JJ, Manwaring KH, Rekate HL. Ventricular shunt removal: the ultimate treatment of the slit ventricle syndrome. J Neurosurg 1998;88:478–84.

20. Corbett JJ. Neuro-ophthalmologic complications of hydrocephalus and shunting procedures. Semin Neurol 1986;6:119–23.

21. Wang SJ, Silberstein SD, Patterson S, et al. Idiopathic intracranial hypertension without papilledema. A case-control study in a headache center. Neurology 1998;51:245–9.

22. Durcan FJ, Corbett JJ, Wall M. The incidence of pseudotumor cerebri. Population studies in Iowa and Louisiana. Arch Neurol 1988;45:875–77.

23. Gideon P, Sorensen PS, Thomsen C, et al. Assessment of CSF dynamics and venous flow in the superior sagittal sinus by MRI in idiopathic intracranial hypertension: a preliminary study. Neuroradiology 1994;36:350–4.

24. Jacobson DM, Wall M, Digre KB, et al. Serum vitamin A concentration is elevated in idiopathic intracranial hypertension. Neurology 1999;53:1114–8.

25. Giuseffi V, Wall M, Siegel PZ, et al. Symptoms and disease associations in idiopathic intracranial hypertension (pseudotumor cerebri): a case control study. Neurology 1991;41:239–44.

26. Weisberg LA. Bening intracranial hypertension. Medicine 1975;54:197–207.

27. Wall M, George D. Idiopathic intracranial hypertension: a prospective study of 50 patients. Brain 1991;114:155–80.

28. Friedman DI, Rausch EA. Headache diagnoses in patients with treated idiopathic intracranial hypertension. Neurology 2002;58:1551–3.

29. Digre KB. Idiopathic intracranial hypertension headache. Curr Pain Headache Rep 2002;6:217–25.

30. Round R, Keane JR. The minor symptoms of increased intracranial pressure: 101 patients with benign intracranial hypertension. Neurology 1988;38:1461–4.

31. Sismanis A, Butts FM, Hughes GB. Objective tinnitus in benign intracranial hypertension: an update. Laryngoscope 1990;100:33–6.

32. Marcelis J, Silberstein SD. Idiopathic intracranial hypertension without papilledema. Arch Neurol 1991;48:392–9.

33. Corbett JJ, Savino PJ, Thompson HS, et al. Visual loss in pseudotumor cerebri: follow up of 57 patients from 5 to 41 years and a profile of 14 patients with permanent severe visual loss. Arch Neurol 1982;39:461–74.

34. Farb RI, Vanek I, Scott JN, et al. Idiopathic intracranial hypertension. The prevalence and morphology of sinovenous stenosis. Neurology 2003;60:1418–24.

35. Johnston PK, Corbett JJ, Maxner CE. Cerebrospinal fluid protein and opening pressure in idiopathic intracranial hypertension (pseudotumor cerebri). Neurology 1991;41:1040–2.

36. Johnson LN, Krohel GB, Madsen RW, et al. The role of weight loss and acetazolamide in the treatment of idiopathic intracranial hypertension (pseudotumor cerebri). Ophthalmology 1998;105:2313–7.

37. Kupersmith MJ, Gamell L, Turbin R, et al. Effect of weight loss on the course of idiopathic intracranial hypertension in women. Neurology 1998;50:1094–8.

38. Corbett JJ, Nerad JA, Tse DT, et al. Results of optic nerve sheath fenestration for pseudotumor cerebri: the lateral orbitotomy approach. Arch Ophthalmol 1988;106:1391–7.

39. Kelman SE, Heaps R, Wolf A, et al. Optic nerve decompression surgery improves visual function in patients with pseudotumor cerebri. Neurosurgery 1992;l30:391–5.

40. Wall M. Idiopathic intracranial hypertension: mechanism of visual loss and disease management. Semin Neurol 2000;20:89–95.

41. Bousser MG, Ross Russell R. Cerebral venous thrombosis. Major problems in neurology. Vol 1. London: WB Saunders; 1997.

42. Fries G, Wallemberg T, Henner T, et al. Occlusion of the pre-superior sagittal sinus, bridging and cortical veins: multistep evolution of sinus-vein thrombosis. J Neurosurg 1992;77:127–33.

43. Bergui M, Bradac GB. Clinical picture of patients with cerebral venous thrombosis and patterns of dural sinus involvement. Cerebrovasc Dis 2003;16:211–6.

44. Bousser MG, Einhaupl K. Cerebral venous thrombosis. In: Olesen J, Tfelt-Hansen P, Welch KMA, editors. The headaches. 2nd ed. Philadelphia: Lippincott, Williams & Wilkins; 2000.

45. Liang L, Korogi Y, Sugahara T, et al. Evaluation of the intracranial dural sinuses with 3D contrast-enhanced MP-RAGE sequence: prospective comparison with 2D-TOF MR venography and digital subtraction angiography. AJNR Am J Neuradiol 2001;22:481–92.

46. Lee SK, ter Brugge KG. Cerebral venous thrombosis in adults: the role of imaging, evaluation and management. Neuroimaging Clin N Am 2003;13:139–52.

47. Farb RI, Scott JN, Willinsky RA, et al. Intracranial venous system: gadolinium-enhanced three-dimensional MR venography with auto-triggered elliptic centric-ordered sequence-initial experience. Radiology 2003;226:203–9.

48. Horowitz M, Purdy P, Unwin H, et al. Treatment of dural sinus thrombosis using elective catheterization and urokinase. Ann Neurol 1995;38:58–67.

49. Biousse V, Tong F, Newman NJ. Cerebral venous thrombosis. Curr Treat Options Neurol 2003;5:409–20.

50. Schottstaedt MF, Sokolow M. The natural history and course of hypertension with papilledema (malignant hypertension). Am Heart J 1952;331–62.

51. Weiss NS. Relation of high blood pressure to headache, epistaxis, and selected other symptoms. N Engl J Med 1972;287:631–3.

52. Waters WE. Headache and blood pressure in the community. BMJ 1971;1:142–3.

53. Cooper WD, Glover DR, Hormbrey JM, et al. Headache and blood pressure: evidence of close relationship. J Hum Hypertens 1989;3:41–4.

54. Chester EM, Agamanolis DP, Banker BQ, et al. Hypertensive encephalopathy: a clinicopathologic study of 20 cases. Neurology 1978;28:928–39.

55. Hayreh SS. Optic disc edema in raised intracranial pressure. VI. Associated visual disturbances and their pathogenesis. Arch Ophthalmol 1977;95:1566–79.

56. Kaplan PW. The neurologic consequences of eclampsia. Neurologist 2001;7:357–63.

57. Digre KB, Varner MW, Osborn AG, et al. Cranial magnetic resonance imaging in severe preeclampsia and eclampsia. Arch Neurol 1993;50:339–406.

58. Hackett PH, Roach RC. High-altitude illness. N Engl J Med 2001;345:107–14.

59. Silber E, Sonnenberg P, Collier DJ, et al. Clinical features of headache at altitude: a prospective study. Neurology 2003;60:1167–71.

60. Headache Classification Committee, International Headache Society. Classification and diagnostic criteria for headaches disorders, cranial neuralgias and facial pain. Cephalalgia 1988;8:1–96.

61. Burtscher M, Likar R, Nachbauer W, et al. Aspirin for prophylaxis against headache at high altitudes: randomized, double blind, placebo controlled trial. BMJ 1998;316:1057–8.

62. Hackett PH, Yarnell PR, Hill R, et al. High altitude cerebral edema evaluated with magnetic resonance imaging. Clinical correlation and pathophysiology. JAMA 1998;280:1920–5.

# Headaches Associated with Head Trauma (Postconcussion Headache)

William B. Young, MD, Joshua B. Khoury, MD, and Nabih M. Ramadan, MD

Post-traumatic headache (PTH) is a new-onset headache that follows a blunt or open injury to the head, neck, or brain.[1] Post-traumatic (or postconcussion) syndrome (PTS) is a constellation of symptoms, including depression, irritability, memory impairment, alcohol intolerance, dizziness or vertigo, attention and concentration difficulties, and loss of libido, that may follow a mild or moderate closed head injury.

Mild head injury (MHI) and minor traumatic brain injury (TBI) are difficult to define compared with moderate or severe injury in which structural damage is evident. The severity of a TBI is defined using scales such as the Glasgow Coma Scale (GCS).[2,3] Accordingly, MHI criteria are (1) a period of unconsciousness lasting less than 20 minutes, (2) a GCS of 14 or greater without subsequent deterioration, and (3) post-traumatic amnesia lasting less than 48 hours.[3] More recently, the American Congress of Rehabilitation Medicine defined minor TBI as "a traumatically induced physiological disruption of brain function" with at least one of the following: (1) less than 30 minutes of loss of consciousness (LOC), (2) any memory loss for events just before or after the accident, (3) any alteration in mental state at the time of the accident, and (4) focal neurologic deficits that may or may not be transient.[4] The American Academy of Neurology practice parameter criteria define concussion as a "trauma-induced alteration in mental status that may or may not involve LOC."

The revised diagnostic criteria of the International Headache Society (IHS) divide PTH along two dimensions: whether there has been moderate or severe head injury versus MHI and whether the headache lasts less than 3 months (acute) or longer.[1]

Whiplash has become an increasingly popular term used to describe flexion, extension, and lateral movements of the neck causing injury without a necessary injury to the head. The most common etiology of whiplash is cervical spine injury during low-velocity, rear-end collisions. The Quebec Task Force on Whiplash Associated Disorders proposed a classification of whiplash disorders on two axes: a clinical-anatomic axis, which has five grades that correspond roughly to severity, and a time axis, on which patients are classified within each grade as those less than 4 days from the time of the injury, those 4 to 21 days from the date of the injury, those from 22 to 45 days, those from 46 to 180 days, and those with durations more than 6 months. The recent IHS classification of headache disorders included chronic headache attributed to whiplash injury if patients present with a history of whiplash associated at the time with neck pain, headache develops within 7 days after whiplash injury. The whiplash-associated headache is defined as chronic if headache persists for more than 3 months after whiplash injury.[1] Ninety-seven percent of patients who seek help from a physician after whiplash have headaches.[5] The symptomatology that follows whiplash is remarkably similar to that experienced by patients following head injury and includes headaches, dizziness, paresthesias, and cognitive and psychological sequelae.

## EPIDEMIOLOGY

Motor vehicle accidents are the most frequent cause of head injury (48%), and men 15 to 24 years old are at highest risk. Other causes of head injury include falls (21%), assaults (12%), and sports injuries (10%).[6] Many motor vehicle accident victims suffer from PTS and have additional somatic and neuropsychological symptoms. Because many patients with MHIs who subsequently develop PTH are never hospitalized, it is difficult to estimate the true burden of the disorder. Patients with MHI, defined as a GCS score of 13 to 15, are hospitalized at a rate of approximately 200 in 100,000 per year,[7] and 30 to 80% develop PTH.[8–12] Conversely, 79 to 90% of patients with postconcussion symptoms also have headache. The incidence of whiplash injury is estimated to be greater than 1 million cases per year.[9,10]

## CLINICAL FEATURES

Symptoms of postconcussion syndrome may develop immediately or be delayed (or not initially recognized) following trauma. Headache (with or without accompanying neck pain) is the cardinal symptom of PTS. Head, neck, and shoulder pain usually begins within 24 to 48 hours of the injury, whereas local occipital tenderness occurs immediately. Neuralgic symptoms can develop in the frontal or occipital region months after the injury. The IHS criteria for PTH require headache onset within 1 week of head injury or of regaining consciousness. However, in clinical practice, it is often difficult to determine when the headache actually started because head pain may be mild and other pains (particularly neck pain) more prominent. Furthermore, patients may develop chronic headaches as long as 24 months after the trauma that are clinically similar to chronic PTH.[10,13] These late-onset headaches (which do not meet the IHS criteria for PTH) are more prevalent than would be expected by chance, and their relationship to the preceding injury is highly controversial and difficult to establish with certainty. Head injury is a risk factor for chronic daily headache, TM, and cluster headache.[14] Some late-onset headaches may be due to a traumatically lowered headache susceptibility that is not manifest until other factors ultimately push the patient over a headache threshold.

Various headache patterns develop after head injury and resemble primary headaches, most notably tension-type headache, which occurs in 85% of patients. The pain is generalized, persistent, bilateral, and mild to moderate[15] and may be exacerbated by very mild physical or mental activity.[16] In one study, headaches were mild in 30% of patients, moderate in 52%, and severe in 18%, and the pain was occipital in 51% of patients, frontal in 44%, and generalized in 11% of patients.[17] Studies have not specified the frequency of headaches, their tempo, or associated symptoms.

Thirty PTH patients were categorized using the 1988 IHS criteria for primary headache disorder. Eight patients' headaches were classified as migraine, 12 as chronic tension-type headache, 2 as analgesic-abuse headache, and 7 as "probable analgesic abuse headache," and 1 was unclassifiable.[18] Couch and colleagues compared 106 patients with post-traumatic chronic daily headache with a similar number of patients with idiopathic chronic daily headache and found no significant differences among 19 headache characteristics.[19]

An otherwise typical migraine with or without aura may be triggered by impact.[20] Alternatively, a pattern of recurring migraine-like headaches may begin some time after a head injury.[8,15,21–23] In one study, 35 patients (27 women and 8 men) had newly acquired migraine with or without aura, beginning within a few days of MHI or whiplash injury.[24] Most patients experienced two or three attacks per week. Amitriptyline or propranolol was dramatically effective in 71% of patients.

Neuralgic pain may occur in the frontal or occipitocervical region and may be associated with other headache types. Several reports indicated that cluster headache–like syndrome may follow head injury,[8,15,25,26] but others found them to be quite rare.[21] These headaches may not undergo remissions.

The symptoms of PTS may be unreported. Only 59% of patients who were hospitalized with head injury complained spontaneously of their headaches; the rest required prompting or direct questioning. At 6 months, only 33% of patients with headache after head injury volunteered this information. Similar percentages of spontaneous complaints of dizziness were noted, whereas the percentages of patients reporting symptoms of depression, anxiety, and irritability were much smaller.[13]

## RARE TYPES OF PTH

Post-traumatic intracranial hypotension and post-traumatic pseudotumor cerebri, with or without papilledema, have been reported.[27] Rarely, dysautonomic cephalalgia occurs following injury to the anterior area of the carotid sheath.[28] This severe, unilateral headache is localized to the frontotemporal area and is associated with ipsilateral pupillary dilation and increased facial sweating.

Temporomandibular joint injury may occur in conjunction with MHI. Symptoms include jaw pain with mastication or prolonged talking, incomplete jaw opening, clicking or lateral movements (which by themselves are not clinically relevant), and pain on palpation of the jaw joint or the muscles of mastication. Many experts believe that actual temporomandibular joint injury at the time of head injury or whiplash injury is rare. Temporomandibular joint dysfunction is thought to be a trigger for headache.

Trauma may also cause a fracture of the styloid process and symptoms that resemble Eagle's syndrome: unilateral pain in the throat or neck or referred pain in the shoulder, chest, tongue, eye, cheek, temporomandibular joint, or ear. The pain is usually dull and continuous, but it may be neuralgic. There may be a foreign body sensation in the throat. Symptoms of carotid artery insufficiency may also occur.[29,30]

## NONHEADACHE SYMPTOMS

Most patients who have PTS have impaired memory and difficulty concentrating.[31] A survey of high school and university students demonstrated that those with self-reported head injury had more cognitive and emotional symptoms than those without such injury.[32] Many PTH patients have difficulty processing different stimuli simultaneously and appear to be absentminded because they must devote full concentration to the task at hand. If the information-processing capacity is overtaxed, the patient will appear to be forgetful.[33] Patients with head injury often seem distracted owing to their inability to disregard irrelevant stimuli.

Other frequently reported symptoms include anger, depression, and personality changes. Irritability, which may be immediate or delayed, is commonly reported after TBI.[34] Constitutional abnormalities include changes in appetite, alterations in sexual drive, weight loss or gain, and menstrual irregularities. Patients may meet the criteria for post-traumatic stress disorder[35] with uncertain frequency.[36,37] Post-traumatic stress disorder often requires aggressive intervention.

Nonspecific dizziness and episodic and positional vertigo are common among patients with PTS.[38] Sleep disturbances, including insomnia and daytime drowsiness, are frequent. Nonrestorative sleep and hypersomnolence are common complaints, with polysomnographic studies showing increased fragmentation of nocturnal sleep.[39] Seizure-like events may occur, although few events appear to be epileptic, and the electroencephalogram (EEG) is usually normal. Nonspecific staring episodes, nonvestibular dizziness, and periodic LOC have been reported. Epilepsy or true syncope is rare. Narcolepsy- or cataplexy-like spells, episodic disorientation, and fugue-like states can occur.[40,41] The attacks are more common when there has been a LOC at the time of the initial injury.[42]

## RISK FACTORS

Age, gender, and certain mechanical factors are risks for a poor outcome after head injury or whiplash injury. Compared with men, women have a 1.9-fold increased risk of PTH[43] and PTS.[44] Increased age is associated with a less rapid and less complete recovery.[13,44–46] In one study, the risk of PTH did not vary with age.[37] Children under 15 years of age may develop acute, but not chronic, PTH.[47]

Mechanical factors may be important. PTH is more likely if the head is inclined or rotated prior to impact. A rear-end collision and an unprepared occupant are other factors that increase the likelihood of PTS.[48]

The relationship between the severity of the injury and that of PTS has not been established conclusively. Several studies have indicated a higher incidence, almost 6:1, of PTHs in patients who suffered only MHIs when compared with those who suffered significant head or neck injuries.[49] In general, the persistence of headache does not correlate with the duration of unconsciousness or the presence of post-traumatic amnesia, skull fracture, EEG abnormalities, or bloody cerebrospinal fluid.[17,38] Two studies, which included patients with moderate and severe head injury, found an inverse relationship between the severity of the injury and the severity of the PTH.[50,51] In another study, initially hospitalized MHI patients had symptoms similar to those who were discharged from the emergency room, but hospitalized patients recovered more quickly.[52]

On the other hand, one study indicated that LOC is predictive of depression and anger-control problems.[42] Also, diplopia, anosmia, and the presence of central nervous system abnormality at 24 hours correlated with persistence of symptoms 6 weeks after injury.[53] High multiple-symptom scores shortly after whiplash injury have a significantly greater chance of persistent symptoms 2 years after the injury.[54] Perhaps individual vulnerability is as important as the severity of injury in determining whether an individual develops PTH or postwhiplash symptoms. The nature of this vulnerability (if it exists) remains elusive.

A history of prior headache could increase the risk of PTH. In one study, pretraumatic migraine was not a risk factor for developing PTH after hospitalization for cerebral concussion.[37] This study suffered from recall bias because the patients were interviewed 9 to 12 months after the injury. Several studies are not in accord with this finding. In another study, 31% of patients who developed migraine-like attacks following mild head or neck trauma had a history of migraine in first-degree relatives, and the authors suggested that head or neck trauma triggers the migraine process in susceptible individuals.[24] When patients were interviewed immediately following whiplash injury, pretraumatic headache was a significant risk factor for developing PTH.[54]

A lack of education may not be a risk factor for acute PTS, but unskilled laborers are more likely to develop symptoms.[38] Likewise, socioeconomic status may predict employment 3 months after MHI. Business managers and executives and persons with a higher education were all employed 3 months after injury, but only 57% of the unskilled laborers were still employed.[31] These studies do not differentiate between the premorbid effect of a lack of education, poor motivation to return to a menial job, poor resources to adjust to the effects of the injury, or employer intolerance.[31]

In one study, patients were assessed for premorbid psychopathology by interviewing the patients and their relatives within 1 month of head injury. The patient's psychological state prior to the injury correlated with the subjective symptomatology. However, physical and social dysfunction correlated with the severity of the injury, not with preexisting factors.[47] Another study showed that patients with pretraumatic emotional problems had higher scores on scales of cognitive and emotional-vegetative dysfunction after MHI, but disability was not measured.[45] These studies might suggest that preexisting psychopathology influences symptoms presentation. However, some symptoms are reported rather than impacting on disability.

Three studies do not support these conclusions. One found no difference in premorbid personality adjustment between chronic PTS sufferers and patients whose symptoms resolved.[46] Another found no differences in pretraumatic neuroticism or adjustment to work between similarly injured patients who developed PTS and those who did not.[38] A third found no differences between premorbid social adjustment, life events, and chronicity of symptoms.[44] In a study assessing subjects shortly after whiplash injury, scores on the nervousness, depression, openness, neuroticism, and masculinity scales did not correlate with outcome 2 years after injury. In contrast, poor well-being scale scores correlated with the persistence of symptoms, but not with disability, among patients who were symptomatic 2 years after injury.[55]

Disparities in the above-described studies could be due to differences in studied cohorts. Alternatively, methodologic problems might have led to erroneous results. For example, some pathologic assessments were retrospective, and the methods used to ascertain preexisting psychopathology were often not well described.

## PATHOPHYSIOLOGY

PTS is probably not a single pathologic entity but a group of traumatically induced disorders with overlapping symptoms. The cognitive, sleep, and psychological deficits of these patients are manifestations of brain injury. Headache is mainly a manifestation of brain dysfunction, with occasional contributions from persistent musculoskeletal injuries.

Neck, jaw, and scalp tissue injuries may contribute to acute PTH; pain originating from these areas can be referred to the head. Most of these injuries heal completely and cannot, by themselves, account for chronic PTH or the associated neurocognitive symptoms of PTH. However, soft tissue or skeletal injuries may initiate or trigger a transformation process in headache-prone patients similar to the process by which daily intermittent migraine or tension-type headache evolves into chronic daily headache. Postconcussion headache patients have more upper cervical segment joint dysfunction, less endurance of the neck flexor muscle, and a higher incidence of moderately tight neck musculature, yet the neck range of motion is normal.[56] These findings could be due to adaptive, and sometimes maladaptive, phenotypic central nervous system changes similar to the phenomenon of central sensitization that is observed in experimental models of chronic pain. One model, based on the kindling phenomenon in experimental epilepsy, could explain the evolution of peripheral injuries into chronic centrally maintained pain.[57] Nerve or musculoskeletal injuries could induce windup and sensitization, which could ultimately result in permanently altered neuronal function. Because these changes occur post- and presynaptically, neuronal function may be altered at distant brain sites involved in the production or experience of pain.[57]

Head injury usually involves a combination of translational and rotational forces. In studies using windows in cadaver skulls, the brain has been demonstrated to lag behind the skull, owing to inertia, when the head is accelerated. Restricted rotation makes it more difficult to produce a concussion in animals.[58] Rotational forces occur even when movement is primarily translational, which can cause shearing and diffuse axonal injury, which is observed histologically. As a result of translational forces, the brain is compressed near the point of impact while negative pressures develop opposite to the site of impact. Animal models using fluid percussion emphasize this kind of injury and demonstrate loss of cholinergic forebrain neurons but little brainstem injury.[59–61] The relative contribution of shear, compression, and stretching remains a subject of debate. In experimental models and computational models,[58,62,63] direct impact is not necessary to produce significant diffuse axonal injury.[64]

Diffuse axonal injury is most common in the corpus callosum, internal capsule, fornices, dorsolateral midbrain, and pons.[65] Gennarelli and colleagues suggested that there is a continuum of diffuse axonal injury that varies from functional abnormalities alone to structural lesions that become increasingly severe and result in widespread injury.[66] Immunohistochemical studies demonstrate similar, although less severe, histologic findings in the rat fluid percussion model in MHI compared with moderate head injury.[67] The relevance and extent of diffuse axonal injury in human MHI are not fully elucidated, but it can occur.[68]

Because of unsynchronized rotations that may develop between the cerebral hemispheres and the cerebellum,[58] axons in the upper brainstem may be particularly vulnerable to shear and thus to diffuse axonal injury and could affect arousal, vigilance, sleep, and pain modulation.[69] Reactive synaptogenesis, a process of axonal sprouting that restores synaptic contact on denuded dendrites, has been demonstrated in at least one model of head injury.[70] Although not yet demonstrated in human head injury, this could account for both physiologic improvement through appropriate healing and new or worsening symptoms as aberrant connections are made.

Ischemic brain injury is common following severe head injury.[71] Post-traumatic vasospasm, which can occur in moderate or severe head injury, correlates with a lower GCS.[72] Abnormal cerebrovascular autoregulation may also occur.[73] Forty-eight hours after MHI, 28% of patients and none of the controls had poorly functioning or absent autoregulation. There was no correlation with the GCS score.[73] Because long-term clinical outcomes were not studied, the role of this observation in chronic PTH or PTS is unknown.

A series of neurochemical changes might occur with head injury, including a shift of electrolytes between intra- and extracellular compartments and the release of excitatory neurotransmitters.[74] The relevance of these alternatives to human head injury and the role of such changes in the evolution of PTS are unknown. However, an altered chemical or electrical environment could account for immediate impact headache or aura. It could result in cellular injury and in PTS. The similarity between the biochemical changes of migraine headaches and those that are seen after head injury suggest a shared physiology and possibly a role for similar treatment strategies.[75]

Over a more prolonged time frame, the effectiveness of treatments such as repetitive intravenous dihydroergotamine (and amitriptyline) in PTH suggests a similar or shared mechanism with the primary headache disorders. This could be due to a "final common pathway" of symptom expression, perhaps with central serotoninergic dysfunction and trigeminovascular activation.[76,77] PTH may be due to a disinhibition or "release phenomenon" of modules that are involved in producing primary headaches but have been inactive prior to the head injury.[78]

Many authors uphold the "psychogenesis" of chronic PTH and PTS, but few point out specific mechanisms to account for it. Some authors used a "path analysis," a directional multiple regression analysis, to examine the relationship between post-traumatic pain, disability, depression, and anger, concluding that depression might cause disability and that expressed and unexpressed anger contribute to depression.[79] However, other explanations for the correlation between depression and disability could be equally valid. Other authors suggest that nonvalidation of cognitive and physically painful symptoms by medical, legal, and employment authorities leads to an anxious or depressive reaction that results in the persistence of originally organic symptoms.[16]

It is likely that there are at least two processes occurring in patients with PTH or PTS. The first process is likely due to diffuse axonal injury and correlates with the acceleration and deceleration forces. When more severe, it is associated with abnormalities on magnetic resonance imaging (MRI), positron emission tomography (PET), single-photon emission computed tomography (SPECT), and certain neuropsychological tests. A challenge to this hypothesis is the observation that patients with severe closed head injury do not report as many symptoms as those with less severe injuries. It could be argued, however, that symptoms of PTS and PTH are masked only by coexisting illnesses and the sequelae of severe head injury. Clinical improvement of diffuse axonal injury, like PTH, may occur over several months,

with normalization or amelioration of the radiologic tests. Also, neuropsychological testing may indicate full recovery, but tests for attention may still be abnormal.

A second process may be responsible for many of the symptoms that persist after MHI. A preexisting vulnerability may be necessary for the chronic post-traumatic symptoms to manifest because preexisting headache is a risk factor in some. A mechanism similar to the kindling model of epilepsy[57] or, perhaps, aberrant connections made by injured axons may underlie this mechanism and explain most of the symptoms of chronic PTS and PTH. Additional factors, perhaps psychological ones, may magnify the expression of symptoms caused by this second process.

For most patients with PTS, the clinical history of new-onset or changed headache after an injury associated with new cognitive, emotional, and sleep disturbances is so characteristic that, once intracranial pathology is excluded, confirmatory tests are not required to proceed with treatment. Unfortunately, tests are often conducted for medicolegal reasons, which increases patients' anxiety and self-doubt when they are negative. Negative test results are often used to indicate no abnormality. However, no test has the specificity or sensitivity to make or exclude a diagnosis in a particular individual. Similarly, if PTS is not a single entity but a syndrome derived from several pathologic processes initiated by head trauma, no single test would be expected to diagnose all patients.

## TESTING

Although many studies have been performed in an attempt to establish the extent of head injury and the diagnosis of PTS, there is no test that reliably distinguishes patients with PTS from normal controls or from patients with primary headache disorders.

### Computed Tomography and MRI

Few studies specifically evaluated brain imaging in PTS. Most series included patients with head injury who might have required neurosurgical intervention. One study found no MRI abnormalities among the subgroup of head injury patients with PTS.[80] On the other hand, another found MRI abnormalities within several weeks of injury in 17 of 20 hospitalized patients with mild or moderate head injury.[81] In this study, MRI was clearly superior to computed tomography (CT) in identifying these abnormalities. Mean parenchymal lesion size decreased or resolved with the passage of time.[81,82] Most of the resolutions occurred within the first month, and lesions that were present at 1 month remained at 3 months. Patients who had an abnormal MRI had more cognitive deficits than did those with normal studies. Although speculative in the absence of pathologic confirmation, these lesions may represent diffuse axonal injury with resolving edema. In another study of MRI of 20 consecutively hospitalized head injury patients, two blinded readers concurred that diffuse axonal injury was present in 30% of patients.[83]

There are no prospective studies that establish the value of brain imaging in patients with PTH or PTS. In the acute setting, it is prudent to image all patients with mild behavioral abnormalities, abnormal findings on clinical examination, or a GCS score of less than 15 because of the risk of subsequent deterioration. With subacute or chronic PTS, there is little information to guide the clinician. Neuroimaging should be guided by findings on clinical examination, medical history, and symptom evolution.

### Functional Imaging

SPECT has not been used specifically in PTH or PTS. In the acute phase of head injury, technetium 99m hexamethylpropyleneamineoxine SPECT may be more useful than CT in identifying brain lesions that CT cannot, in demonstrating abnormalities of function, and in predicting outcome.[84–86] Also, one study showed that the number of lesions on SPECT correlated with the extent of disability.[87] These studies involved relatively small numbers of subjects. The Academy of Neurology's Therapeutics and Technology Assessment Subcommittee determined the use of SPECT for the evaluation of head trauma to be "investigational" based on class II evidence (one or more well-designed clinical studies).[88] Abnormal sites on SPECT studies include the basal ganglia and thalamus in 55.2% of patients, the frontal lobes in 23.8%, the temporal lobes in 13%, the parietal lobes in 3.7%, and the insular and occipital regions together in 4.8%.[89] A more recent study has shown significant orbitofrontal hypoperfusion in 67% of patients with post-traumatic anosmia.[90]

Studies using xenon-inhalation cerebral blood flow (CBF) have suggested a correlation between regional blood flow asymmetries and headache disability.[91] Also, the same investigators reported that patients with chronic PTH have lower mean initial slope indices, significant regional interhemispheric flow differences, and more interhemispheric asymmetries compared with migraineurs and nonheadache controls.[92] The authors concluded that the xenon-inhalation CBF findings are indicators of neurovascular instability that persists months to years after the initial head injury.

Like SPECT, PET examines physiologic activity within the brain. In head trauma, PET has revealed widespread abnormalities in cerebral glucose metabolism[93,94] and areas of diminished perfusion that tend to improve with clinical recovery.[94] In one study, these areas of perfusion abnormality corresponded to the areas of abnormality that had been identified by neuropsychological testing.[95]

One month after head injury, patients with minor TBI and control subjects showed different functional MRI brain activation patterns in response to increasing working memory processing loads. Patients with minor TBI had significantly more cognitive symptoms but performed as well as controls on a neuropsychological battery, differing only in response speed, sample reaction time, and distractibility tasks of the continuous performance test. The presence of headache was not commented on.[96]

### Electroencephalography

EEG is usually of little value in evaluating PTS in patients with head injury. Although it may be abnormal immediately after injury, it generally normalizes within minutes to weeks.[97]

Quantitative EEG may or may not be useful in head injury. In one small study, quantitative EEG showed a statistically significant increase in both slow and fast activity over the temporal region of the skull.[98] However, the authors concluded that this test offers little benefit to the patient with PTH because of variability within the PTH group, and similar findings are common in some control patients. Another study examined the ability of power spectrum analysis to discriminate between 608 head injury patients and 108 age-matched controls and found that head injury could be discriminated from age-matched controls with more than 90% accuracy without correlating the symptoms of PTH or PTS to abnormal test results.[99] Therefore, the predictive value of this study is uncertain at this time. In general, these studies indicate that PTH patients, as a group, differ from nonheadache controls, but unlike the xenon CBF,[92] they cannot reliably differentiate an individual PTH patient from a patient with an idiopathic headache.

### Magnetic Source Imaging

Magnetic source imaging combines MRI and magnetoencephalography. One study showed abnormalities in 5% of a normal control group, 10% of an asymptomatic MHI group, and 65% of a group of patients with persistent symptoms ($p < .01$).[100] These abnormal findings improve as the patient improves. Like the xenon CBF studies,[101] this study demonstrates an organic abnormality in patients with postconcussion syndrome.

### Evoked Potentials and Electronystagmography

Short-latency somatosensory evoked potentials have not been shown to be of value in testing patients with head injury or PTS.[102] On the other hand, brainstem auditory evoked potentials (BAEPs) were abnormal in 10 to 20% of patients with head injury and postconcussion syndrome, correlating with the duration of unconsciousness.[97] BAEP does not correlate with symptomatic dizziness and can either improve or deteriorate from 2 days to 1 month after injury.[103] Like quantitative EEG, BAEP does not differentiate between patients with head injury and PTS and those with injury but without PTS.

The electronystagmogram (ENG) is abnormal in 40 to 50% of patients with head injury or "whiplash" in clinic-based studies. Toglia examined 150 patients who complained of vestibular symptoms following either head injury or whiplash injury and reported abnormal caloric tests (including both canal paresis and directional preponderance) in 63% of those with whiplash injury and 68% of head injury patients.[104] Another study of 19 patients with postconcussion dizziness following head injury found that 11 patients (58%) had abnormalities consisting of latent or positional nystagmus or caloric-induced nystagmus.[105] The study found that in patients with dizziness an ENG more likely detects brainstem pathway abnormalities than BAEP.[105] More recently, ENG abnormalities were found in patients with whiplash injury and MHI, but not in whiplash injury alone, although the symptoms of dizziness were similar in both groups.[106] In the same study, computerized dynamic posturography was abnormal in dizzy patients after whiplash injury, whether or not it was accompanied by MHI.[106]

Studies of P300, an event-related potential correlated with cognitive functions, such as memory information delivery and decision-making, have yielded mixed results in head injury patients. One study demonstrated significant abnormalities of P300 amplitude and latency in 20 head injury patients compared with 20 control subjects,[107] whereas another found an abnormal response in only 1 of 18 patients.[108] A third study found a correlation between an abnormal P300 and an abnormal MRI.[109] Yet another study demonstrated that hearing accident-related words (ie, "stressful") produced a significantly larger P300 than hearing neutral words in patients with MHI but not in nonhead injury controls. These amplitude differences correlated with the patient's state anxiety scores.[110]

Brainstem-mediated antinociceptive inhibitory reflexes of the temporalis muscle were investigated in 82 patients with acute PTH following whiplash injury but without neurologic deficits or skeletal injury. Highly significant reflex alterations were found in patients with PTH.[111] These findings were believed to be due to transient dysfunction of the brainstem-mediated reflex circuit pointing to an altered central pain control as a cause of the PTH.

## Blood Testing: S-100

The S-100B protein is a small dimeric cytosolic protein initially felt to be nervous system specific in glial and schwann cells and was recently studied extensively as a marker of brain injury in head trauma patients. In hospitalized MHI patients, S-100 was detectable in 28% of patients, 36% of whom had MRI signs of contusions.[112] In patients with detectable S-100 levels, there was a trend toward impaired neuropsychological functioning on measures of attention, memory, and information processing speed.[112] More recently, the question of tissue specificity was raised for the S-100B marker, finding increased titers in trauma patients without head injuries, suggesting non-neural sources.[113]

## Neuropsychological Testing

Neuropsychological testing in head injury often shows marked early abnormalities that improve or resolve with time. These include information processing, auditory vigilance, reaction time, sustained divided and distributed attention, visual and verbal memory, design fluency, imagination, and analytic capacity. Tests of design fluency and verbal memory may improve and normalize over 1 to 3 months in parallel with MRI findings.[114]

The paced auditory serial addition test is a widely used test of information processing that is often abnormal shortly after head injury. Patients are presented with a random series of digits at intervals of either 1 to 2 or 2 to 4 seconds (the same interval for the entire test) and are asked to add the most recently presented number to the one before. The score is expressed as the percentage correct at each rate or as the mean correct response per second. It has been given serially over 8 weeks postinjury and demonstrates cognitive recovery to normal. Paced auditory serial addition test recovery, however, was delayed in head injury patients with PTS compared with a non-PTS control group.[115]

Within 8 weeks of head injury, a test of auditory vigilance in which patients had to detect the rare instances in which the interval between elements in a string of numbers was longer than in the others showed normalization.[116] However, these deficits may reappear under physiologic stress.[117] Several measures of reaction time are also impaired in patients with head injury at various times after injury.[118]

In a test of selective attention, head injury patients were significantly slower but not less accurate than controls 3 months after injury.[119] Sustained and divided attention showed significant differences from controls at 1 month but were inconclusive 3 months after injury.[119] On the other hand, patients with MHI and PTS perform less well on a test of sustained attention than MHI controls (without PTS) 12 to 34 months after injury.[120] Similarly, tests of distributed attention show deficits 1 and 3 months after head injury.[119] The authors pointed out that the most sensitive tools for revealing cerebral dysfunction test the function of the greatest number of cortical and subcortical areas simultaneously.[119] Only one study has been shown to distinguish PTH or PTS from MHI alone.[120]

Repeated neuropsychological tests on 30 patients with PTS after whiplash injury demonstrate a hierarchy of functional recovery occurring over a period of greater than 12 weeks after apparently mild injury.[121] Attention and concentration deficits recover first; visual memory, imagination, and analytic capacity recover within the next 6 to 12 weeks; and verbal memory abstraction, cognitive selectivity, and information processing speed take more than 12 weeks to recover.[121]

Patients with PTH were compared with patients with chronic "combination headache" and low-back pain and with pain-free controls.[122] PTH patients had the highest scale elevations on the Symptom Checklist 90-Revised. The findings suggest that PTH patients exhibit more psychopathology than individuals with other headache types and normal controls. On some tests, patients with PTH had more psychopathology than patients with low-back pain. In general, these tests do not demonstrate any specific pattern of psychopathology.[122]

## DIAGNOSIS

The diagnosis of PTH and PTS is established by symptoms consistent with this syndrome, trauma-related onset, and the exclusion of other conditions that can present similarly (Table 16–1). The IHS criteria for PTH require the headache to occur within 7 days after regaining consciousness (or after the trauma if there is no LOC). There are no IHS criteria for late-onset PTH. The IHS differentiates between acute PTH, which lasts less than 3 months, and chronic PTH, which lasts longer and is likely to be permanent. A worsening of a preexisting headache disorder does not qualify as PTH. A substantial difference between headache features before and after injury must be present for the designation of PTH.

Many patients diagnosed with PTS are portrayed as malingerers or are thought to profoundly embellish their symptoms. Most experts believe that this is uncommon. The diagnosis of malingering should be actively made by surreptitiously observing a patient

**Table 16–1  Differential Diagnosis**

| |
|---|
| Subdural or epidural hematoma |
| Cerebrospinal fluid hypotension |
| Cerebrospinal fluid hypertension |
| Cerebral vein thrombosis |
| Cavernous sinus thrombosis |
| Cervical or carotid artery dissection |
| Cerebral hemorrhage |
| Epilepsy |
| Hydrocephalus |

performing a task that he stated he could not accomplish.[22] Simulators have been shown to perform worse on sensorimotor tests[123] and memory tests[124] than would be expected. Performance that is significantly worse than chance on a forced-choice memory test can be interpreted as the deliberate production of wrong answers but may not distinguish between malingering and conversion reactions.[125] Other clues of malingering include antisocial or borderline personality, a poor work record, prior claims for injury, random test performance, and excessive endorsement of symptoms.[126]

## TREATMENT

Patients with PTS are often distressed and misunderstood, and they require an objective and comprehensive treatment approach. Treating them inappropriately may create pathologic resentment and disability that is refractory to treatment. The comprehensive approach to treatment uses medications, physical modalities, and biofeedback or counseling. One study showed that 85% of patients returned to work after being treated aggressively in individualized programs that included medication, biofeedback, stress management, exercise, and neuromuscular relaxation.[127]

In the absence of any known remediable mechanism, treatment should be directed at the identifiable components of the PTS. Headache is treated as if it had arisen as a primary headache disorder. Cervical and soft tissue injury should be identified and treated. Anxiety and depression should be meticulously identified and addressed. Cognitive dysfunction should also be addressed.

Few studies have evaluated specific drug treatments for PTH, and most have involved the use of the antidepressant amitriptyline. In an uncontrolled study, 75 to 250 mg of amitriptyline was effective in 90% of PTH patients, not distinguishing between various headache patterns of PTH.[128] On the other hand, a study of two groups of psychiatrically hospitalized patients with depression, one with PTH, the other with idiopathic headaches, used amitriptyline at an average dose of 175 mg/d. Amitriptyline was effective for the uninjured patients but not for the PTS patients.[129] This study is likely to have selected a particularly intractable subgroup of PTS patients and may not apply to all patients with PTH.

Other antidepressants, including imipramine, doxepin, nortriptyline, selective serotonin reuptake inhibitors, venlafaxine, and mirtazapine, may be effective in select patients with PTH (unpublished observations). Donepezil is used for the cognitive symptoms of major head injury but has not been studied after MHI or postconcussion syndrome.

Abortive medications are widely used for patients with PTS but can lead to development of medication-overuse headache. Sumatriptan is effective for the migrainous exacerbation of PTH but not for the baseline headache.[130] Repetitive intravenous dihydroergotamine is effective for PTH that meet the criteria of chronic daily headache.[76,77] Intravenous chlorpromazine has been effective in acute PTH.[131] In patients with daily or near-daily headache, preventive medications should be used preferentially, and the use of abortive medications should be limited.

In the presence of true epilepsy, anticonvulsant therapy is indicated. Divalproex sodium and perhaps topiramate are drugs of choice if the patient has PTH and a seizure disorder. The many other spells seen in this population rarely respond to anticonvulsant treatment. Even in nonepileptic patients, divalproex sodium has shown a 60% improvement rate in patients with chronic PTH.[132]

Biofeedback and psychotherapy or behavior modification may be helpful for many patients. Biofeedback enables the patient to recognize muscle tension and bring it under voluntary control. A recent study found that biofeedback enabled 53% of patients to moderately increase their ability to relax and cope with pain, and 80% of patients felt that it was at least moderately helpful.[133] Behavior modification or cognitive therapy is often helpful in providing support and education and improving the patient's ability to cope. For patients with more severe psychopathology, long-term psychotherapy may be needed. Medication may be valuable to treat anxiety and depression.

If a whiplash type of injury has occurred, or if there is significant persistent neck pain with a suggestive physical examination, cervical zygapophyseal joint pain should be searched for and treated if identified. Lord and colleagues found the prevalence of zygapophyseal joint pain in patients with chronic neck pain after whiplash injury to be 60%.[134] Among patients with whiplash injury who rated their headaches more severe than their neck pain, the incidence of C2–3 zygapophyseal joint pain (based on diagnostic blocks) was 50%.[134] When initially successful, the benefits of radiofrequency neurotomy last an average of 422 days, and repeat procedures are successful.[135]

Cognitive retraining exercises, counseling, adaptive strategy programs, and vocational rehabilitation are accepted treatments for neurocognitive dysfunction. However, Alexander suggested that programs that allege to treat attention and memory problems are of uncertain value in head injury in general and are inappropriate for MHI.[136] One study demonstrated greater improvement in neuropsychological function in patients with MHI who were treated with CDP-choline for the month after injury than in placebo-treated controls.[137] The role for this treatment in the long-term management of postconcussion syndrome is uncertain.

Physical modalities, such as physical therapy and exercise, chiropractic treatment, and massage, have been beneficial for some patients, particularly when headache is related to or occurs in association with cervical trauma. Cold, heat, electrotherapy, and cervical orthoses have been used successfully, particularly in the acute stage, to improve functioning. In one open study, manual therapy was more successful than cold packs in relieving chronic PTS.[43] After the initial, acute phase, exercise programs are important to prevent deconditioning with a decrease in the overall level of functioning.

## OUTCOME

Various studies have demonstrated gradual resolution of acute PTH symptoms in most, but long-term symptoms occur in almost one-quarter of subjects presenting for treatment (Table 16–2). Approximately one-third of patients are unable to return to work after head injury.[138] In one study, 34% of previously employed patients who were admitted to a hospital had not returned to work 3 months after injury.[31] Older patients with higher levels of education and employment, greater income, and higher socioeconomic status were more likely to return to work.

Patients with mild TBI have 1.8 times the risk of behavioral discharge from the armed services compared with the total discharge population.[139] Mild and moderate head injury patients have 2.6 and 5.4 times the risk of discharge for alcohol and drug abuse, respectively, compared with the total population.[139] An alternate explanation for these findings could be that the behavioral abnormalities are the risk factor for MHI (although previous studies [see "Risk Factors"] in other populations have failed to show that behavioral abnormalities have such a strong effect on outcome).

**Table 16-2** Recovery from Acute Post-traumatic Headache

| Time since Injury | % with Post-traumatic Headache | Reference |
| --- | --- | --- |
| 1 mo | 31–90 | Munderhoud et al,[148] Denker[149] |
| 2–3 mo | 32–78 | Rimel et al,[31] Denny-Brown[150] |
| 1 yr | 8–35 | Dencker and Lofving,[118] Rutherford et al[138] |
| 2–4 yr | 20–24 | Dencker,[149] Edna and Cappelen[151] |

## CONTROVERSIES SURROUNDING THE DIAGNOSIS OF PTH AND PTS

Patients with PTS are often told, either by physicians, insurers, or employers, that they are embellishing or malingering, that they have a primary psychiatric disorder, or that their condition is not related to their injury. This belief is not substantiated, however, because (1) patients with chronic PTH rarely engage in such behavior, (2) the presence of litigation does not appear to influence outcome, (3) patients are not cured by a verdict,[31,48,140] and (4) symptoms of litigants are similar to those of nonlitigants.[141] Nonetheless, physicians are often placed in a position of justifying an accurate diagnosis of PTS.

Miller published a series of lectures in which he ascribed chronic PTS to a desire for compensation or a desire not to work.[142] These arguments continue to be used today. However, a prospective study demonstrated that poor work adjustment did not predict PTS but that patients with PTS subsequently demonstrated poor work adjustment.[38]

Arguing for nonorganicity, one study demonstrated that a control population identified the symptoms of PTS from a checklist in a similar manner to patients who complained of PTS.[143] The authors concluded that the symptoms of PTS are due to patients expecting to experience the symptoms. These findings suggest that most people are familiar with PTS, perhaps because they previously experienced the symptoms of a minimal concussion or because they have heard about head injuries in sports figures.

Another argument against organicity is that sports injuries rarely cause complaints of PTS. However, the velocities and forces experienced during most sports injuries are much less than those that result from motor vehicle accidents and falls, which are the injuries that commonly cause PTS. In sports injuries, the head is often held fixed and the athlete is prepared for impact, whereas in automobile accidents, the head is freely mobile, which results in more severe damage. Many recent studies have demonstrated subtle neurocognitive injury among athletes in sports in which head injury may occur.

One of the arguments used against the organicity of PTS is that patients do not have abnormal studies and there are no abnormal signs on examination: "Failure to understand the problem is no proof of psychogenicity."[144] Many neurologic diseases, such as migraine with and without aura, have no abnormal signs on examination. Several paraclinical studies show group differences between uninjured MHI patients without chronic PTS and PTS patients (see below). They do not yet have the sensitivity to distinguish individuals with "organic" PTH from those with psychological or other causes of PTH.

Work factors have been hypothesized to cause prolonged disability. Miller stated that unskilled workers and less intelligent persons suffer more prolonged disability owing to PTS.[142,145] The group that was studied consisted of patients sent by an insurance company and, hence, had a significant referral bias. Furthermore, jobs that require certain cognitive skills are particularly difficult for patients suffering from PTS. Laborers whose jobs depend on sustained physical effort and mental vigilance have particular difficulty performing their jobs, whereas patients whose jobs allow more flexibility and do not require physical activity may be better able to cope with their symptoms. Other authors noted that patients who blamed their employer as a large impersonal body had more symptoms than those who did not. This was felt to show "clear evidence of nervous and emotional factors at work in the production of symptoms."[146] The possibility that patients who are anxious, depressed, and irritable and have more symptoms owing to their PTS are more likely to blame others was not addressed. Many kinds of brain injuries, including stroke and neurodegenerative disease, produce psychiatric symptoms. Chronic pain, by itself, can induce depression and abnormal behavior; this does not mean that an organic pathology does not exist. Having a disabling illness that is not accepted by medical professionals, employers, and family is a legitimate cause of anxiety, depression, and abnormal behaviors.

In a study of Lithuanian automobile accident victims, Obelieniene and colleagues failed to show an increased incidence of headache or neck pain years after injury.[147] This finding was attributed to the fact that insurance was not available to compensate Lithuanian accident victims for lost work and to the general lack of recognition of whiplash-associated disorder or postconcussion syndrome in the community. In contrast to Lithuania, postconcussion headache and postconcussion syndrome are recognized in many countries in the Americas, Europe, and East Asia.

## CONCLUSION

Chronic PTH and PTS are common and frequently disabling conditions. There is no specific symptom cluster or reliable diagnostic test to unequivocally establish a diagnosis. The diagnosis is thus most reliably made by establishing the onset of symptoms soon after injury. The absence of a generally accepted mechanism for the genesis of chronic symptoms has led to an unfortunate skepticism about the validity of these symptoms, which has hindered the development of more effective treatments. The search for better treatment should continue; if new treatments can be based on interfering with a putative mechanism of symptom genesis (ie, windup, kindling, aberrant reinnervation, neurochemical cascade), they may provide insight into the causes of PTS. Relying on psychogenesis as the sole explanation of the syndrome feeds into a culture that could be harmful to individuals who have already been injured.

## REFERENCES

1. Headache Classification Committee, International Headache Society. The international classification of headache disorders, 2nd edition. Cephalalgia 2004;24:1–160.

2. Teasdale G, Jennett B. Assessment of coma and impaired consciousness: a practical scale. Lancet 1984;ii:81–4.

3. Rimel RW. Disability caused by minor head injury. J Head Trauma Rehabil 1981;6:86–7.

4. American Congress of Rehabilitation Medicine. Definition of mild traumatic brain injury. J Head Trauma Rehabil 1993;6:87.

5. Machado EB, Michet CJ, Ballard DJ, et al. Trends in incidence and clinical presentation of temporal arteritis in Olmsted County, Minnesota, 1958–1985. Arthritis Rheum 1988;31:745–9.

6. Kraus JF, Black MA, Hessol N, et al. The incidence of acute brain injury and serious impairment in a defined population. Am J Epidemiol 1984;119:186–201.

7. Kraus JF, McArthur DL, Silberman TA. Epidemiology of mild brain injury. Semin Neurol 1994;14:1–7.

8. Evans RW. The postconcussion syndrome and the sequelae of mild head injury. Neurol Clin 1992;10:815–47.

9. Raskin NH. Posttraumatic headache: the postconcussion syndrome. In: Raskin NH, editor. Headache. New York: Churchill Livingstone; 1988.

10. Brenner C, Friedman AP. Posttraumatic headache. J Neurosurg 1944;1:379–91.

11. Elkind AH. Posttraumatic headache. In: Diamond S, Dalessio DJ, editors. The practicing physician's approach to headache. 5th ed. Baltimore: Williams & Wilkins; 1992. p. 146–61.

12. Speed WG. Psychiatric aspects of posttraumatic headaches. In: Adler C, Adler S, Packard R, editors. Psychiatric aspects of headache. Baltimore: Williams & Wilkins; 1987. p. 210–7.

13. Cartlidge N, Shaw D. In: Cartlidge N, Shaw D, editors. Head injury. Philadelphia: WB Saunders; 1981. p. 95–154.

14. Scher AI, Lipton RB, Stewart W. Risk factors for chronic daily headache. Curr Pain Headache Rep 2002;6:486–91.

15. Mandel S. Minor head injury may not be "minor." Postgrad Med J 1989;85:213–5.

16. Kelly R. Headache after cranial trauma. In: Hopkins A, editor. Headache: problems in diagnosis and management. London: Saunders; 1988. p. 219.

17. DeBenedittis G, DeSantis A. Chronic posttraumatic headache: clinical, psychopathologic features and outcome determinants. J Neurosurg Sci 1983;27:177.

18. Haas DC. Classification of chronic posttraumatic headache. Cephalalgia 1995;15:162.

19. Couch JR, Samuel S, Leviston T, Teagram H. Can head injury by itself produce the syndrome of chronic daily headache? Presented at the American Headache Society 42nd Annual Scientific Meeting; 2000 June 23–25.

20. Haas DC, Lourie T. Trauma-triggered migraine: an explanation for common neurologic attacks after mild head injury. Neurosurgery 1988;68:181–8.

21. Packard RC, Ham LP. Incidence of cluster-like posttraumatic headache: an inconsistency. Headache Q 1996;7:139.

22. Binder LM. Persisting symptoms after mild head injury: a review of the postconcussive syndrome. J Clin Exp Neuropsychol 1986;8:323–46.

23. Winston KR. Whiplash and its relationship to migraine. Headache 1987;27:452–7.

24. Weiss HD, Stern BJ, Goldbert J. Posttraumatic migraine: chronic migraine precipitated by minor head or neck trauma. Headache 1991;31:451–6.

25. Saper JR. Headache disorders: current concepts in treatment strategies. Littleton: Wright-PSG; 1983.

26. Gfeller JD, Chibnall JT, Duckro PN. Postconcussion symptoms and cognitive functioning in posttraumatic headache patients. Headache 1994;34:503–7.

27. Silberstein SD, Marcelis J. Pseudotumor cerebri without papilledema. Headache 1990;30:304.

28. Vijayan N. A new posttraumatic headache syndrome. Headache 1977;17:19–22.

29. Montalbetti L, Ferrandi D, Pergami P, Savoldi F. Elongated styloid process and Eagle's syndrome. Cephalalgia 1995;15:80.

30. Wong E, Lee G, Mason DT. Temporal headaches and associated symptoms relating to the styloid process and its attachments. Ann Acad Med 1995;24:124.

31. Rimel RW, Giordani B, Barth JT, et al. Disability caused by minor head injury. Neurosurgery 1981;9:221–8.

32. Segalowitz SJ, Lawson S. Subtle symptoms associated with self-reported mild head injury. J Learn Disabil 1995;28:309.

33. Andrasik F, Wincze JP. Emotional and psychologic aspects of mild head injury. Semin Neurol 1994;14:60.

34. Kim SH, Manes F, Kosier T, et al. Irritability following traumatic brain injury. J Nerv Ment Dis 1999;187:327–35.

35. Hickling EJ, Blanchard EB, Silverman DJ, Schwarz SP. Motor vehicle accidents, headaches, and posttraumatic stress disorder. Headache 1992;32:147.

36. Sbordone RJ, Liter JC. Mild traumatic brain injury does not produce posttraumatic stress disorder. Brain Injury 1995;9:405.

37. Jensen OK, Nielson FF. The influence of sex and pretraumatic headache on the incidence and severity of headache after injury. Cephalalgia 1990;10:285–93.

38. Lidvall HF, Linderoth B, Norlin B. Causes of the postconcussional syndrome. Acta Neurol Scand 1974;40:1–143.

39. Prigatano GP, Stahl ML, Orr WC, et al. Sleep and dreaming disturbances in closed head injury patients. J Neurol Neurosurg Psychiatry 1982;45:78.

40. Silberstein SD, Lipton RB, Saper JR, et al. Headache and facial pain: part A. Continuum 1995;1:8.

41. Lankford DA, Wellman JJ, O'Hara C. Posttraumatic narcolepsy in mild to moderate closed head injury. Sleep 1994;25.

42. Lake AE, Branca B, Lutz T, et al. Comorbid symptoms in chronic posttraumatic headache. I: comparison to intractable migraine. II: relationship to severity of injury and litigation [abstract]. Headache 1995;35:302.

43. Jensen OK, Nielsen FF, Vosmar L. An open study comparing manual therapy with the use of cold packs in the treatment of posttraumatic headache. Cephalalgia 1990;10:241–50.

44. Fenton GW. The postconcussional syndrome reappraised. Clin Electroencephalogr 1996;27:174–82.

45. Bohnen N, Twinjnstra A, Jolles J. Posttraumatic and emotional symptoms in different subgroups of patients with mild head injury. Brain Injury 1992;6:481–7.

46. McClelland RJ, Fenton GW, Rutherford W. The postconcussional syndrome revisited. J R Soc Med 1994;87:508–10.

47. Keshavan MS, Channabasavanna SM, Reddy GN. Posttraumatic psychiatric disturbances: patterns and predictors of outcome. Br J Psychiatry 1981;131:157.

48. Mendelson G. Not "cured by a verdict." Med J Aust 1982;2:132–4.

49. Landy PJB. Neurological sequelae of minor head and neck injuries. Injury 1998;29:199–206.

50. Yamaguchi M. Incidence of headache and severity of head injury. Headache 1992;32:422.

51. Wilkinson M, Gilchrist E. Posttraumatic headache. Ups J Med Sci 1980;31:48.

52. Barrett K, Ward AB, Boughey A, et al. Sequelae of minor head injury: the natural consciousness and followup. J Accid Emerg Med 1994;11:79.

53. Rutherford WH. Postconcussion symptoms. In: Levin HS, Eisenberg HM, Beriton AZ, editors. Mild head injury. New York: Oxford University Press; 1989. p. 217.

54. Radanov BP, Sturzeneger M, DiStefano G. Long-term outcome after whiplash injury: a 2-year followup considering features of injury mechanism and somatic, radiologic, and psychosocial findings. Medicine 1995;74:281.

55. Sturzenegger M. Ultrasound findings in spontaneous carotid artery dissection. Arch Neurol 1991;48:1057–63.

56. Treleaven J, Jull G, Atkinson L. Cervical musculoskeletal dysfunction in postconcussional headache. Cephalalgia 1994;14:273–9.

57. Post RM, Silberstein SD. Shared mechanisms in affective illness, epilepsy, and migraine. Neurology 1994;44:S37–47.

58. Elson LM, Ward CC. Mechanisms and pathophysiology of mild head injury. Semin Neurol 1994;14:8–18.

59. Jane JA, Steward O, Gennarelli TA. Axonal degeneration induced by experimental noninvasive minor head injury. J Neurosurg 1985;62:96.

60. Povlishock JT, Coburn TH. Morphopathologic change associated with mild head injury. In: Levin HS, Eisenberg HM, Benton AL, editors. Mild head injury. New York: Oxford University Press; 1989.

61. Schmidt RH, Grady MS. Loss of forebrain cholinergic neurons following fluid-percussion injury: implications for cognitive impairment in closed head injury. J Neurosurg 1995;83:496.

62. Ward CC, Nahum AM. Correlation between brain injury and intracranial pressures in experimental head impacts. In: Proceedings of the 4th International Conference on the Biomechanics of Trauma. 133. 1979.

63. Ward CC. Finite element modeling of the head and neck. In: Ewing R, et al, editors. Impact injury of the head and spine. Springfield: Thomas; 1982. p. 421.

64. Gennarelli TA. Mechanisms of brain injury. J Emerg Med 1993;1:5–11.

65. Blumbergs PC, Jones NR, North JB. Diffuse axonal injury in head trauma. J Neurol Neurosurg Psychiatry 1989;52:838–41.

66. Gennarelli TA, Thibault LE, Adams JH, et al. Diffuse axonal injury and traumatic coma in the primate. In: Dacey RG,

et al, editors. Trauma of the central nervous system. New York: Raven Press; 1975. p. 169.

67. Saatman KE, Graham DI, McIntosh TK. The neuronal cytoskleton is at risk after mild and moderate brain injury. J Neurotrauma 1998;15:1047–58.

68. Blumbergs PC, Scott G, Manavis J, et al. Staining of amyloid precursor protein to study axonal damage in mild head injury. Lancet 1994;344:1055.

69. Servadei P, Vergoni G, Pasini A, et al. Diffuse axonal injury with brainstem localization: report of a case in a mild head injured patient. J Neurosurg Sci 1994;38:129.

70. Erb DE, Povlishock JT. Neuroplasticity following traumatic brain injury: a study of GABAergic terminal loss and recovery in the cat dorsal lateral vestibular nucleus. Exp Brain Res 1991;83:253.

71. Goodman JC. Pathologic changes in mild head injury. Semin Neurol 1994;14:19.

72. Zubkov AY, Pilkington AS, Bernanke DH, et al. Posttraumatic cerebral vasospasm: clinical and morphological presentations. J Neurotrauma 1999;16:763–70.

73. Junger EC, Newell DW, Grant GA, et al. Cerebral autoregulation following minor head injury. J Neurosurg 1997;86:425–32.

74. Packard RC, Ham LP. Pathogenesis of posttraumatic headaches and migraine: a common headache pathway? Headache 1997;37:142–52.

75. Packard RC. Epidemiology and pathogenesis of posttraumatic headache. J Head Trauma Rehabil 1999;14:9–21.

76. McBeath JG, Nanda A. Use of dihydroergotamine in patients with postconcussion syndrome. Headache 1994;34:148–51.

77. Young WB, Hopkins MM, Janyszek B, Primavera JP. Repetitive intravenous DHE in the treatment of refractory posttraumatic headache [abstract]. Headache 1994;34:297.

78. Young WB, Peres MF, Rozen TD. Modular headache theory: a unified approach to headaches [abstract]. Cephalalgia 2001;21:384.

79. Duckro PN, Chibnall JT, Tomazic TJ. Anger, depression, and disability: a path analysis of relationships in a sample of chronic posttraumatic headache patients. Headache 1995;35:7.

80. Kelly AB, Zimmerman RD, Gandy SE, Deck MD. Comparison of magnetic resonance imaging and computed tomography in the evaluation of head injury. Neurosurgery 1986;18:45.

81. Levin HS, Amparo E, Eisenberg HM. Magnetic resonance imaging and computerized tomography in relation to the neurobehavioral sequelae of mild and moderate head injuries. J Neurosurg 1987;66:706–13.

82. Levin HS, Williams DH, Eisenberg HM, et al. Serial MRI and neurobehavioral findings after mild to moderate head injuries. J Neurol Neurosurg Psychiatry 1992;55:255.

83. Mittle RL, Grossman RI, Hiehl JF, et al. Prevalence of MR evidence of diffuse axonal injury in patients with mild head injury and normal head CT findings. AJNR Am J Neuroradiol 1994;15:1583.

84. Abdel-Dayem HM, Sadek SA, Kouris K. Changes in cerebral perfusion after acute head injury: comparison of CT with Tc-99m-PAO SPECT. Radiology 1987;165:221–6.

85. Reid RH, Gulenchyn K, Ballinger JR. Cerebral perfusion imaging with Tc-HM-PAO following cerebral trauma. Clin Nucl Med 1990;15:383–8.

86. Abdel-Dayem HM, Masdeu J, O'Connell R. Brain perfusion abnormalities following minor/moderate closed head injury: comparison between early and late imaging in two groups of patients. Eur J Nucl Med 1994;21:750.

87. Newton MR, Greenwood RJ, Britton KF, et al. A study comparing SPECT with CT and MRI after closed head injury. J Neurol Neurosurg Psychiatry 1992;55:92.

88. American Academy of Neurology. Assessment of brain SPECT. Report of the Therapeutics and Technology Assessment Subcommittee of the American Academy of Neurology. Neurology 1996;46:278.

89. Abdel-Dayem HM, Abu-Judeh H, Kumar M, et al. SPECT brain perfusion abnormalities in mild or moderate traumatic brain injury. Clin Nucl Med 1998;23:309–17.

90. Varney NR, Bushnell D. NeuroSPECT findings in patients with posttraumatic anosmia: a quantitative analysis. J Head Trauma Rehabil 1998;13:63–72.

91. Ramadan NM, Norris LL, Shultz LR. Abnormal cerebral flood flow correlates with disability to chronic posttraumatic headache [abstract]. J Neuroimaging 1995;5:68.

92. Gilkey SJ, Ramadan NM, Aurora TK, Welch KM. Cerebral blood flow in chronic posttraumatic headache. Headache 1997;37:583–7.

93. Alavi A, Fazekas T, Alves W, et al. Positron emission tomography in the evaluation of head injury. J Cereb Blood Flow Metab 1987;7:646.

94. George JK, Alavi Z, Zimmerman RA, et al. Metabolic (PET) correlates of anatomic leads (CT/MRI) produced by head trauma [abstract]. J Nucl Med 1989;30:802.

95. Rao N, Turski PA, Polcyn RE, et al. [18]F positron emission computed tomography in closed head injury. Arch Phys Med Rehabil 1984;65:780.

96.  McAllister TW, Saykin AJ, Flashman LA, et al. Brain activation during working memory 1 month after mild traumatic brain injury: a functional MRI study. Neurology 1999;53:1300–8.

97.  Schoenhuber R, Gentilini M. Neurophysiologic assessment of mild head injury. In: Levin HS, Eisenberg HM, Benton AL, editors. Mild head injury. New York: Oxford University Press; 1989. p. 142–50.

98.  Hughes JR, Robbins LD. Brain mapping in migraine. Clin Electroencephalogr 1990;21:14.

99.  Thatcher RW, Walker RA, Gerson I, et al. EEG discriminant analyses of mild head trauma. Electroencephalogr Clin Neurophysiol 1989;73:1989.

100. Lewine JD, Davis JT, Sloan JH, et al. Neuromagnetic assessment of pathophysiologic brain activity induced by minor head trauma. AJNR Am J Neuroradiol 1999;20:857–66.

101. Ramadan NM, Schultz LL, Gilkey SJ. Migraine prophylactic drugs: proof of efficacy, utilization, and cost. Cephalalgia 1997;17:73–80.

102. Bricolo AP, Turella GS. Electrophysiology of head injury. In: Braakman R, editor. Handbook of clinical neurology. New York: Elsevier; 1990. p. 181–206.

103. Geets W, Louette N. EEG et potentiels évoqués du tronc cérébral dans 125 commotions récentes. Electroencephalogr Neurophysiol Clin 1983;13:253.

104. Toglia JU. Dizziness after whiplash injury of the neck and closed head injury. In: Walker WF, Caveness WF, Critchley M, editors. The late effects of head injury. Springfield: Thomas; 1969. p. 72.

105. Rowe MJ, Carlson C. Brainstem auditory evoked potentials in postconcussion dizziness. Arch Neurol 1980;37:679.

106. Mallinson AI, Longridge NS. Dizziness from whiplash and head injury: differences between whiplash and head injury. Am J Otol 1998;19:814–8.

107. Pratap-Chand R, Sinniah M, Salem FA. Cognitive evoked potential (P300): a metric for cerebral concussion. Acta Neurol Scand 1988;78:185.

108. Werner RA, Vanderzant CW. Multimodality evoked potential testing in acute mild closed head injury. Arch Phys Med Rehabil 1991;72:31.

109. Kobylare EJ, Dunford J, Jabbari B, et al. Auditory event-related potentials in head injury patients. Neurology 1995;45:358P.

110. Granovsky Y, Sprecher E, Hemli J, Yarnitsky D. P300 and stress in mild head injury patients. Electroencephalogr Clin Neurophysiol 1998;108:554–9.

111. Keidel M, Rieschke P, Stude P, et al. Antinociceptive reflex alteration in acute posttraumatic headache following whiplash injury. Pain 2001;92:319–26.

112. Ingebrigtsen T, Waterloo K, Jacobsen EA, et al. Traumatic brain damage in minor head injury: relation of serum S-100 protein measurements to magnetic resonance imaging and neurobehavioral outcome. Neurosurgery 1999;45:468–75.

113. Anderson RE, Hansson LO, Nilsson O, et al. High serum S100B levels for trauma patients without head injuries. Neurosurgery 2001;48:1255–60.

114. Eisenberg HM. CT and MRI finding in mild to moderate head injury. In: Levin HL, Eisenberg HM, Benton AL, editors. Mild head injury. New York: Oxford University Press; 1989. p. 133.

115. Gronwall D, Wrightson P. Delayed recovery of intellectual function after minor head injury. Lancet 1974;ii:605–9.

116. McCarthy D. Memory and vigilance after concussion. Auckland: University of Auckland; 1977.

117. Ewing R, McCarthy D, Gronwall D, Wrightson P. Persisting effects of minor head injury observable during hypoxic stress. J Clin Neuropsychol 1980;2:147.

118. Dencker SJ, Lofving BA. A psychometric study of identical twins discordant for closed head injury. Acta Psychiatr Neurol Scand 1958;33.

119. Gentilini TM, Michelli P, Schoenhuber R. Assessment of attention in mild head injury. In: Levin HS, Eisenberg HM, Benton AL, editors. Mild head injury. New York: Oxford University Press; 1989. p. 163.

120. Bohnen NI, Jolles J, Twijnstra A, et al. Late neurobehavioural symptoms after mild head injury. Brain Injury 1995;9:27.

121. Keidel M, Yaguez L, Wilhelm H, Diener HC. Prospective followup of neuropsychologic deficiency after cervicocephalic acceleration trauma. Neurol Klin PoliklinUniversitat Essen Nervenarzt 1992;63:731.

122. Ham LP, Andrasik F, Packard RC, Bundrick CM. Psychopathology in individuals with posttraumatic headaches and other pain types. Cephalalgia 1994;14:118.

123. Heaton RK, Smith HH, Lehman RA, Vogt AJ. Prospects for faking believable deficits on neuropsychologic testing. J Consult Clin Psychol 1978;46:892.

124. Benton AL, Spreen O. Visual memory test: the simulation of mental incompetence. Arch Gen Psychiatry 1961;4:79.

125. Binder LM. Malingering following minor head trauma. Clin Neuropsychol 1990;4:25.

126. Ruff MR, Willie T. Malingering and malingering-like aspects of mild closed head injury. J Head Trauma Rehabil 1993;8:60.

127. Medina JL. Efficacy of an individualized outpatient program in the treatment of chronic posttraumatic headache. Headache 1992;32:180–3.

128. Tyler GS, McNeely HE, Dick ML. Treatment of posttraumatic headache with amitriptyline. Headache 1980;20:213.

129. Saran A. Antidepressants not effective in headache associated with minor closed head injury. Int J Psychiatry Med 1988;18(1):75–83.

130. Gawel MJ, Rothbart P, Jacobs H. Subcutaneous sumatriptan in the treatment of acute episodes of posttraumatic headache. Headache 1993;33:96–7.

131. Herd A, Ludwig L. Relief of posttraumatic headache by intravenous chlorpromazine. J Emerg Med 1994;12:849–51.

132. Packard RC. Treatment of chronic daily posttraumatic headache with divalproex sodium. Headache 2000;40:736–9.

133. Ham LP, Packard RC. A retrospective, followup study of biofeedback-assisted relaxation therapy in patients with posttraumatic headache. Biofeedback Self Regulation 1996;21:93–104.

134. Lord SM, Barnsley L, Wallis BJ, Bogduk N. Chronic cervical zygapophysial joint pain after whiplash: a placebo-controlled prevalence study. Spine 1996;21:1737–44.

135. McDonald GJ, Lord SM, Bogduk N. Long-term followup of patients treated with cervical radiofrequency neurotomy for chronic neck pain. Neurosurgery 1999;45:61.

136. Alexander MP. Mild traumatic brain injury: pathophysiology, natural history, and clinical management. Neurology 1995;45:1253.

137. Levin HS, Williams D, Eisenberg HM. Treatment of postconcussional symptoms with CDP-choline. Neurology 1990;40:326.

138. Rutherford WH, Merrett JD, McDonald JR. Symptoms of one year following concussion from minor head injuries. Injury 1978;10:225–30.

139. Ommaya AK, Salazar AM, Dannenberg AL, et al. Outcome after traumatic brain injury in the U.S. military medical system. J Trauma 1996;41:972–5.

140. Packard RC. Posttraumatic headache: permanency and relationship to legal settlement. Headache 1992;32:496–500.

141. Davis RA, Luxon LM. Dizziness following head injury: a neurotologic study. J Neurol 1995;242:222.

142. Miller H. Accident neurosis: lecture II. BMJ 1961;1:992.

143. Mittenberg W, DiGiulio D, Perrin S, Bass A. Symptoms following mild head injury: expectation as etiology. J Neurol Neurosurg Psychiatry 1992;55:200.

144. Strauss I, Savitsky N. Head injury. Arch Neurol Psychiatry 1934;31:893.

145. Miller H. Accident neurosis: lecture I. BMJ 1961;1:918.

146. Rutherford WH, Merrett JD, McDonald JR. Sequelae of concussion caused by minor head injuries. Lancet 1977;i:1–4.

147. Obelieniene D, Bovim G, Schrader H, et al. Headache after whiplash: a historical cohort study outside the medicolegal context. Cephalalgia 1998;18:559–64.

148. Munderhoud JM, Boclens ME, Huizenga J. Treatment of minor head injuries. Clin Neurol Neurosurg 1980;82:127–40.

149. Denker PG. The postconcussion syndrome: prognosis and evaluation of the organic factors. N Y State J Med 1944;44:379–84.

150. Denny-Brown D. Disability arising from closed head injury. JAMA 1945;127:429–36.

151. Edna T-H, Cappelen J. Late postconcussional symptoms in traumatic head injury. An anlysis of frequency and risk factors. Acta Neurochir 1987;86:12–7.

# CHAPTER 17

# Temporomandibular Disorders and Headache

Steven B. Graff-Radford, DDS

Chronic daily headache (CDH) is now cosidered to have primary and secondary causes (Table 17–1). The temporomandibular joint (TMJ) and associated orofacial structures should be considered as triggering or perpetuating factors for CDH. It is important that the clinician considers both peripheral and central processes that may contribute to persistent headache. Often, ignoring the TMJ, muscles, or other orofacial structures as a peripheral trigger will result in a poor clinical outcome in managing CDH. The trigeminal nerve is the final conduit of face, neck, and head pain. Owing to the central connections, it is possible for referral to occur between divisions.[1] The management of pain in the first division may be influenced by therapy aimed at structures innervated by the second or third trigeminal division. This chapter discusses the relationship between the TMJ, muscles, or other orofacial structures and headache.

**Table 17–1  Classification of Chronic Daily Headache**

*Primary*

Chronic migraine

Chronic tension-type headache

Hemicrania continua

New daily persistent headache

Chronic post-traumatic headache

*Secondary*

Chronic headache attributed to whiplash

Chronic headache attributable to other trauma

Medication-overuse headache

Chronic postinfection headache

## TEETH AND HEADACHE

The pathology associated with dental disease is not a common cause of headache. Dental disease may be summarized as pulpal or periodontal. Pulpal pain may be characterized as an irreversible pulpitis in which pulpal tissue death is inevitable, resulting in root canal therapy. Reversible pulpitis may be resolved by eliminating the inciting pathology (eg, caries). Periodontal disorders involve the supporting teeth structures, bone, periodontal ligament, and cementum. Periodontal disease triggers tissue inflammation, producing pain and often swelling in the affected site. When acute pain occurs in the dental structures, patients will often describe referred pain and tenderness to adjacent structures, including headache. The frequency and epidemiology of headache and tooth pain are unknown. Headache is usually a secondary phenomenon and does not pose a significant diagnostic dilemma. Possibly, pericoronitis is the most frequent periodontal inflammation causing headache. Pericoronitis, as its name implies, results from infection or traumatic irritation around a partially erupted tooth, usually a wisdom tooth.

The dental problems are best managed with conventional dental therapies and rarely produce any long-term or significant disability. Chronic dental pains are, however, different. Atypical odontalgia (AO) has been linked with headache and described as possibly secondary to a migrainous etiology.[2,3] Unfortunately, atypical facial pain has become a wastebasket term for all pains in the face that are not readily diagnosed. Harris first described AO as slightly more specific because it is localized to the tooth site.[4] Graff-Radford and Solberg defined AO as pain in a tooth or tooth site for which no organic cause is obvious.[5,6] They emphasized that prior to making a diagnosis, positive inclusionary criteria are required rather than arriving at the diagnosis by exclusion. Graff-Radford and Solberg suggested a deafferentation mechanism, either peripheral, central, or sympathetically maintained pain.[7,8] The relationship of psychopathology and AO was also explored by Graff-Radford and Solberg, and no positive relationship was found.[9] It is most likely that these pains are neuropathic, follow some neural injury or sensitization, and can be divided into pains mediated by the sensory system versus the sympathetic system.[8] Criteria are therefore proposed for defining neuropathic facial pain. The correct term should be "trigeminal deafferentation." The criteria for trigeminal deafferentation are listed in Table 17–2.

---

**Table 17–2    Suggested Diagnostic Criteria for Trigeminal Deafferentation**

Continuous pain punctuated with sharp electric pains Requires four of the following:

Known trauma

Presence of neurosensory deficit (numbness)

Allodynia

Hyperalgesia

Temperature change

Block effect

    Somatic

    Sympathetic

---

## MIGRAINE AND FACIAL PAIN

Lovshin was the first to describe migraine as a facial pain problem that could occur without pain in the first division of the trigeminal nerve.[10] The pain in facial migraine is described as dull pain with superimposed throbbing occurring once to several times per week. Each attack may last minutes to hours. Raskin and Prusiner described ipsilateral carotid tenderness in facial migraine, a finding also seen when migraine occurs in the head.[11] This condition has also been referred to as carotidynia. Treatment of facial migraine is no different than that for migraine presenting in the head. All treatments should include an understanding that the disorder is genetic and that the goals should be to reduce pain frequency and intensity and restore function, as well as provide a sense of self-control. Therapy may involve nonpharmacologic and pharmacologic approaches. In general, addressing triggering factors through diet, exercise, and sleep is first-line care. The acute attack is treated by early administration of the most effective therapy. Analgesics, anti-inflammatories, ergots, and triptans are most commonly used. If the headache is frequent, preven-

tive medications may be considered. The groups of medications that may be considered are β-blockers, calcium channel blockers, antidepressants, antiepileptic drugs, and antiserotonin drugs.[12]

## TEMPOROMANDIBULAR DISORDERS AND HEADACHE

Scientific investigation has described the pathways and mechanisms for pain referral from the head to the TMJ and vice versa.[13]

Headache may result from temporomandibular structures, or pain may be referred to the TMJ, secondary to a primary headache diagnosis. Functional disorders and pain in the anatomic region of the TMJ and associated musculature are referred to as temporomandibular disorders (TMDs). This overlap is primarily related to the anatomy and neural innervations. It is essential not to confuse the issue and suggest a cause-and-effect relationship based on treatment responses. The trigeminal nerve is the final pathway for both head pain and TMD, making the relationship between TMD and headache confusing. It is suggested that the two are separate but may be aggravating or perpetuating factors for each other. Patients with primary headache can see their pain worsened or triggered when there is a coexisting TMD.

### EPIDEMIOLOGY

TMD epidemiology has not specifically differentiated headache from facial pain. In nonpatient population studies, 75% have at least one joint dysfunction sign (clicking, limited range of motion) and about 33% have at least one symptom (pain, pain, on palpation). Of the 75% with a sign or symptom, fewer than 5% require treatment, and even fewer have headache as the primary pain location.

### ETIOLOGY

Inflammation within the joint accounts for TMD pain, and the dysfunction is due to a disk-condyle incoordination. Muscle pain disorders may include spasm, myositis, muscle splinting, and myofascial pain. The most frequent muscle disorder included in TMD classification is myofascial pain. Although each may be a trigger for headache and occur together, they are discussed separately.

**Inflammation**

Primary inflammatory conditions of the TMJ include capsulitis, synovitis, and the polyarthritides. Polyarthritides are relatively uncommon and are associated primarily with rheumatologic disease. Inflammatory conditions such as synovitis or capsulitis frequently occur secondary to trauma, irritation, or infection and often accompany other TMDs.[14]

Several proinflammatory cytokines have been detected in painful TMDs, which suggests that they may play a role in pain.[15] Capsulitis, an inflammation of the capsule related to sprain of capsular ligaments, is clinically difficult, if not impossible, to differentiate from synovitis. However, the pain related to capsulitis increases during all translatory movements and joint distraction but not usually during clenching.[16] Both conditions may be accompanied by a fluctuating swelling (owing to effusion) that decreases the ability to occlude on the ipsilateral posterior teeth. Pain associated with inflammation is localized to the TMJ capsule and the intracapsular tissues. The pain is typically dull and achy but may be throbbing. It is frequently described as sharp on movements. The pain is continuous but worsens with jaw function.

## Disk Derangement Disorders

Articular disk displacement is the most common TMJ arthropathy and is characterized by several stages of clinical dysfunction that involve the disk-condyle relationship. The usual direction for displacement is in an anterior or anteromedial direction,[17,18] although other directions have been described. Pain or mandibular movement symptoms are not specific for disk derangement disorders,[19] and disk position may not be related to any presenting symptom.[20,21]

The causes of disk displacement are not agreed on; however, it is postulated that in a majority of cases, stretched or torn ligaments that bind the disk to the condyle permit the disk to become displaced.[22] An increased horizontal angle of the mandibular condyle has been associated with more advanced TMJ internal derangement.[23,24] Lubrication impairment has also been suggested as a possible etiologic factor of disk displacement.[25] Disk displacement is subdivided into disk displacement with reduction or disk displacement without reduction.

Disk displacement with reduction is described when a temporarily misaligned disk reduces or improves its structural relation with the condyle when mandibular translation occurs during opening. This produces a joint noise (sound) described as clicking or popping. Disk displacement with reduction is usually characterized by what is termed reciprocal clicking, a reciprocal noise that is heard during the opening movement and again before the teeth occlude during the closing movement. Because disk displacement with reduction is so common, it may represent a physiologic accommodation without clinical significance.[26,27] In fact, clicking in reducing disk displacement is not pathologic because over one-third of an asymptomatic sample can have moderate to severe derangement and as many as one-quarter of clicking joints show normal or only slightly displaced disk positions. Disk displacement may or may not be a painful condition. If the condition is painful, inflammation of the retrodiskal tissue, the synovial tissues, the capsule, or the ligaments and pressure and traction on the disk attachments are more likely causes of the pain.[28] TMJ disk displacement with reduction may persist for several years up to decades without progression or complication.[29] De Leeuw and colleagues reported that if clicking in patients with disk displacement with reduction does not respond to treatment and is still present 2 to 4 years afterward, it is likely to persist for several decades.[29] Disk displacement with reduction may progress to disk displacement without reduction. This condition is characterized by sudden cessation of clicking and sudden onset of restricted mouth opening and is frequently accompanied by pain. This condition is described in detail below.

Disk displacement without reduction is described as having a permanently displaced disk that does not improve its relationship with the condyle on translation. When acute, it is characterized by sudden and marked limited mouth opening because of a jamming or fixation of the disk secondary to disk adhesion, deformation, or dystrophy. Pain is often present and especially related to the patient's attempt to open the mouth. The acute stage is manifested clinically as a straight-line deflection to the affected side on opening, a marked limited laterotrusion to the contralateral side, and a lack of joint noise in the affected joint. As the condition becomes chronic, the pain is markedly reduced from the acute stage to the point of becoming nonpainful in many cases, and the opening range may approach normal dimensions over time.[30] If chronic, there usually is a history of joint noise and/or limitation of mandibular opening,[31] and the condition may progress to reveal radiographically visible osteoarthritic changes. Disk displacement is generally treated with reassurance and education, rest, instructions to avoid loading, control of contributing factors, and mobility exercises within the pain-free range. In the presence of pain, mild analgesics or anti-inflammatory medications are the drugs of choice. Additional management may consist of splint therapy, physical therapy, arthrocentesis, or arthroscopy to restore range of motion. In an acute disk displacement without reduction, one may try to manually reduce the disk and temporarily maintain the disk-condyle relationship by means of an anterior repositioning splint. This splint serves to hold the lower jaw forward of its resting position, thereby translating it with the objective of keeping the disk in a favorable position. The outcome is very poor. When the disk cannot be reduced, a stabilization appliance can be part of the treatment for painful disk displacement with or without reduction. The high degree of spontaneous reduction of symptoms has to be taken into account before recommending any kind of treatment. Surgical treatments, such as arthroscopy and open joint surgeries, may be considered but only after reasonable nonsurgical efforts have failed and when the patient's quality of life is significantly affected.[32]

## MYOFASCIAL PAIN

Myofascial pain is characterized as a regional muscle pain, described as dull and/or achy and associated with the presence of trigger points in muscles, tendons, or fascia.[33–35] Myofascial pain is a common cause of persistent regional pain such as neck pain, shoulder pain, headaches, and orofacial pain.[36] The major characteristics of myofascial pain include trigger points in muscles and local and referred pain. A trigger point is identified as a localized spot of tenderness in a nodule in a palpable taut band of muscle, tendon, or ligament. The trigger points may be active or latent. Active trigger points are hypersensitive and display continuous pain in the zone of reference that can be altered with specific palpation. Latent trigger points display other characteristics of trigger points, as increased muscle tension or muscle shortening, but do not produce spontaneous pain. The pain is usually dull and deep in quality, diffuse in nature, and present in subcutaneous tissues, including muscles and joints.

Myofascial therapy can be directed peripherally or centrally. The emphasis must be on management and controlling perpetuating factors while enhancing central inhibition. Active relaxation exercises, Fluori-Methane spray and passive stretching, acupressure, ultrasonography, deep massage, moist heat, electrical stimulation, transcutaneous electrical nerve stimulation, biofeedback, relaxation techniques, cognitive-behavioral techniques, occlusal stabilization appliances, myofascial release, pharmacotherapy (such as nonsteroidal anti-inflammatory drugs, muscle relaxants, and tricyclic antidepressants), and needling and infiltration of taut bands with a local anesthetic alone or combined with botulinum toxin have been used.[37–40]

Increased tenderness in pericranial muscles is the most prominent clinical finding in patients with tension-type headache and migraine. The relationship between local tenderness, as seen in trigger points, and general tenderness, as seen in allodynia associated with migraine, must be differentiated. The first indications that there may be a correlation with the muscle tenderness and pain were experiments by Kellgren.[41] He injected an algesic substance (hypertonic saline) into the muscle and asked the subjects to define the area in which they perceived pain. The subjects receiving the hypertonic saline injections mapped out patterns of referral similar to those seen in tension-type headache. Further, he injected local anesthetic into similar areas after the pain was initiated and could abolish the pain. These tender points became known as myofascial trigger points. The question that may be asked is under what circumstances could referral take place in the patterns described?

Mense described a hypothesis for muscle pain referral to other deep somatic tissues remote from the original muscle stimulation site. He criticized the convergence-projection pain referral theory because there is little convergence evident at the dorsal horn from deep tissues.[42–44] Mense's hypothesis adds two new components to the convergence-projection theory. First, the convergent connections from deep tissues to dorsal horn neurons are opened only after nociceptive inputs from muscle are activated. The connections opened after muscle stimuli are called silent connections. Second, the referral to muscle beyond the initially activated site is due to central sensitization and spread to adjacent spinal segments. The initiating stimulus requires a peripheral inflammatory process (neurogenic inflammation). In the animal model described by Mense[41], the noxious stimulus was bradykinin injected into the muscle. In the work by Kellgren, a hypertonic saline solution was used to trigger the referred pain.[41] This seems to mimic what is seen in the animal model. It is unclear what triggers the muscle referral in the clinical setting where there is usually no obvious inflammation-producing incident. Mense's theory was used by Simons to discuss a neurophysiologic basis for trigger-point pain.[45] Simons hypothesized that when the tender area in the muscle is palpated, there is a neurotransmitter release in the dorsal horn (trigeminal nucleus), resulting in previously silent nociceptive inputs becoming active. This, in turn, causes distant neurons to produce a retrograde referred pain. This model accounts for most of the clinical presentation and therapeutic options seen in myofascial pain but does not account for what initiates the peripheral tenderness that must be present to activate the silent connections. Perhaps a central nervous system–activated neurogenic inflammation, similar to migraine, stimulates nociceptors in muscle rather than around the blood vessel. Calcitonin gene–related peptide, neurokinin A, and substance P have been used to demonstrate their contribution in myofascial pain.[46] Fields and Heinricher described a means whereby the central nervous system may switch on nociception.[47] They described the presence of "on" cells, which, when stimulated, may produce activation of trigeminal nucleus nociceptors.[47]

The first people to suggest a relationship between myofascial pain and tension-type headache were Olesen and Jensen in 1991.[48] They proposed a vascular-supraspinal-myogenic model for headache pain. This model hypothesizes that perceived pain (headache) intensity is modulated by the central nervous system. In tension-type headache, the inputs are primarily myofascial, whereas in migraine, these inputs are vascular. This model helps explain why the clinical presentation and treatment options are often similar for migraine and tension-type headache and why there is only temporary relief with peripheral treatments, such as trigger-point injections. The resultant hyperalgesia or trigger-point sensitivity in myofascial pain may represent a peripheral sensitization to serum levels of serotonin. Ernberg and colleagues showed a significant correlation with serum serotonin levels and allodynia associated with muscular face pain.[49] Based on this information, it is proposed that in patients presenting with dull, aching head pain and related muscle tenderness, the etiology may be myofascial pain. In other words, myofascial pain and tension-type headache may be the same problem. Bendtsen hypothesized that central neuroplastic changes may affect the regulation of peripheral mechanisms leading to increased pericranial muscle activity or release of neurotransmitters in the muscle tissues.[50] By these mechanisms, the central sensitization can be maintained even after the initial eliciting factors are gone. This may account for conversion of episodic into chronic tension-type headache.

## TREATING HEADACHE BY TARGETING TMDS

In that there are thought to be several etiologic factors involved in TMD, it is to be expected that there are several different therapeutic approaches. Unfortunately, most of the literature concerning the treatment methods of TMD consists of uncontrolled observations; less than 5% of treatment studies have been controlled clinical trials.[51] Even these are sometimes compromised by weaknesses in their design. Thus, only general conclusions can be drawn regarding treatment effectiveness. When the effects of different treatments are compared, the results seldom reveal major advantages of one method over another. Elimination of the cause would be the most effective treatment. However, if the cause cannot be identified, symptomatic treatment has to be provided. The goals of treatment are to decrease pain, decrease adverse loading, and restore normal function. Because the signs and symptoms of TMD can be transient and self-limiting, simple and reversible treatments must be preferred over complicated and irreversible procedures.

### Nonsurgical Treatment

In an uncontrolled study, 33 TMD patients were treated with occlusal splint therapy.[52] Following 4 weeks of therapy, 64% of patients reported a decrease in the number of weekly headaches, with 30% showing a complete remission of headache. Patients with a high frequency of headaches (four or more per week) seemed to respond more favorably to occlusal splint therapy.

In another uncontrolled study with TMD patients, changes in headache were followed 1 year after the start of TMD treatment.[53] The treatment consisted of occlusal splints, therapeutic exercises for masticatory muscles, or occlusal adjustment, most often combinations of these measures. Seventy percent of these patients reported less frequent headache than 1 year earlier. Forty percent reported less severe head pain. The results achieved seemed to be lasting at a 2.5-year follow-up.[54] These studies, however, did not control for the placebo effect, and the definition for the type of headache being treated was not clearly stated. Furthermore, one cannot know what part of the treatment was actually necessary.

Vallon and colleagues assessed the effects of occlusal adjustment on headache in TMD patients.[55–57] Fifty patients were randomly assigned to a treatment group and a control group receiving only counseling. The treatment outcome was evaluated after 1, 3, and 6 months and 2 years by a blinded examiner. No significant differences were found at follow-ups regarding changes in the frequency of headache. The problem with the study was the great dropout of patients from the original treatment groups, ranging from 20% at the 3-month follow-up to 66% at 2 years.

A new form of splint therapy has been suggested to effectively manage headache. Shankland suggested an intraoral Nociceptive Trigeminal Inhibition Tension Suppression System (NTI-tss) device for the reduction of frequency and severity of tension-type and migraine headaches compared with the known efficacy of the non–commercially available full-coverage occlusal splint.[58] A multicenter open-label trial was conducted to determine the response in migraine. The NTI-tss is a small intraoral device that is fitted over the two maxillary central incisors and has a dome-shaped protrusion, which extends lingually. The dome is customized by the provider to act as a single-point contact at the incisal embrasure of the two mandibular central incisors, thereby preventing posterior or canine tooth contact. Following a 4-week pretreatment baseline observation, patients were instructed to insert and wear their device during sleep and as required during perceived stressful times during the day for 8 consecutive weeks. A control device, a mandibular full-coverage occlusal splint, was used. Ninety-four patients were studied and randomized to the NTI-tss ($n = 43$) or full-coverage occlusal splint ($n = 51$). Although this was a migraine study, it appears that patients had chronic tension-type headache. The statistical analysis is confusing because no information is given on pretreatment days of headache and the outcome is reported in the number of headaches reduced. An example is the reduction in the numbers of migraine per month, which is reported as the same (2 migraines per month) in weeks 4 to 7, but at week 8, the NTI-tss reduced migraine to 2.5 events per month and the occlusal splint to 1.6 episodes per month, when the week before it was a reduction of 2 episodes per month. As with many other intraoral appliance studies, it is difficult to correlate outcome with pharmacologic studies of prevention because the patient selection, outcome criteria, and statistical analysis are confusing. This is not to detract from the concept that managing TMD in a migraine patient may reduce headache frequency.

Given that TMD is believed to have a multifactorial etiology, it is assumed that the best treatment results are achieved by using several different treatment methods to eliminate as many predisposing and perpetuating factors as possible. This assumption was addressed in a randomized controlled study comparing the effects of occlusal equilibration and other forms of TMD therapy in patients with signs and symptoms of TMD, including headache.[59] The TMD therapy consisted of occlusal splints, as well as muscle exercises and minor occlusal adjustment in some cases, whereas the comparison group received only occlusal equilibration therapy. The reduction in the symptoms of TMD and in the frequency and intensity of headache was significantly greater in the combined-therapy group versus the comparison group.

Some studies focusing on signs and symptoms attributable to TMD have been performed on general headache patients. In a series of studies, 100 recurrent headache patients, referred for neurologic examination, were invited for a functional examination of the stomatognathic system.[60] Fifty-five patients displayed pain caused by TMD. In 51 patients, the pain was determined to be of myogenous origin and in 4 patients of arthrogenous origin. The 55 patients were divided at random into two groups.[61] One group was treated by the neurologist according to conventional headache treatment regimens, and the other group was treated with stabilization splints for 6 weeks and, in some cases, with physical therapy. In the TMD treatment group, headache frequency decreased in 56% of patients compared with 32% in the neurologic treatment group. There is also a reported significant difference in the reduction of headache intensity and in the symptomatic medication taken to control headache. Thus, the clinical result of TMD therapy exceeded the results of the neurologic treatment in patients in whom headache was assumed to be related to TMD. The confounding factor is that the TMD group had a much greater exposure to the treating clinician, which could, in part, account for the difference.

A randomized controlled trial by Forssell and colleagues evaluated the effect of occlusal adjustment versus a mock adjustment on tension-type headache using a double-blind study design.[62] The study consisted of 56 patients with tension-type headache (20 of them also had migraine, ie, combination headache) from a neurologic clinic. Most of them reported subjective symptoms of TMD, and in all patients, signs of TMD were registered. Patients were randomly assigned to active and placebo groups, and after a 4- to 8-month follow-up period, a neurologist evaluated the treatment outcome. The headache frequency was reduced in 80%

and the intensity in 47% of patients in the active group and in 50% and 16% in the placebo group, respectively. Some of the patients from the placebo group with moderate to severe TMD symptoms were afterward treated with occlusal therapy.[63] A significant reduction in headache frequency was also observed in these patients. Except for the possible confounder that the same clinician performed both treatments (active and placebo) unblinded, this study again supports the value of TMD treatment for tension-type headache associated with TMD signs and symptoms.

Contradictory results were reported by Quayle and colleagues in an uncontrolled study of headache patients who were treated with soft occlusal splints for 6 weeks.[64] Many patients with migraine-type headache improved, but most patients suffering from tension-type headache failed to benefit from splint therapy. The small number of patients ($n = 9$) in the tension-type headache group may reduce the significance of the result.

In a double-blind trial by Karppinen, 44 patients seeking treatment for chronic headache and neck and shoulder pain received a routine battery of physical therapy.[65] In addition, 23 of the patients were randomly allocated to an occlusal adjustment group and 21 to a mock adjustment group. Patients were followed up for 6 weeks and 12 months. The short-term response to physical therapy was good and was not associated with the type of occlusal treatment. At 12 months, the effects of treatment began to subside in the mock adjustment group, but further improvement was evident in the real adjustment group. A statistically significant decrease in the occurrence of headache was observed in the real adjustment group compared with the mock adjustment group. In a qualitative systematic review of randomized controlled trials of analysis of occlusal therapies for TMD, Forssell and colleagues concluded that there was insufficient evidence to support the use of occlusal adjustments and suggestive evidence of splint therapy.[66]

Given that several controlled clinical trials seem to suggest that TMD treatment can be effective for headache, the question arises as to whether there are some special features that could, in practice, help single out patients whose headache is related to TMD from other headache patients. Reik and Hale suggested that patients with continuous unilateral headache were patients with TMD.[67] This was not supported by Schokker and colleagues, who found that headaches responsive to TMD treatment were mainly bilateral and showed only a tendency to be present permanently.[68] In that study, patients with headaches linked to TMD showed a greater difference between passive and active mouth opening recorded before treatment. This is considered to be a sign of myogenous origin of TMD. Another study showed that patients who had reported pain while chewing responded more favorably in terms of headache reduction following TMD therapy.[69] Pain while chewing is one of the most common subjective symptoms of TMD.

### Surgical Treatment

TMJ surgery is considered to be useful treatment for certain TMDs. Very few studies examine surgery and the response to headache. Vallerand and Hall reported on 50 patients diagnosed with internal TMJ derangements, myalgia, and headaches who had not responded to nonsurgical management.[70] The surgical procedures they underwent included disk repositioning, repair of disk perforation, disk recontouring, lysis of adhesions, and diskectomy. In the retrospective evaluation, the majority of patients reported decreases in headache in addition to decreases in joint pain and noise. The surgeons offer the explanation that the change in head pain is a secondary result of decreasing joint pain, which allowed the patients to cope better with other pains. In another study, Montgomery and colleagues reported significant changes in TMJ, ear, neck, and shoulder pain, whereas headaches were less consistently changed following arthroscopy of the TMJ.[71]

## CONCLUSION

Much can be learned by trying to identify and understand pain mechanisms and apply current therapeutic options based on these concepts. This allows a broad approach to an often complex and challenging problem. Our primary goal must be to help alleviate the pain and suffering our patients with head, neck, and facial pain experience. We are therefore obliged to approach pain management using all therapies at our disposal, with specific care not to worsen the situation. Sometimes therapy can be aimed specifically at the source of nociception, but in chronic situations, dealing with behavior and suffering may be more important than altering the nociception. To this end, all clinicians are not only encouraged to understand the mechanisms causing pain but also to remember that attached to every joint and nerve is a human being.

## REFERENCES

1. Bartsch T, Goadsby PJ. Increased responses in trigeminocervical nociceptive neurons to cervical input after stimulation of the dura mater. Brain 2003;126:1801–13.

2. Brooke RI. Periodic migrainous neuralgia: a cause of dental pain. Oral Surg Oral Med Oral Pathol 1978;46:511–5.

3. Sicuteri F, Nicolodi M, Fusco BM, Orlando S. Idiopathic headache as a possible risk factor for phantom tooth pain. Headache 1991;31:577–81.

4. Harris M. Psychosomatic disorders of the mouth and face. Practioner 1975:214:372.

5. Graff-Radford SB, Solberg WK. Atypical odontalgia. California Dental Association 1986;14:27–31.

6. Graff-Radford SB, Solberg WK. Atypical odontalgia. J Craniomandib Disord Oral Facial Pain 1992;6:260–6.

7. Graff-Radford SB, Solberg WK. Differential neural blockade in atypical odontalgia. Cephalalgia 1991;Suppl 11:289–91.

8. Graff-Radford SB. Facial pain. Curr Opin Neurol 2000;13:291–6.

9. Graff-Radford SB, Solberg WK. Is atypical odontalgia a psychological problem? Oral Surg Oral Med Oral Pathol 1993;75:579–82.

10. Lovshin LL. Carotidynia. Headache 1977;17:192–5.

11. Raskin NH, Prusiner S. Carotodynia. Neurology 1977;27:43–6.

12. Silberstein SD. Practice parameter. Evidence-based guidelines for migraine headache: report of the Quality Standards Subcommittee of the American Academy of Neurology. Neurology 2000;55:754–62.

13. Cairns BE, Sessel BJ, Hu JW. Evidence that excitatory amino acid receptors within the temporomandibular joint region are involved in the reflex activation of jaw muscles. J Neurosci 1998;18:8056–64.

14. Schille H. Injuries of the temporomandibular joint: classification, diagnosis and fundamentals of treatment. In: Kruger E, Schilli W, editors. Oral and maxillofacial traumatology. Vol 2. Chicago: Quintessence; 1986. p. 121–125.

15. Takahashi T, Kondoh T, Fukuda M, et al. Proinflammatory cytokines detectable in synovial fluids from patients with temporomandibular disorders. Oral Surg Oral Med Oral Pathol Oral Radiol Endod 1998;85:135–41.

16. Okeson JP. Diagnosis of temporomandibular disorders. In: Okeson JP, editor. Temporomandibular disorder and occlusion. 4th ed. St. Louis: Mosby; 1998. p. 310–51.

17. Isberg-Holm AM, Westesson PL. Movement of the disc and condyle in temporomandibular joints with clicking: an arthrographic and cineradiographic study on autopsy specimens. Acta Odontol Scand 1982;40:151–64.

18. Farrar WB, McCarty WL. A clinical outline of the temporomandibular joint diagnosis and treatment. Edited by NS Group, Montgomery, 1983. p. 19.

19. Tallents RH, Hatala M, Katzberg RW, Westesson PL. Temporomandibular joint sounds in asymptomatic volunteers. J Prosthet Dent 1993;69:298–304.

20. Kozeniauskas JJ, Ralph WJ. Bilateral arthrographic evaluation of unilateral temporomandibular joint pain and dysfunction. J Prosthet Dent 1988:60:98–105.

21. Davant TS, Greene CS, Perry HT, Lautenschlager EP. A quantitative computer-assisted analysis of disc displacement in patients with internal derangement using sagittal view magnetic resonance imaging. J Oral Maxillofac Surg 1993:51:974–9.

22. Stegenga B, de Bont LG, Boering G, van Willigen JD. Tissue responses to degenerative changes in the temporomandibular joint: a review. J Oral Maxillofac Surg 1991;49:1079–88.

23. Westesson PL, Bifano JA, Tallents RH, Hatala MP. Increased horizontal angle of the mandibular condyle in abnormal temporomandibular joints. A magnetic resonance imaging study. Oral Surg Oral Med Oral Pathol 1991;72:359–63.

24. Nilner M, Petersson A. Clinical and radiological findings related to treatment outcome in patients with temporomandibular disorders. Dentomaxillofac Radiol 1995;24:128–31.

25. Nitzan DW. The process of lubrication impairment and its involvement in temporomandibular joint disc displacement: a theoretical concept. J Oral Maxillofac Surg 2001;59:36–45.

26. Scapino RP. The posterior attachment: its structure, function, and appearance in TMJ imaging studies. Part 1. J Craniomandib Disord 1991;5:83–95.

27. Scapino RP. The posterior attachment: its structure, function, and appearance in TMJ imaging studies. Part 2. J Craniomandib Disord 1991;5:155–66.

28. Dolwick MF. Intra-articular disc displacement. Part I: its questionable role in temporomandibular joint pathology. J Oral Maxillofac Surg 1995;53:1069–72.

29. de Leeuw R, Boering G, Stegenga B, de Bont LG. Clinical signs of TMJ osteoarthrosis and internal derangement 30 years after nonsurgical treatment. J Orofacial Pain 1994;8:18–24.

30. Stegenga B, de Bont LG, Dijkstra PU, Boering G. Short-term outcome of arthroscopic surgery of temporomandibular joint osteoarthrosis and internal derangement: a randomized controlled clinical trial. Br J Oral Maxillofac Surg 1993;31:3–14.

31. Choi BH, Yoo JH, Lee WY. Comparison of magnetic resonance imaging before and after non-surgical treatment of closed lock. Oral Surg Oral Med Oral Pathol 1994;7:301–5.

32. de Bont LG, Dijkgraaf LC, Stegenga B. Epidemiology and natural progression of articular temporomandibular disorder. Oral Surg Oral Med Oral Pathol 1997;83:72–6.

33. Rivner MH. The neurophysiology of myofascial pain syndrome. Curr Pain Headache Rep 2001;5:432–40.

34. Gerwin RD. Classification, epidemiology, and natural history of myofascial pain syndrome. Curr Pain Headache Rep 2001;5:412–20.

35. Simons DG, Travell JG, Simons LS. The trigger point manual. Vol 1, 2nd ed. Baltimore: Lippincott Williams & Wilkins; 1998.

36. Fricton JR. Masticatory myofascial pain: an explanatory model integrating clinical, epidemiological and basic science research. Bull Group Int Res Sci Stomatol Odontol 1999;41:14–25.

37. Graff-Radford SB, Reeves JL, Jaeger B. Management of chronic head and neck pain: effectiveness of altering factors perpetuating myofascial pain. Headache 1987; 27:186–90.

38. Solberg WK. Temporomandibular disorders: masticatory myalgia and its management. Br Dent J 1986;160:351–6.

39. Dao TT, Lavigne GJ, Charbonneau A, et al. The efficacy of oral splints in the treatment of myofascial pain of the jaw muscles: a controlled clinical trial. Pain 1994;56:85–94.

40. Cheshire WP, Abashian SW, Mann JD. Botulinum toxin in the treatment of myofascial pain syndrome. Pain 1994;59:65–9.

41. Kellgren JH. Observations on referred pain arising from muscle. Clin Sci 1938;3:175–90.

42. Mense S. Referral of muscle pain: new aspects. Pain Forum 1994;3(1):1–9.

43. Mense S. Considerations concerning the neurobiological basis of muscle pain. Can J Physiol Pharm 1991;9:610–6.

44. Mense S. Nociception from skeletal muscle in relation to clinical muscle pain. Pain 1993;54:241–89.

45. Simons DG. Neurophysiological basis of pain caused by trigger points. APS J 1994;3(1):17–9.

46. Pedersen-Bjergaard U, Nielsen LB, Jensen K, et al. Calcitonin gene related peptide, neurokinin A and substance P on nociception and neurogenic inflammation in human skin and temporal muscle. Peptides 1991;12:333–7.

47. Fields HL, Heinricher M. Brainstem modulation of nociceptor-driven withdrawal reflexes. Ann N Y Acad Sci 1989;563:34–44.

48. Olesen J, Jensen R. Getting away from simple muscle contraction as a mechanism of tension-type headache. Pain 1991;46:123–4.

49. Ernberg M, Hadenberg-Magnusson B, Alstergren P, et al. Pain, allodynia, and serum serotonin level in orofacial pain of muscular origin. J Orofacial Pain 1999;13:56–62.

50. Bendtsen L. Central sensitization in tension-type headache—possible pathophysiological mechanisms. Cephalalgia 2000;20:486–508.

51. Antczak-Bouckoms A. Epidemiology of research for temporomandibular disorders. J Orofacial Pain 1995;9:226–34.

52. Kemper JT, Okeson JP. Craniomandibular disorders and headaches. J Prosthet Dent 1983;49:702–5.

53. Magnusson T, Carlsson GE. Changes in recurrent headache and mandibular dysfunction after various types of dental treatment. Acta Odontol Scand 1980;38:311–20.

54. Magnusson T, Carlsson GE. A $2^1/_2$-year follow-up of changes in headache and mandibular dysfunction after stomatognathic treatment. J Prosthet Dent 1983;49:398–402.

55. Vallon D, Ekberg EC, Nilner M, Kopp S. Short-term effect of occlusal adjustment on craniomandibular disorders including headaches. Acta Odontol Scand 1991;49:89–96.

56. Vallon D, Ekberg EC, Nilner M, Kopp S. Occlusal adjustment in patients with craniomandibular disorders including headaches. A 3- and 6-month follow-up. Acta Odontol Scand 1995;53:55–9.

57. Vallon D, Nilner M. A longitudinal follow-up of the effects of occlusal adjustment in patients with craniomandibular disorders. Swed Dent J 1997;21:85–91.

58. Shankland WE. Nociceptive trigeminal inhibition–tension suppression system: a method of preventing migraine and tension headaches. Compend Contin Educ Dent 2002;23:105–8.

59. Wenneberg B, Nyström T, Carlsson G. Occlusal equilibration and other stomatognathic treatment in patients with mandibular dysfunction and headache. J Prosthet Dent 1988;59:478–83.

60. Schokker RP, Hansson TL, Ansink BJJ. Craniomandibular disorders in headache patients. J Craniomandib Disord Facial Oral Pain 1989;3:71–4.

61. Schokker RP, Hansson TL, Ansink BJJ. The results of treatment of the masticatory system of chronic headache patients. J Craniomandib Disord Facial Oral Pain 1990;4:126–30.

62. Forssell H, Kirveskari P, Kangasniemi P. Changes in headache after treatment of mandibular dysfunction. Cephalalgia 1985;5:229–36.

63. Forssell H, Kirveskari P, Kangasniemi P. Response to occlusal treatment in headache patients previously treated by mock occlusal adjustment. Acta Odontol Scand 1987;45:77–80.

64. Quayle AA, Gray RJM, Metcalfe RJ, et al. Soft occlusal splint therapy in the treatment of migraine and other headaches. J Prosthet Dent 1990;18:123–9.

65. Karppinen K. Purennan hoito osana kroonisten pää-, niska- ja hartiakipujen hoitoa [dissertation]. Annales Universitatis Turkuensis Series C,114. 1995.

66. Forssell H, Kalso E, Koskela P, et al. Occlusal treatments in temporomandibular disorders: a qualitative systematic review of randomized clinical trials. Pain 1999;83:549–60.

67. Reik L, Hale M. The temporomandibular joint pain-dysfunction syndrome: a frequent cause of headache. Headache 1981;21:111–6.

68. Schokker RP, Hansson TL, Ansink BJJ. Differences in headache patients regarding their response to treatment of the masticatory system. J Craniomandib Disord Facial Oral Pain 1990;4:228–32.

69. Forssell H, Kirveskari P, Kangasniemi P. Distinguishing between headaches responsive and irresponsive to treatment of mandibular dysfunction. Proc Finn Dent Soc 1986;82:219–22.

70. Vallerand WP, Hall MB. Improvement in myofascial pain and headaches following TMJ surgery. J Craniomandib Disord Facial Oral Pain 1991;5:197–204.

71. Montgomery MT, Van Sickels JE, Harms SE, Thrash WJ. Arthroscopic TMJ surgery: effects on signs, symptoms, and disc position. J Oral Maxillofac Surg 1989;47:1263–71.

# New Daily
# Persistent Headache

—

# CHAPTER 18

# New Daily Persistent Headache

Todd D. Rozen, MD

New daily persistent headache (NDPH) was first described by Vanast in 1986 as a benign form of chronic daily headache (CDH) that improved without therapy.[1] In the headache specialist's office, NDPH is anything but benign and is felt to be one of the most treatment refractory of all headache conditions. Very little is known about this syndrome. It is unique in that the headache begins daily from onset, typically in a patient with no headache history, and can continue for years, without any sign of alleviation, despite aggressive treatment. It seems that only in the last several years has NDPH been recognized as a distinct headache syndrome by the headache community. NDPH is one of the primary headache disorders in that no underlying secondary cause can be identified. However, several secondary conditions can present as NDPH, which must be ruled out before a diagnosis of primary NDPH can be made.

## DIAGNOSTIC CRITERIA

NDPH has been included in the second edition of the International Classification of Headache Disorders (Table 18–1). Given that only a few studies have looked at the clinical characteristics of NDPH, these consensus criteria may not reflect what is seen in everyday practice and may need to be modified as more data on this syndrome are published. The International Headache Society (IHS) criteria reflect almost a daily form of tension-type headache, although migrainous features have certainly been identified in this patient population (see below). Alternative criteria for NDPH based on previous investigation are as follows:

A. Acute onset of constant unremitting headache (daily from onset)

B. Daily head pain without significant pain-free time for > 3 months

C. Average headache duration of > 4 hours per day (if untreated); frequently, constant pain without medication

D. No history of migraine or tension-type headache that is increasing in frequency before the onset of NDPH

E. History of any headache disorder is uncommon

F. At least two of the following pain characteristics:

1. Pulsating or pressing/tightening quality
2. Mild, moderate, or severe pain intensity
3. Bilateral pain location
4. Can be aggravated by walking stairs or similar routine physical activity

**Table 18–1** International Headache Society Criteria for New Daily Persistent Headache

A. Headache for > 3 mo fulfilling criteria B–D

B. Headache is daily and unremitting from onset or < 3 d from onset

C. At least 2 of the following pain characteristics:

1. Bilateral location

2. Pressing/tightening (nonpulsating) quality

3. Mild or moderate intensity

4. Not aggravated by routine physical activity, such as walking or climbing stairs

D. Both of the following

1. No more than 1 of photophobia, phonophobia, or mild nausea

2. Neither moderate or severe nausea nor vomiting

E. Not attributed to another disorder

G.  At least one of the following can be present:
    1. Nausea and/or vomiting
    2. Photophobia or phonophobia
H.  Does not fit the criteria for hemicrania continua

It appears that there may be two subtypes of NDPH: a self-limited form, which typically goes away within several months without any therapy, and the individual never presents to a physician's office (at least a neurologist's or a headache specialist's office), and a refractory form, which is basically resistant to aggressive outpatient and inpatient treatment schemes. In Vanast's original description of NDPH, he described the self-limited subtype and referred to NDPH as a benign daily headache.[1]

NDPH should not be difficult to diagnose in a physician's office based on its profile of headache onset. Problems can arise in a patient who presents with CDH and has overused medication. It is important when taking any CDH headache history to ask about onset of headache. In NDPH, the headache starts daily from onset in an individual who is not progressively taking more and more analgesics to combat an ever-increasing headache frequency; that history is consistent with a diagnosis of chronic migraine from analgesic overuse. By the time many NDPH patients reach the physician's office, they are overusing analgesics, but the overuse started after daily headache onset, not before.

## EPIDEMIOLOGY

Even though NDPH has probably been around for centuries, it has only recently been diagnosed as an entity separate from chronic tension-type headache, hemicrania continua, and chronic migraine. The prevalence of CDH from population-based studies in the United States, Asia, and Europe is about 4%.[2] In those epidemiologic investigations, primary CDH types are sometimes not mentioned in the analysis and NDPH is rarely stratified from the data. Several studies have documented the prevalence of NDPH: Castillo and colleagues looked at the prevalence of CDH in 2,252 subjects in Spain and found that 4.7% of the population had CDH, of whom 0.1% had NDPH.[3] Bigal and colleagues noted that 10.8% of 638 patients with CDH in a headache specialty clinic had NDPH,[4] whereas Koenig and colleagues found that 13% of a pediatric CDH population, surveyed from selected pediatric headache specialty clinics, had NDPH.[5]

## CLINICAL FEATURES

Only three case series in the literature are dedicated to describing the clinical characteristics of NDPH: Vanast's initial description in 1986,[1] Li and Rozen's article in 2002,[6] and Takase and colleagues' recent study

from Japan.[7] Vanast noted in 45 patients, whom he identified with NDPH over a 2-year period, a female predominance to the syndrome (26 women and 19 men).[1] There was an earlier age at onset of NDPH in women compared with men, and the age at onset of NDPH in women ranged from 16 to 35 years and in men from 26 to 45 years. Seventy-two percent of the patients stated that the pain of NDPH was constant. Pain location was temporal in 9 of 45 patients, temporal plus other areas in 14 patients, occipital and extra sites in 20 patients, and holocranial in 5 patients. "Migrainous" associated symptoms were noted in a large percentage of patients: nausea, 55%; vomiting, 12%; photophobia, 34%; and phonophobia, 37%. Other associated symptoms included drowsiness and lethargy in 15%, vertigo in 13%, and near fainting spells in 1%.

The Li and Rozen article reports the largest study to date describing the syndrome of NDPH.[6] A retrospective chart review was carried out using a computerized database of patients from the Jefferson Headache Center (a large university-based headache specialty unit). All patients who were seen between August 1997 and May 2000 and diagnosed with NDPH were included. Secondary headache disorders were excluded (via laboratory and neuroimaging studies) before a diagnosis of primary NDPH was made. Patients with other forms of CDH, including hemicrania continua, chronic migraine, and chronic tension-type headache, were excluded from the study.

Forty women and 16 men were identified (the female to male gender ratio was 2.5:1). The age at onset ranged from 12 to 78 years. The peak age at onset was the second and third decade in women and the fifth decade in men (Figure 18–1). Eighty-two percent of patients were able to pinpoint the exact day their headache started. Headache onset occurred in relation to an infection or flu-like illness in 30%, extracranial surgery (eg, hysterectomy) in 12%, and a stressful life event in 12%. Over 40% of patients could not identify any precipitating event. A headache history was found in 38% of patients (episodic migraine, 19%; episodic tension-type headache, 2%; unspecific headache, 17%). No patient had a history of CDH or an increasing frequency of episodic headache just prior to the onset of NDPH. The duration of the daily headache ranged from 1.5 to 24 hours. In 79% of patients, the pain was continuous throughout the day, with no pain-free time noted. Baseline average pain intensity was moderate (4 to 6 of 10 on a visual analog pain scale) in 61% of patients, whereas 21% experienced severe pain ($\geq$ 7 of 10) all of the time. Headache location was bilateral in 64% of patients. Almost 60% of patients had some pain localized to the occipital-nuchal region, whereas 44% experienced retro-orbital pain and 18% had holocranial pain. Headache quality was described as a throb-

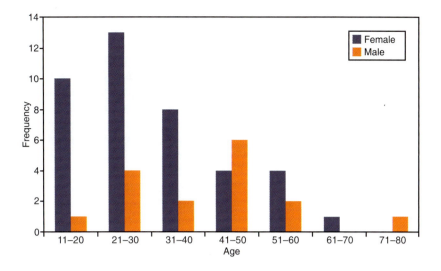

**Figure 18–1** Age at onset of men and women with new daily persistent headache.

bing sensation in 55% and pressure-like in 54%; other descriptions included stabbing, 45%; achy, 43%; dull, 37%; tightness, 36%; burning, 23%; and searing, 4%. Headaches were aggravated by stress in 40%, physical exertion in 32%, and bright light in 29%. Headaches were relieved by lying down in 66%, by being in a dark room in 48%, with massage in 23%, and with sleep in 9%. In regard to associated symptoms, nausea occurred in 68% of patients, photophobia in 66%, phonophobia in 61%, lightheadedness in 55%, sore or stiff neck in 50%, blurred vision in 43%, vomiting in 23%, osmophobia in 23%, and vertigo in 11%. Aura-type symptoms also were present in some patients, including visual photopsias in 9% and seeing zigzag lines in 5%. A family history of headache was documented in 29% of patients. Takase and colleagues looked at the clinical characteristics of NDPH in 30 Japanese patients.[7] In this study, there was a male predominance (17 men and 13 women). The age at onset of NDPH ranged from 13 to 73 years. Headache onset was associated with a stressful life event in 20%, whereas the remainder could not identify a probable cause. The headache was of severe intensity in all patients. Headache was present throughout the entire day with little if any headache-free time. Headache quality was pressure or tightening in 73%, pulsating in 10%, and both pressing and pulsating in 5%. Associated symptoms were rare, with mild nausea occurring in 10 patients, whereas only 1 patient had photophobia.

## ETIOLOGY

Given that a number of NDPH patients state that they had a cold or flu-like illness when their headache began, an infectious etiology for NDPH can be hypoth-

esized. Some authors have linked Epstein-Barr virus (EBV) infection with NDPH. Diaz-Mitoma and colleagues identified oropharyngeal secretions of EBV in 20 of 32 patients with NDPH compared with 4 of 32 age- and gender-matched controls.[8] A history of mononucleosis was identified in 12 of the patients with NDPH. Almost 85% of the NDPH patients were found to have an active EBV infection as opposed to 8 in the control group. The authors hypothesized that activation of a latent EBV infection may have been the trigger for the development of a CDH from onset. EBV titers were tested in 7 patients from the Li and Rozen investigation, of whom 5 had positive titers indicating past but not active infection.[6] Santoni and Santoni-Williams demonstrated evidence of systemic infection in 108 patients with NDPH, including *Salmonella*, adenovirus, toxoplasmosis, herpes zoster virus, EBV, and *Escherichia coli* urinary tract infections.[9] How an infection can induce NDPH is unknown. One may hypothesize an activated immune response to a new or reactivated viral infection leading to an autoimmune triggered headache, possibly by setting up a state of continuous neurogenic inflammation. The virus itself could in some way activate and damage the trigeminal system, leading to daily pain. Chronic meningitis is not present in patients with NDPH because cerebrospinal fluid (CSF) studies are usually normal.

An infectious etiology is not the presumed cause of NDPH in every patient because almost 40 to 60% of NDPH sufferers have no recognized trigger.[6] A stressful life event has been shown to trigger NDPH in a subset of patients. Recently, Stewart and colleagues documented that stressful life events are a risk factor for CDH in the general population.[10] In the year before or the same year of onset of CDH, individuals who developed headache compared with controls more likely had a change in personal relationships, had moved, had a problem with their children, or had an extremely stressful ongoing situation. The study did not define CDH subtypes, so the number of patients who developed NDPH after a stressful life event could not be ascertained.

The only study to date looking at the cause of NDPH in children was completed at the Mayo Clinic in 2003. Mack identified 41 children with NDPH, of whom 15 patients had their onset of headache during a viral infection.[11] A positive EBV titer was found in 60% of these patients. Of the remaining children, 8 had their headaches begin after mild head injury, 3 patients after a surgical procedure, and 1 patient during high-altitude camping. In 5 patients, no inciting event was identified, whereas in 4 patients, an initial diagnosis of intracranial hypertension was made, but the headache persisted after treatment and normalization of pressures.

## LABORATORY STUDIES

In most instances, laboratory and neuroimaging studies in NDPH are normal. Elevation of EBV titers has been identified, but the significance of this is unknown. In the Li and Rozen investigation, brain magnetic resonance imaging (MRI) or computed tomography was completed in 49 patients, of whom 66% had normal studies, whereas the remainder had nonspecific imaging findings that were felt not to be related to the headache condition (eg, nasal polyps). CSF data are scant but appear to be normal in adults with NDPH. Rozen and colleagues recently reported the first observation of CSF from adolescents with NDPH.[12] A lumbar puncture was completed in four adolescent patients with NDPH who were admitted to an inpatient headache unit. CSF evaluation included opening pressures, cell count, total protein, glucose, Gram stain, and bacterial cultures. A low and almost nonexistent CSF protein level was documented in 4 of 4 adolescent patients with NDPH. The cause of the low CSF protein level was unknown. Low CSF protein has been associated with hyperthyroidism, leukemia, and intracranial hypertension (recent reports have refuted this) and in children between the ages of 6 months and 2 years. One patient did have an elevated opening pressure but had no papilledema and no response to CSF-lowering agents. No other pertinent medical conditions were identified in any patient. Serum protein levels were normal in all patients (CSF protein does not decrease if serum protein levels are above 4 g/dL). The authors stated that further study looking into the cause of the low CSF protein is needed, and elucidation of the cause may lead to a better understanding of the pathogenesis of NDPH.

## SECONDARY MIMICS

A diagnosis of primary NDPH is made only after secondary causes have been ruled out. Two disorders in particular can mimic the presentation of NDPH: spontaneous CSF leak and cerebral venous sinus thrombosis. Spontaneous CSF leaks typically present as a daily headache with a positional component. However, the longer a patient suffers with a CSF leak–induced headache, the less pronounced the positional component becomes. Thus, if a patient is seen in a physician's office months to years after onset of a CSF leak, that patient may not even divulge a history of positional headaches because that trigger may not have been evident to the patient for a very long time. In this setting, the CSF leak headache may mimic a primary NDPH picture.

In the patients who present with new daily headache and are subsequently found to have cerebral venous thrombosis, in many instances, none of the typical features recognized of cerebral venous thrombosis are present, including no history of new-onset seizures, focal neurologic deficits, change of consciousness, cranial nerve palsies, bilateral cortical signs, and no evidence of papilledema on fundoscopic examination. A recent patient of mine presented with a daily headache from onset of 4 months duration with mostly occipital-nuchal discomfort. Her examination was normal, and she had no history of coagulopathy. She obtained complete headache relief with occipital nerve blockade, and the headache never returned after only a single nerve block. On subsequent magnetic resonance venography (MRV), she was found to have an extremely large transverse sinus thrombosis. The presentation of NDPH is so unique that even if patients readily improve with therapy, investigative studies still must be completed.

The evaluation of an NDPH patient should include neuroimaging, specifically brain MRI with and without gadolinium and MRV. Gadolinium must be given to look for the pachymeningeal enhancement associated with spontaneous CSF leaks, whereas MRV will help make the diagnosis of venous sinus thrombosis. If those studies are negative, then a lumbar puncture should be considered, especially in a patient who is treatment refractory. The lumbar puncture can rule out an indolent infection and can also determine CSF pressures. In some instances, a patient may have a CSF leak without typical MRI changes and with a loss of a positional headache; thus, an opening CSF pressure on a lumbar puncture is the only way in which to diagnose a low CSF pressure syndrome. A syndrome of idiopathic intracranial hypertension may also mimic NDPH. Papilledema on fundoscopic examination would be a major reason to search for this diagnosis, although some individuals may have elevated spinal pressure without papilledema and may not resemble the typical pseudotumor cerebri patient of a young obese woman with CDH, tinnitus, and visual obscurations.[13] CSF analysis would be the only way to determine the presence of elevated spinal pressure.

Daily headaches from onset may present as unilateral head pain. This is not typical of the primary syndrome of NDPH. The differential diagnosis of a unilateral headache from onset should include hemicrania continua, cluster headache, chronic paroxysmal hemicrania, SUNCT syndrome (short-lasting, unilateral, neuralgiform headache with conjunctival infection and tearing), and secondary conditions, such as carotid dissection, cervicogenic headache, and cortical mass lesion–induced headache. Trigemino-autonomic cephalalgias should be easy to distinguish from primary NDPH based on headache duration, associated symptoms and triggering, and relieving maneuvers. Hemicrania continua is a unilateral or one-sided headache that is continuous (always present) and is usually of mild intensity, with added pain exacerbation periods of varying frequency consisting of severe headache that lasts for hours to days with associated migrainous and/or autonomic symptoms. Hemicrania continua is one of the indomethacin-responsive headache syndromes. If a patient presents with a one-sided headache, with normal investigative studies and no contraindication to taking indomethacin, then a trial of this nonsteroidal anti-inflammatory drug should be completed to assess for indomethacin responsiveness.

The most common site of arterial dissection in the cerebral circulation is the extracranial internal carotid artery (ICA), followed by the vertebral artery (VA). Vertebral artery dissections are about one-third as common as ICA dissections. Dissection of cranial vessels is often spontaneous but can also be secondary to major trauma (whiplash injury) or mild trauma, such as coughing, sleeping in an abnormal position, or normal flexion or extension of the neck. Underlying connective tissue disorders, such as Marfan's syndrome, fibromuscular dysplasia, and Ehlers-Danlos syndrome, can predispose the patient to arterial dissection. Migraine may also be a risk factor for cervical arterial dissection. Most individuals who develop ICA or VA dissections are younger than 50 years of age. ICA dissections usually present with pain involving the face, neck, or head. Headache, the most common symptom of ICA dissection, occurs in 84% of patients; this is followed in decreasing frequency by focal ischemic symptoms (61%), oculosympathetic paresis (Horner's syndrome) (53%), neck pain (23%), and lightheadedness (21%).[14] Mokri and colleagues found that stroke-like spells can occur minutes or up to 11 days after the onset of hemicrania.[15] Bruits, either objective or subjective, are present in about 45% of patients. Less common symptoms include amaurosis fugax, scintillating scotomas, trigeminal nerve palsy, and dysgeusia. The headaches are usually one sided and focal, most commonly involving the anterior head region in the orbit or periorbit. The head pain is usually nonthrobbing and constant and is the initial symptom in 47% of cases. Headache onset is usually gradual but can be of sudden onset (thunderclap) in 10% of patients.[16]

If a new daily headache begins after the age of 50 years, then giant cell arteritis must be ruled out. Headache is the most commonly reported symptom of the disorder, occurring in up to 90% of individuals.[16] The pain can be throbbing in quality, although it can also be described as a dull, burning, sharp, or lancinating disturbance. The pain can be continuous or intermittent and can be of any varying intensity. The location of the headache can be variable, typically in a temporal distribution, but certainly can be generalized. Even strictly occipital pain has been noted in some patients with biopsy-proven temporal arteritis. Other common symptoms outside headache in giant cell arteritis include fever, weight loss, night sweats, visual loss, temporal artery tenderness, jaw claudication, mononeuropathies, ischemic events, and sometimes associated depression and confusion. Criteria for the diagnosis for temporal arteritis set out by the American College of Rheumatology include needing to satisfy three of the five following criteria: (1) age at least 50 years; (2) new onset of localized headache; (3) temporal artery tenderness or decreased pulse; (4) a sedimentation rate of at least 50 mm/h; and (5) a positive biopsy.[17] If three or more of the five criteria are present, this is associated with a sensitivity of 93.5% and a specificity of 91.2%.

## TREATMENT

NDPH can continue for years to decades after onset and be extremely disabling to the patient. Even with aggressive treatment, many NDPH patients do not improve. In many circles, primary NDPH is felt to be the most treatment refractory of all headache disorders. Many patients with NDPH will fail every possible class of abortive and preventive medications without any sign of pain relief. Typically, NDPH patients will start to overuse medications because they have a CDH, but unlike with chronic migraine from analgesic overuse, getting NDPH patients out of analgesic rebound typically does nothing to help in relieving their pain. Recently, I presented five patient cases in which successful treatment of NDPH was obtained with gabapentin or topiramate.[18] This was the first published study recognizing positive treatment response for the refractory form of NDPH (the self-limited form will alleviate without any therapy). Two of the cases are presented.

## Case 1

An 18-year-old woman presented with a 2-year holocranial headache that was daily from onset, with no inciting event. Imaging and laboratory investigations were normal. On presentation, she was overusing over-the-counter medication. After removal of the rebounding compounds, she showed no improvement. She failed various preventive medications, including amitriptyline, fluoxetine, valproic acid, and propranolol. She was placed on gabapentin, and on reaching a dose of 2,700 mg/d, her daily headache broke, and she had very infrequent episodic headaches through 2-year follow-up. Her episodic headaches were easily aborted with indomethacin.

## Case 2

An 18-year-old woman with a history of infrequent headaches presented with a headache of 7 months duration that was daily from onset. She may have had a flu-like illness at the time of headache initiation. For a brief time, she was overusing over-the-counter medications but stopped without any change in headache. Imaging and laboratory testing were negative. On topiramate 75 mg twice daily, she became headache free. She developed mood changes on the medication, so she decreased the dosage to 15 mg twice daily, with resolution of the mood changes and still remaining headache free through 4-month follow-up.

At present, no specific treatment strategy can be recognized for primary NDPH. Most headache specialists will treat NDPH with the same acute and preventive medications that are used to treat chronic migraine, although based on the response to these medications, NDPH and chronic migraine are two disparate syndromes. If gabapentin and/or topiramate have not yet been used in the treatment regimen, they should be tried because there is at least some evidence that they may help this basically treatment-refractory syndrome.

Because a number of NDPH patients appear to have cervicogenic signs on examination (even without a history of head or neck trauma), sending them for anesthesiology or pain clinic evaluation for nerve blocks and facet blocks is recommended when medication is not helping. Anecdotally, I have had several NDPH patients achieve significant pain relief after cervical facet blocks or selective nerve blocks (greater occipital, auriculotemporal, supraorbital). Because this can be a refractory syndrome, any pain relief is welcomed by the patient. At present, no one has looked at the use of long-term opiate therapy for the NDPH patient, and this should be considered only on an individual basis.

## PROGNOSIS

The self-limited form of NDPH has a good prognosis because patients appear to improve without any intervention. In Vanast's initial description of NDPH, 30% of the men affected were headache free at 3 months and 86% were headache free at 2 years.[1] In women, 30% were headache free at 3 months, whereas 73% were pain free at 2 years. In the patients who have the refractory form of NDPH, their syndrome can continue unabated for years to decades even with aggressive treatment. Takase and colleagues evaluated the effect of treatment using muscle relaxants, tricyclic and selective serotonin reuptake inhibitor antidepressants, and valproic acid on NDPH.[7] In 8 of 30 patients, treatment was deemed very effective (daily headache intensity 3 of 10 or less), 1 patient had a moderately effective response (daily headache intensity 4 to 5 of 10), and 6 patients had a mildly effective response (daily headache intensity 6 to 7 of 10), whereas 15 patients showed no response to treatment. Only 2 patients developed headache-free time after therapy; the remainder continued with daily head pain, although some had an improved quality of life. The authors concluded that, overall, NDPH is unresponsive to typical headache treatment.

## CONCLUSION

NDPH is a newly recognized form of CDH. It is unique in its presentation and course. Many NDPH patients can state the exact date when their headache began. NDPH is marked by continuous daily head pain of varying intensity that may be associated with migrainous symptoms. Further research must be invested into studying NDPH because it is becoming more prevalent in the physician's office and, in many instances, is refractory to many of the known CDH preventive and abortive treatment strategies.

## REFERENCES

1.  Vanast WJ. New daily persistent headaches: definition of a benign syndrome. Headache 1986;26:317.

2   Silberstein SD, Lipton RB. Chronic daily headache, including transformed migraine, chronic tension-type headache and medication overuse. In: Wolff's headache and other head pain. Oxford (UK): Oxford University Press; 2001. p. 247–82.

3.  Castillo J, Munoz P, Guitera V, Pascual J. Epidemiology of chronic daily headache in the general population. Headache 1999;38:497–506.

4.  Bigal ME, Sheftell FD, Rapoport AM, et al. Chronic daily headache in a tertiary care population: correlation between the International Headache Society diagnostic criteria and proposed revisions of criteria for chronic daily headache. Cephalalgia 2002;22:432–8.

5. Koenig MA, Gladstein J, McCarter RJ, et al, and the Pediatric Committee of the American Headache Society. Chronic daily headache in children and adolescents presenting to tertiary headache clinics. Headache 2002;42:491–500.

6. Li D, Rozen TD. The clinical characteristics of new daily persistent headache. Cephalalgia 2002;22:66–9.

7. Takase Y, Nakano M, Tatsumi C, Matsuyama T. Clinical features, effectiveness of drug based treatment and prognosis of new daily persistent headache: thirty cases in Japan. Cephalalgia 2004;24:955–9.

8. Diaz-Mitoma F, Vanast WJ, Tyrell DL. Increased frequency of Epstein-Barr virus excretion in patients with new daily persistent headaches. Lancet 1987;i:411–5.

9. Santoni JR, Santoni-Williams CJ. Headache and painful lymphadenopathy in extracranial or systemic infection: etiology of new daily persistent headaches. Intern Med 1993;32:530–3.

10. Stewart WF, Scher AI, Lipton RB. Stressful life events and risk of chronic daily headache: results from the frequent headache epidemiology study. Cephalalgia 2001;21:278–80.

11. Mack K. What causes new daily persistent headache in children? Cephalalgia 2003;23:609.

12. Rozen T, Haynes G, Range C, Swidan S. Low cerebrospinal fluid protein levels in adolescents with new daily persistent headache. Neurology 2004;62 Suppl 5: A336.

13. Marcelis J, Silberstein SD. Idiopathic intracranial hypertension without papilledema. Arch Neurol 1991;48:392–9.

14. Mokri B. Traumatic and spontaneous extracranial internal carotid artery dissections. J Neurol 1990; 237:356–61.

15. Mokri B, Sundt TM, Houser W, Piepgras DG. Spontaneous dissection of the cervical internal carotid artery. Ann Neurol 1986;19:126–30.

16. Mokri B. Headache in spontaneous carotid and vertebral artery dissections. In: Goadsby PJ, Silberstein SD, editors. Headache. Boston: Butterworth-Heinemann; 1997. p. 327–54.

17. Hunder GG, Bloch DA, Michel BA, et al. The American College of Rheumatology 1990 criteria for the classification of giant cell arteritis. Arthritis Rheum 1990;33:1122–8.

18. Rozen TD. Successful treatment of new daily persistent headache with gabapentin and topiramate. Headache 2002;42:433.

# Index